Essential Manual of 24-Hour Blood Pressure Management

Essential Manual of 24-Hour Blood Pressure Management

From Morning to Nocturnal Hypertension

Second Edition

Kazuomi Kario, MD, PhD, FACC, FAHA, FESC

Professor and Chairman, Department of Cardiovascular Medicine
Jichi Medical University School of Medicine, Tochigi, Japan

WILEY Blackwell

Registered Offices
John Wiley & Sons, Inc., 111 River Street, Hoboken, NJ 07030, USA
John Wiley & Sons Ltd, The Atrium, Southern Gate, Chichester, West Sussex, PO19 8SQ, UK

Editorial Office
9600 Garsington Road, Oxford, OX4 2DQ, UK

For details of our global editorial offices, customer services, and more information about Wiley products visit us at www.wiley.com.

Wiley also publishes its books in a variety of electronic formats and by print-on-demand. Some content that appears in standard print versions of this book may not be available in other formats.

Library of Congress Cataloging-in-Publication Data

Names: Kario, Kazuomi, author.
Title: Essential manual of 24-hour blood pressure management: from morning to nocturnal hypertension / Kazuomi Kario.
Other titles: Essential manual of twenty four-hour blood pressure management
Description: Second edition. | Hoboken, NJ : Wiley-Blackwell, 2022. | Includes bibliographical references and index.
Identifiers: LCCN 2021028709 (print) | LCCN 2021028710 (ebook) | ISBN 9781119799368 (paperback) | ISBN 9781119799382 (adobe pdf) | ISBN 9781119799405 (epub)
Subjects: MESH: Hypertension–drug therapy | Blood Pressure Monitoring, Ambulatory | Blood Pressure–physiology | Blood Pressure Determination | Circadian Rhythm–physiology
Classification: LCC RC685.H8 (print) | LCC RC685.H8 (ebook) | NLM WG 340 | DDC 616.1/32061–dc23
LC record available at https://lccn.loc.gov/2021028709
LC ebook record available at https://lccn.loc.gov/2021028710

Cover Design: Wiley
Cover Images: © Creations/Shutterstock

Set in 9/12pt Meridien by Straive, Pondicherry, India

SKY1B1B37B9-CAF2-4B44-8D2F-AB1FEF6DF0F3_012822

Contents

Author biography

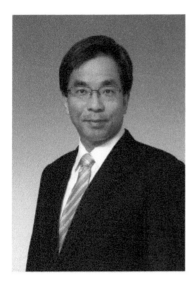

Kazuomi Kario, MD, PhD, FACC, FAHA, FESC
Professor
Division of Cardiovascular Medicine,
Department of Medicine,
Center of Excellence, Cardiovascular
Research and Development (JCARD),
Jichi Medical University School of Medicine;
Hypertension Cardiovascular Outcome
Prevention and Evidence (HOPE)
Asia Network/World Hypertension League

3311-1, Yakushiji, Shimotsuke, Tochigi
329-0498, JAPAN
Tel: +81-285-58-7538;
Fax: +81-285-44-4311;
E-mail: kkario@jichi.ac.jp

Professor Kazuomi Kario graduated from Jichi Medical School in 1986. He is currently professor and chairman of cardiovascular medicine, Jichi Medical University School of Medicine, Japan; staff visiting professor, Institute of Cardiovascular Science, University College London, London, UK; visiting professor, Shanghai Jiao Tong University School of Medicine, Shanghai, China; adjunct professor, Yonsei University School of Medicine, Seoul, Korea; and distinguished professor, Fu Wai Hospital, National Center for Cardiovascular Diseases, Chinese Academy of Medical Sciences, Beijing, China.

In 2003, Professor Kario and his team were the first to report that the **morning surge in blood pressure** (BP) was an independent risk factor for cardiovascular disease [1, 2]. He first used "morning hypertension," defined as morning BP ≥135/85 mmHg, regardless of office BP, and stressed its clinical relevance in his book Clinician's Manual on Early Morning Risk Management in Hypertension in 2004 (Science Press, London, UK, 2004) [3]. He has also proposed the **Resonance hypothesis of BP surge** [4], and the concept of **systemic hemodynamic atherothrombotic syndrome** (SHATS) as a vicious cycle of BP variability and vascular disease [5]. These stress the importance and clinical implications of the **perfect 24-hour BP management from morning to nocturnal hypertension** concept (2004, 2015, 2018) (Figure 1).

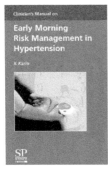

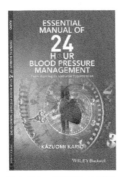

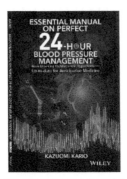

Kario K, Clinician's Manual on Early Morning risk Management in Hypertension, Science Press, London, UK, pp.1–68, 2004

Kario K, Essential Manual of 24-hour Blood Pressure Management from Morning to Nocturnal Hypertension, John Wiley & Sons Ltd., Oxford,UK, pp.1–138, 2015.

Kario K. Essential Manualon Perfect 24-hour BloodPressureManagement from Morning to Nocturnal Hypertension. Up-to date for Anticipation Medicine, Wiley Publishing Japan KK, Tokyo, pp.1–309, 2018.

Figure 1 Books written by the author.

(a)

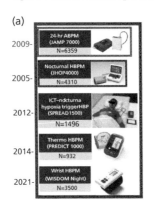

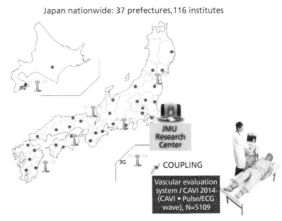

(b)

Prospective Cohort study
1. Jichi Medical School ABPM Wave 1 (1992–1998)
2. JHOP (Japan Morning Surge-Home Blood Pressure, 2005–2014)
3. JAMP (Japan Ambulatory Blood Pressure Prospective Study) / HI-JAMP / HI-JAMP-V (2009-)
4. COUPLING (Cardiovascular Prognostic COUPLING Study in Japan, 2015-)
5. WISDOM (Wrist Sleep and CircaDian BlOodPressure Monitoring Program, 2021-)

Intervention study
1. JMS-1 (Japan Morning Surge 1, 2003–2005)
2. JMS-TOP (Japan Morning Surge-Total Organ Protection, 2005–2008)
3. HONEST(Home blood pressure measurement with Olmesartan Naive patients to Establish Standard Target blood pressure, 2009–2012)
4. Nocturne (2015–2016)
5. SACRA (SGLT-2i and ARB combination therapy in patients with T2DM and nocturnal hypertension, 2017)
6. REQUIRE (Renal Denervation on Quality of 24-hr BP Control by Ultrasound In Resistant Hypertension, 2017–2020)
7. HERB DH1 (HERB digital hypertension 1 pivotal, 2018–2019)

Figure 2 (a) Jichi Medical University (JMU), Center of Excellence, Community Medicine Cardiovascular Research and Development (JCARD) Network Program Study for Device Development and Evidence. ABPM, ambulatory blood pressure monitoring; CAVI, cardio-ankle vascular index; HBPM, home blood pressure monitoring; ICT, information and communication technology. (b) Jichi Medical University Hypertension Program – Major Clinical Studies.

Professor Kario is the principal investigator on several clinical studies, including the Japan Morning Surge-Home Blood Pressure (J-HOP), Japan Ambulatory BP Monitoring (JAMP), Home-activity ICT-based Japan Ambulatory Blood Pressure Monitoring Prospective (HI-JAMP), Sleep BP and disordered breathing in Resistant Hypertension and Cardiovascular Disease (SPREAD), Cardiovascular Prognostic Coupling study in Japan (COUPLING Japan), and Wrist Sleep and Circadian Blood Pressure Monitoring study-night (WISDOM Night) studies, among many others (Figure 2).

Professor Kario's research is now focusing on the area of **digital hypertension**, including research and development of new technology-based BP monitoring devices, risk detection algorithms, and digital therapeutics to achieve "Perfect 24-hour Blood Pressure Management from morning to nocturnal hypertension" [6, 7].

He has served as **Editor-in-Chief of** *Hypertension Research,* **an official journal of Japanese Society of Hypertension** since 2021 and *Current Hypertension Reviews*, and as associate editor of the *Journal of Clinical Hypertension*. Professor Kario has published more than 1000 academic papers during his career. In addition, he founded the **Hypertension Cardiovascular Outcome Prevention and Evidence in Asia (HOPE Asia) Network** in 2016.

References

1. Kario K, Pickering TG, Umeda Y, Hoshide S, Hoshide Y, Morinari M, Murata M, Kuroda T, Schwartz JE, Shimada K. Morning surge in blood pressure as a predictor of silent and clinical cerebrovascular disease in elderly hypertensives: A prospective study. Circulation. 2003; 107: 1401–1406.
2. Kario K, Ishikawa J, Pickering TG, Hoshide S, Eguchi K, Morinari M, Hoshide Y, Kuroda T, Shimada K. Morning hypertension: The strongest independent risk factor for stroke in elderly hypertensive patients. Hypertens Res. 2006; 29: 581–587.
3. Kario K. Clinician's Manual on Early Morning Risk Management in Hypertension. Science Press, London, UK, pp.1–68, 2004.
4. Kario K. New insight of morning blood pressure surge into the triggers of cardiovascular disease – synergistic resonance of blood pressure variability. Am J Hypertens. 2016; 29: 14–16.
5. Kario K. Orthostatic hypertension – a new haemodynamic cardiovascular risk factor. Nat Rev Nephrol. 2013; 9: 726–738.
6. Kario K. Nocturnal hypertension: New technology and evidence. Hypertension. 2018; 71:997–1009.
7. Kario K. Management of hypertension in the digital era: small wearable monitoring devices for remote blood pressure monitoring. Hypertension. 2020; 76: 640–650.

Preface – Direction to "Perfect 24-hour Blood Pressure Control"

"Cardiovascular events do not establish in a day, but the onset is non-linear".

Over a lifetime, blood pressure (BP) plays two key roles as a central risk factor for cardiovascular disease (Figure 01) [1]. The first is as chronic risk factor advancing vascular disease and the second is as acute risk factor triggering cardiovascular events.

The benefits associated with the management of hypertension are due to BP lowering per se, highlighting the importance of BP control throughout each 24-hour period. Recent guidelines stress the importance of an out-of-office BP-guided approach using diagnostic and therapeutic thresholds based on home and/or ambulatory BP values. This prompts earlier BP management targeting lower thresholds throughout a 24-hour period, which is the essential pathway hypertension management [2]. Disrupted circadian rhythm (a riser pattern of nighttime BP) and exaggerated morning BP surge contribute to the risk of cardiovascular events [3, 4]. Thus, we hypothesized that "perfect 24-hour BP control," consisting of lowering the average 24-hour BP, maintaining adequate circadian rhythm and stabilizing BP variability, is the ideal BP status (Figure 02) [5].

Practically, the first target is morning hypertension [6]. BP has been shown to increase over the period from night to early morning, and cardiovascular events

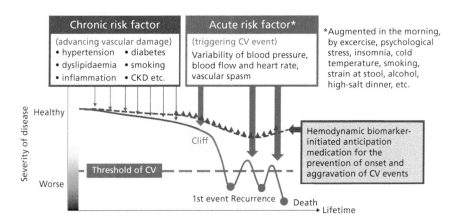

Figure 01 Differential effects of acute versus chronic risk factors and hemodynamic biomarker-initiated cardiovascular anticipation medicine. CKD, chronic kidney disease; CV, cardiovascular. *Source:* Kario [1].

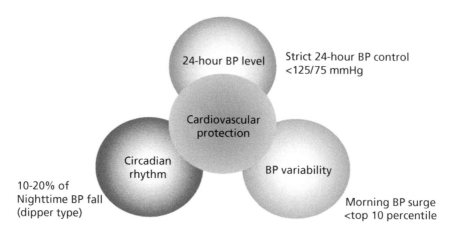

Figure 02 Triad of perfect 24-hour blood pressure (BP) control. *Source:* Kario 2004 [5].

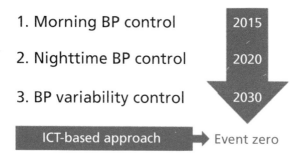

Figure 03 Information and communication technology (ICT)-based strategy for "Cardiovascular Event Zero". BP, blood pressure. *Source:* Kario 2016 [7].

occur more frequently in the morning. The second target is uncontrolled nocturnal hypertension, control of which is a limitation of current antihypertensive medication (Figure 03)[7]. Stabilizing BP variability at the physiological oscillation level is the final goal for achieving zero cardiovascular events.

In the near future, wearable BP monitoring [8] and the new hemodynamic biomarker-initiated "anticipation medicine" approach using real-time information and communications technology (ICT)-based cardiovascular risk prediction and alert system over 24-hours would ideally prevent adverse cardiovascular events, resulting in a healthy life [9].

In this book, I present recent evidence on morning hypertension and nocturnal hypertension, and the technology that will support an individualized approach to hypertension management guided by at-home BP measures. I believe a "perfect 24-hour BP control" strategy using a health information technology (HIT)-based nonpharmacological approach, medication (changing the dose, the class, and timing of drug administration), digital therapeutics, and/or neuromodulation device treatment [10] will achieve the most effective cardiovascular and renal protection. I hope this book will provide good practical advice for the updated treatment of hypertension on a day-to-day basis.

Kazuomi Kario, MD, PhD, FACC, FAHA, FESC
Division of Cardiovascular Medicine
Department of Medicine
Jichi Medical University School of Medicine
Tochigi, Japan
October 1st, 2021

References

1. Kario K. Evidence and perspectives on the 24-hour management of hypertension: Hemodynamic biomarker-initiated "anticipation medicine" for zero cardiovascular. Event. Prog Cardiovasc Dis. 2016; 59: 262–281.
2. Kario K. Global impact of 2017 AHA/ACC hypertension guidelines: A perspective from Japan. Circulation. 2018; 137: 543–545.
3. Kario K. Morning surge in blood pressure and cardiovascular risk – evidence and perspectives – Hypertension. 2010; 56:765–773.
4. Kario K, Hoshide S, Mizuno H, Kabutoya T, Nishizawa M, Yoshida T, Abe H, Katsuya T, Fujita Y, Okazaki O, Yano Y, Tomitani N, Kanegae H, on behalf of JAMP study group. Nighttime blood pressure phenotype and cardiovascular prognosis: The practitioner-based nationwide JAMP Study. Circulation 2020; 142: 1810–1820.
5. Kario K. Clinician's Manual on Early Morning Risk Management in Hypertension. Science Press, London, UK, pp.1–68, 2004.
6. Kario K, Chen CH, Park S, Park CG, Hoshide S, Cheng HM, Huang QF, Wang JG. Consensus document on improving hypertension management in Asian patients, taking into account Asian characteristics. Hypertension. 2018; 71: 375–382.
7. Kario K. Nocturnal hypertension: New technology and evidence. Hypertension. 2018;71:997–1009.
8. Kario K. Management of hypertension in the digital era: small wearable monitoring devices for remote blood pressure monitoring. Hypertension. 2020; 76: 640–650.
9. Kario K, Tomitani N, Kanegae H, Yasui N, Nishizawa M, Fujiwara T, Shigezumi T, Nagai R, Harada H. Development of a new ICT-based multisensor blood pressure monitoring system for use in hemodynamic biomarker-initiated anticipation medicine for cardiovascular disease: The national IMPACT program project. Prog Cardiovasc Dis. 2017; 60: 435–449.
10. Böhm M, Kario K, Kandzari DE, Mahfoud F, Weber MA, Schmieder RE, Tsioufis K, Pocock S, Konstantinidis D, Choi JW, East C, Lee DP, Ma A, Ewen S, Cohen DL, Wilensky R, Devireddy CM, Lea J, Schmid A, Weil J, Agdirlioglu T, Reedus D, Jefferson BK, Reyes D, D'Souza R, Sharp ASP, Sharif F, Fahy M, DeBruin V, Cohen SA, Brar S, Townsend RR; SPYRAL HTN-OFF MED Pivotal Investigators. Efficacy of catheter-based renal denervation in the absence of antihypertensive medications (SPYRAL HTN-OFF MED Pivotal): a multicentre, randomised, sham-controlled trial. Lancet. 2020;395:1444–1451.

Acknowledgments

I would particularly like to thank the three academic fathers of my research, Kazuyuki Shimada, Takefumi Matsuo, and the late Thomas G Pickering, who continuously supported me. I would also like to thank other senior researchers in this field and my colleagues who provided many helpful academic comments and criticism on the contents of this book. They include Ryozo Nagai, Michael Weber, Bryan Williams, Gianfranco Parati, George Stergiou, Jiguang Wang, Daichi Shimbo, Wanpen Vongpatanasin, Alta Schutte, Chen-Huan Chen, Sungha Park, Yook-Chin Chia, Tzung-Dau Wang, Satoshi Hoshide, Tomoyuki Kabutoya, Hiroyuki Mizuno, Takeshi Fujiwara, Keisuke Narita, Naoko Tomitani, Hiroshi Kanegae, Masafumi Nishizawa, Tetsuro Yoshida, Yuichiro Yano, Masahisa Shimpo, Yasushi Imai, Takahide Kohro, Hiroshi Funayama, Kenji Harada, Yukiyo Ogata, Takahiro Komori, Tomonori Watanabe, Kenichi Katsurada, Masashi Kamioka, Katsuaki Yokota, Hayato Shimizu, Shinichi Toriumi, Mizuri Taki, Yusuke Oba, Ayako Yokota, Hiroaki Watanabe, Yukako Ogoyama, Kana Kubota, Yusuke Ishiyama, Hirotaka Waki, Keita Negishi, Takahiro Watanabe, Daisuke Kaneko, Yusuke Suzuki, Hisaya Kobayashi, Takafumi Okuyama, Hajime Shinohara, Tadayuki Mitama, Yutaka Aoyama, Masafumi Sato, Shunsuke Saito, Noriyasu Suzuki, Eri Morita, Naoki Watanabe, Toshiya Kakurai, Yuki Hirata, Sumika Wachi, Tomohisa Sakata, Kenta Fujimura, Tomohide Sato, Daisuke Suzuki, Ayako Kokubo, Taro Fukuda, Yuki Imaizumi, Sirisawat Wanthong, Praew Kotruchin, Kazuo Eguchi, Joji Ishikawa, Yoshio Matsui, Michiaki Nagai, Shizukiyo Ishikawa, Seiichi Shibasaki, Motohiro Shimizu, Ken Kono, Yoshioki Nishimura, Satoshi Niijima, Mitsunori Sugiyama, Mikio Iwashita, Toshikazu Shiga, Noboru Shinomiya, Mitsuo Kuwabara, Nobuhiko Yasui, Shinobu Ozaki, Kyohei Fukatani, Takashi Kuwayama, Takeshi Niho, Kohta Satake, Shin Suzuki, Akihiro Nomura, Kiyose Nakagawa. Last but not least, I would like to thank Noriko Sugawara, Haruna Hamasaki, Yuri Matsumoto, Yukie Okawara, Ryoko Nozue, Hiromi Suwa, Rika Toyoda, Yukiko Suzuki, Chie Iwashita, Tomoko Morimoto, Tomoko Shiga, Noriko Harada, Hisae Shiokawa, Hisako Umeta and Takako Yokoyama for their research coordination, Ayako Okura for editorial assistance, without whom this book would not have been possible. Studies highlighted in this book were partly supported by the ImPACT Program of Council for Science, Technology and Innovation (Cabinet Office, Government of Japan), the Japan Agency for Medical Research and Development (AMED) under Grant Number JP17he1102002h0003, JSPS KAKENHI Grant-in-Aid for Scientific Research B (Grant Number JP26293192) and JSPS KAKENHI Grant-in-Aid for Scientific Research S (Grant Number 17H06151) from the Japan Society for the Promotion of Science, a grant from the Foundation for Development of the Community (Tochigi), MSD Life Science Foundation, Public Interest Incorporated Foundation, Omron Healthcare, Co., A&D, Co.,Fukuda Denshi, Co., Otsuka Medical Device, Co., Terumo, Co., Medtronic plc, and CureApp Inc.

CHAPTER 1

Evidence and scientific rationale for ambulatory blood pressure monitoring (ABPM)

Diurnal BP variation and the concept of "perfect 24-hour BP control"

Blood pressure (BP) always varies over time, including beat-by-beat, trigger-induced, orthostatic, diurnal, day-by-day, weekly, seasonal, and age-related variations. Of these different BP variability components, circadian rhythm is the central component of individual BP variability, and there is a large body of accumulating evidence highlighting the importance of this parameter.

Basic circadian rhythm forms the basis of individual diurnal BP variation (Figure 1.1) [1]. The circadian rhythm of BP is physiologically determined partly by the intrinsic rhythm of central and peripheral clock genes, which regulate the neurohumoral factor and cardiovascular systems, and partly by the sleep-wake behavioral pattern, and is associated with various pathological conditions.

In addition to different patterns of circadian rhythm, short-term BP variability such as morning blood pressure surge (MBPS), physical or psychological stress-induced daytime BP, and nighttime BP surge triggered by hypoxic episodes in obstructive sleep apnea, arousal, rapid-eye-movement sleep, and nocturnal behavior (e.g. nocturia) modulates the circadian rhythm of BP, resulting in the different individual diurnal BP variation.

It is well-known that elevated 24-hour BP is a more important cardiovascular risk factor than office BP. In addition, disrupted circadian rhythm and exaggerated forms of short-term BP variability (e.g. MBPS) are associated with an increased risk of cardiovascular events [2]. We hypothesized that "perfect 24-hour BP control," which includes lowering the average 24-hour BP (quantity of BP control), maintaining adequate circadian rhythm, and stabilizing BP variability (quality of BP control), is the ideal goal (Figure 02) [3]. In particular, control of 24-hour BP to <130/80 mmHg is important to minimize organ damage, independent of any regional differences in the risk of cardiovascular disease (Figure 1.2) [4].

Essential Manual of 24-Hour Blood Pressure Management: From Morning to Nocturnal Hypertension,
Second Edition. Kazuomi Kario.

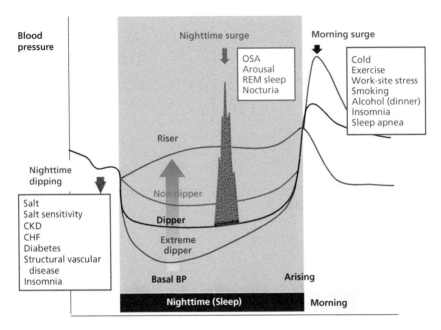

Figure 1.1 Components of nocturnal hypertension and determinants—nocturnal dipping status and surge in blood pressure. BP, blood pressure; CHF, chronic heart failure; CKD, chronic kidney disease; OSA, obstructive sleep apnea; REM, rapid eye movement. *Source*: Kario. Hypertension. 2018; 71: 997–1009 [1].

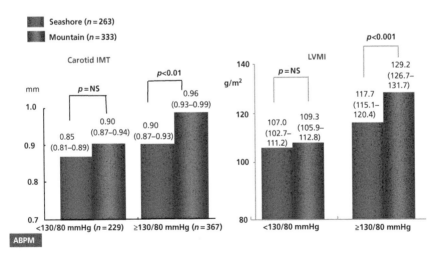

Figure 1.2 Regional differences in the impact of 24-hour blood pressure control on cardiovascular remodeling and target organ damage (*n* = 596). IMT, intima-media thickness; LVMI, left ventricular mass index; NS, not statistically significant. *Source*: Created based on data from Yano et al. Am J Hypertens. 2011; 24: 437–443 [4].

Nocturnal hypertension and nocturnal BP dipping status

Nocturnal BP dipping status

Different patterns of the circadian rhythm of BP can be determined using ambulatory BP monitoring (ABPM). Population-based and clinical studies using ABPM have shown that nighttime BP is a better predictor of cardiovascular diseases than daytime BP [5, 6]. Nocturnal hypertension (where nighttime BP is high) and a non-dipper/riser pattern (where nighttime BP is higher than daytime BP, even if office and 24-hour BP readings are within the normal range) both increase the risk of target organ damage and subsequent cardiovascular events [7–10].

In healthy subjects, nighttime BP falls by 10–20% from daytime BP (normal dipper pattern). Patients with hypertension who do not have target organ damage also show the dipper pattern. However, those with organ damage tend to exhibit a non-dipper pattern with diminished nighttime BP fall. Recent guidelines on the management of hypertension defined four different dipping patterns of nighttime BP: dipper, non-dipper, riser, and extreme dipper based on the magnitude of the nighttime BP fall (Figure 1.3) [7, 8]. The terms "riser" and "extreme dipper" patterns describe the extremes on a continuum of circadian BP variability and represent the most pathologically relevant forms of disrupted circadian BP rhythm [11].

Non-dipper patterns of BP and pulse rate

O'Brien et al. first demonstrated that an abnormal, non-dipping pattern of nighttime BP, with a <10% reduction in nocturnal BP compared with daytime BP, is associated with advanced organ damage [12]. The magnitude of the nighttime BP

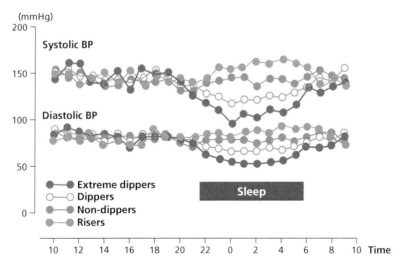

Figure 1.3 Four different dipping status of nighttime blood pressure (BP) in hypertensive patients. *Source*: Created based on data from Kario et al. Hypertension. 2001; 38: 852–857 [8].

fall tends to diminish with advancing age. Shimada et al. first demonstrated that a non-dipper pattern of nighttime BP in elderly patients with hypertension was associated with advanced silent cerebral disease (such as silent cerebral infarcts and deep white matter lesions) detected using brain magnetic resonance imaging (MRI) [13].

Non-dipping of the pulse rate pattern is also associated with poor cardiovascular prognosis, and synergistically increases the risk associated with a non-dipper pattern of nighttime BP fall. In a prospective study of elderly patients with hypertension, those with a non-dipper pulse rate pattern showed a increase in cardiovascular events compared with a dipping pattern, independent of BP. In addition, non-dippers of both nighttime BP and nighttime pulse rate were found to have the worst cardiovascular prognosis, showing a synergistic 7.9-fold increase in the risk of cardiovascular events compared to those with a dipping profile for both parameters (Figure 1.4) [14].

Riser pattern of BP and cardiovascular disease risk
The "riser" pattern is defined as higher BP during nighttime vs. daytime BP (i.e. no nocturnal BP fall), and the term "extreme dippers" refers to patients with an exaggerated nighttime BP fall (≥20%) compared with the daytime BP reading [7]. Some authors use the term "reverse dipper" or "inverted dipper" instead of "risers," but these refer to the same lack of nocturnal BP fall.

A study in elderly patients with hypertension was the first to demonstrate that both extreme forms of disrupted circadian BP pattern (i.e. riser and extreme dipper) were associated with advanced silent cerebral disease evaluated on brain MRI (Figure 1.5) and were significantly associated with the occurrence of stroke

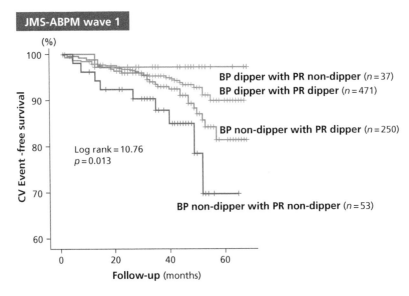

Figure 1.4 Cardiovascular (CV) prognosis in non-dippers of blood pressure (BP) and pulse rate (PR) (JMS-ABPM study wave 1). *Source*: Kabutoya et al. Am J Hypertens. 2010; 23: 749–755 [14].

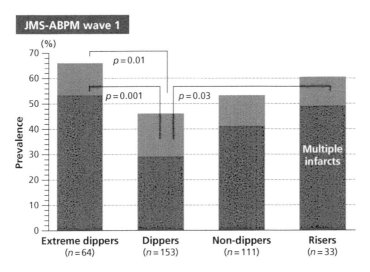

Figure 1.5 Silent cerebral infarcts detected by brain magnetic resonance imaging and nighttime blood pressure dipping in elderly patients with hypertension (JMS ABPM study wave 1). Green area indicates single infarct per person. *Source*: Kario et al. Hypertension. 2001; 38: 852–857 [8].

(Figure 1.6) [8]. In particular, the riser pattern appears to have a particularly poor prognosis with respect to stroke and cardiac events (Figure 1.7) [15].

The multicenter, prospective, practitioner-based, Japan Ambulatory Blood Pressure Monitoring Prospective (JAMP) study used the same ABPM device across all study centers to investigate the impact of nocturnal hypertension and nighttime BP dipping patterns on the occurrence of cardiovascular events, including heart failure (HF), in patients with hypertension (Figure 1.8) [16]. The results

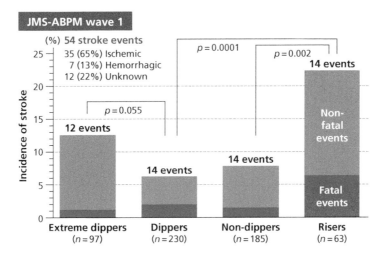

Figure 1.6 Nighttime blood pressure dipping status and stroke prognosis in older patients with sustained hypertension. *Source*: Kario et al. Hypertension. 2001; 38: 852–857 [8].

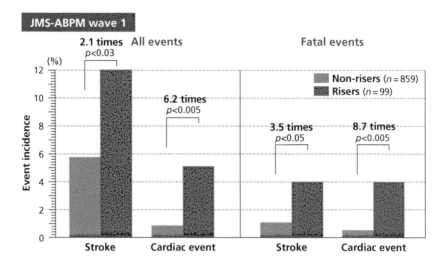

Figure 1.7 Fatal and non-fatal cardiovascular events in patients with a riser vs. non-riser pattern. *Source*: Kario and Shimada Clin Exp Hypertens. 2004; 26: 177–189 [15].

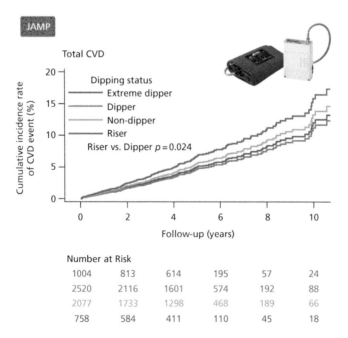

Figure 1.8 Nighttime blood pressure phenotype and heart failure (HF): JAMP study (*n* = 6359, 4.5 years' follow-up, 88 HF events). Cumulative incidence of different cardiovascular disease (CVD) events by dipping status (adjusted for age, sex, body mass index, smoking, alcohol use, diabetes, dyslipidemia, history of CVD, use of antihypertensive drugs, bedtime antihypertensive dosing, office systolic blood pressure, and 24-hour systolic blood pressure, with dipper status as the reference). *Source*: Kario et al. Circulation. 2020; 142: 1810–1820 [16].

showed that both higher nighttime BP values and a riser pattern were signifi-cantly associated with the risk of developing atherosclerotic cardiovascular dis-ease. The multivariable-adjusted hazard ratio (HR) value for the risk of atherosclerotic cardiovascular disease associated with a 20 mmHg increase in nighttime systolic blood pressure (SBP) was 1.21 (95% confidence interval [CI] 1.03–1.41; p = 0.017) [16].

A riser pattern has also been shown to significant increase the risk of cardio-vascular disease events in very elderly patients (age ≥80 years) [17]. Even after adjustment for covariates and mean nighttime SBP, patients with a riser pattern of nighttime BP were at significantly higher risk of experiencing a cardiovascular event than those with a dipper pattern (HR 3.11; 95% CI 1.10–8.88) (Figure 1.9) [17].

The elevated cardiovascular risk associated with a riser pattern might be fur-ther increased when sleep duration is short. Data from a prospective study showed that a riser pattern and shorter sleep duration combined to synergistically increase cardiovascular risk in patients with hypertension; those with a riser pat-tern and short sleep duration had the worst cardiovascular prognosis (Figure 1.10) [18].

Chronic kidney disease (CKD) is likely to be associated with nocturnal hyper-tension and the non-dipper/riser pattern. The fall in nighttime BP is attenuated in parallel with decreases in the glomerular filtration rate and increases in urinary albumin excretion. Although CKD increases the risk of future cardiovascular events in both dippers and non-dippers/risers, non-dippers with CKD have the highest level of cardiovascular risk (Figure 1.11) [19].

Riser pattern and HF

The JAMP study was one of the first to separately evaluate the risk of HF associ-ated with nocturnal hypertension and disrupted circadian BP patterns [16]. Both higher nighttime BP values and a riser pattern were significantly associated with the risk of developing HF (multivariable adjusted HR: 2.45 [95% CI 1.34–4.48]; p =0.004) (Figure 1.12). The relationship between a riser pattern and HF risk was independent of nighttime BP, and patients with a riser pattern was found to be at increased risk of developing HF even when 24-hour SBP was well controlled (Figure 1.13) [16]. The risk of coronary artery disease and HF was highest in individuals with a riser pattern and higher nighttime SBP (Figure 1.12) [16].

Additional data come from a follow-up study of patients hospitalized with HF, which showed an association between a non-dipper or riser pattern and a higher rate of cardiovascular events in HF patients who had preserved ejection fraction (HFpEF), but not in those with a reduced ejection fraction (HFrEF) (Figure 1.14) [20]. Furthermore, inpatients with HF who had a riser pattern of nighttime BP were more likely to have HFpEF than HFrEF (Figure 1.15) [21].

Circadian BP pattern appears to be important even in normotensive community-dwelling populations (24-hour BP <125/80 mmHg), with non-dippers and risers showed an increased frequency of concentric cardiac hypertrophy and higher plasma levels of atrial and B-type natriuretic peptides (BNP) compared to

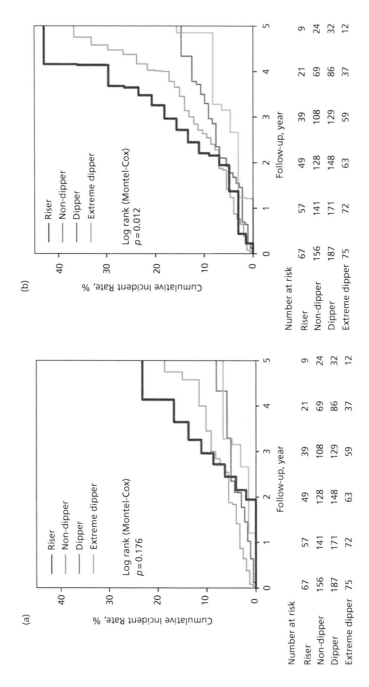

Figure 1.9 Cardiovascular disease (CVD) events in patient subgroups based on patterns of nighttime blood pressure change. (a) CVD event. 41 events (23.6/1000 person-years); (b) Composite outcomes. 72 events (41.5/1000 person-years). *Source:* Fujiwara et al. Am J Hypertens. 2020; 33:520–527 [17].

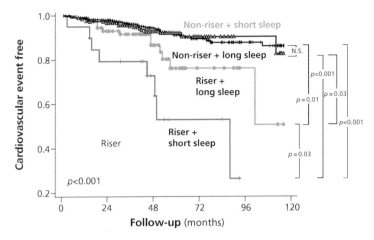

Figure 1.10 Synergistic effect of a riser pattern and short sleep duration on cardiovascular prognosis (n = 1255; 70 years; follow-up 50 months). *Source*: Eguchi et al. Arch Intern Med. 2008; 168: 2225–2231 [18].

individuals with a dipper profile (Table 1.1) [9]. These changes are precursors to the development of HF.

In addition, a pulse rate non-dipper pattern was significantly associated with higher plasma BNP level, especially in those with a non-dipping profile for both BP and pulse rate (Figure 1.16) [22]. A non-dipper pulse rate profile combined with high N-terminal pro-brain natriuretic peptide (NT-proBNP) levels was associated

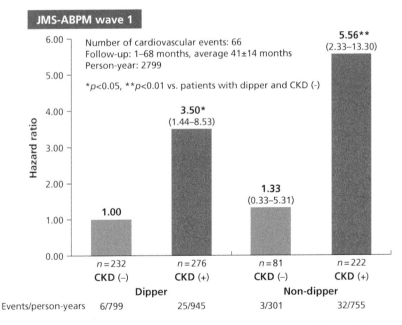

Figure 1.11 Effect of chronic kidney disease (CKD) and dipping status on the rate of cardiovascular events (Jichi Medical University ABPM study). *Source*: Ishikawa et al. J Clin Hypertens (Greenwich). 2008; 10: 787–794 [19].

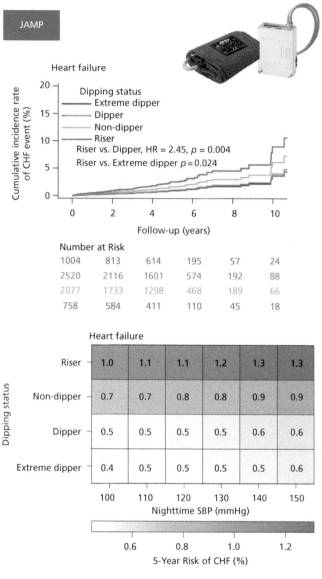

Figure 1.12 Heart failure risk associated with nighttime systolic blood pressure (SBP) and nocturnal dipping status. JAMP Study ($n = 6359$, 4.5 years' follow-up, 88 HF events). Upper: Cumulative incidence of heart failure events by dipping status (adjusted for age, sex, body mass index, smoking, alcohol use, diabetes, dyslipidemia, history of cardiovascular disease, use of antihypertensive drugs, bedtime antihypertensive dosing, office SBP, and 24-hour SBP, with dipper status as the reference). Lower: Heat map showing 5-year risk of heart failure events by nighttime SBP and dipping status (adjusted for age, sex, body mass index, smoking, alcohol use, diabetes, dyslipidemia, history of cardiovascular disease, use of antihypertensive drugs, bedtime antihypertensive dosing, and office SBP). CHF, chronic heart failure; HR, hazard ratio. *Source:* Kario et al. Circulation. 2020; 142: 1810–1820 [16].

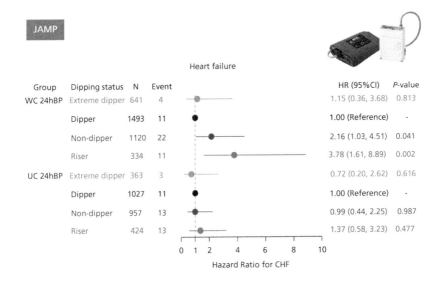

Figure 1.13 Risk of congestive heart failure (CHF) by nocturnal blood pressure (BP) dipping status and 24-hour systolic blood pressure control status. JAMP Study (*n* = 6359, 4.5 years follow-up, 88 HF events). CI, confidence interval; HR, hazard ratio; UC 24hBP, uncontrolled 24-hour BP (24-hour SBP>130 mmHg); WC 24hBP, well-controlled 24-hour BP (24-hour SBP ≤130 mmHg). Values are adjusted for age, sex, body mass index, smoking, alcohol intake, diabetes, dyslipidemia, prevalent cardiovascular disease, use of antihypertensive drugs, bedtime antihypertensive drug dosing, and office and 24-hour systolic blood pressure. *Source*: Kario et al. Circulation. 2020; 142: 1810–1820 [16].

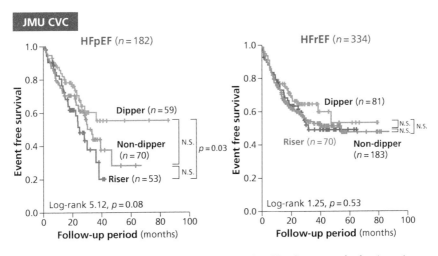

Figure 1.14 Cardiovascular events and disrupted circadian blood pressure rhythm in patients with heart failure (Jichi Medical University Cardiovascular Center, *n* = 516). HFpEF, heart failure with preserved ejection fraction; HFrEF, heart failure with reduced ejection fraction. *Source*: Komori et al. Circ J. 2017; 81: 220–226 [20].

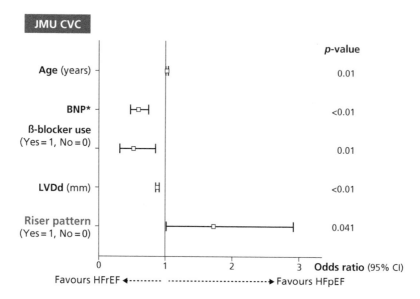

Figure 1.15 Predicting ejection fraction in patients with heart failure (Jichi Medical University Cardiovascular Center, n = 508). *Geometric mean. BNP, brain natriuretic peptide; HFpEF, heart failure with preserved ejection fraction; HFrEF, heart failure with reduced ejection fraction; LVDd, left ventricular diastolic diameter. *Source*: Komori et al. J Clin Hypertens (Greenwich). 2016; 18: 994–999 [21].

with a substantial increase in cardiovascular risk in patients with cardiovascular risk factors undergoing ABPM (p = 0.002 vs. dipper pulse rate + high NT-proBNP, and p < 0.001 vs. the other three groups) (Figure 1.17) [23].

BNP levels have potential for use as a biomarker to assist in achieving perfect 24-hour BP control. Even in patients receiving antihypertensive therapy who have well-controlled office BP, the causes of an increase in wall stress (resulting in elevated

Table 1.1 Cardiac overload in normotensive community-dwelling individuals (n = 74) with a non-dipper nighttime blood pressure (BP) profile (office BP <140/90 mmHg, 24-hour BP <125/80 mmHg).

	Dipper	Non-dipper + riser	
	n = 49	n = 25	p
Office SBP (mmHg)	122 ± 14	123 ± 10	NS
24-hr SBP (mmHg)	112 ± 7.1	111 ± 6.1	NS
LV mass index (g/m²)	103 ± 26	118 ± 34	<0.05
LV relative wall thickness	0.38 ± 0.07	0.43 ± 0.09	<0.01
Concentric hypertrophy (%)	10	28	<0.05
ANP (pg/mL)	14 ± 10	36 ± 63	<0.01
BNP (pg/mL)	16 ± 12	62 ± 153	<0.05

ANP, atrial natriuretic peptide; BNP, B-type natriuretic peptide; LV, left ventricular; NS, not statistically significant; SBP, systolic BP.
Source: Created based on data from Hoshide et al. Am J Hypertens. 2003; 16: 434–438 [9].

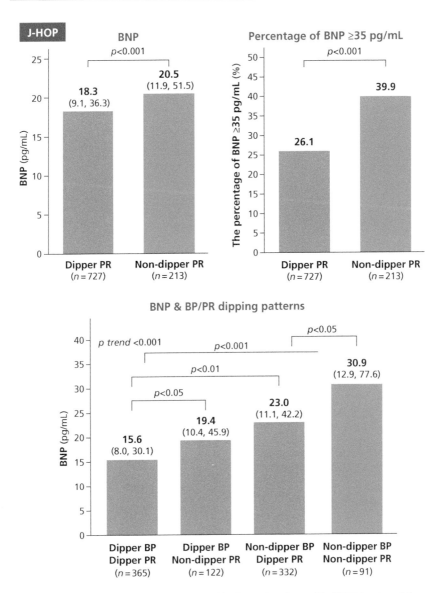

Figure 1.16 Pulse rate (PR) dipping patterns and brain natriuretic peptide (BNP) levels and the percentage of BNP ≥35 pg/mL in high-risk patients from the J-HOP study who underwent ambulatory blood pressure monitoring (*n* = 940); data are presented as median values (25%, 75%). BP, blood pressure. *Source*: Oba et al. J Clin Hypertens (Greenwich). 2017; 19: 402–409 [22].

BNP levels) should be examined because nocturnal hypertension and/or sleep apnea might be present (Figure 1.18) [24]. An increase in NT-proBNP levels during antihypertensive treatment suggests an increase in left ventricular wall stress [25] because serum NT-proBNP is a major determinant of left ventricular wall stress, especially during systole (Figure 1.19). Given that wall stress is determined by both cavity

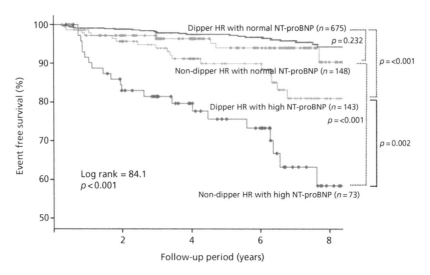

Figure 1.17 Kaplan–Meier curves for cardiovascular events in patient subgroups ($n = 1039$) based on different heart rate (HR;dipping or non-dipping) and N-terminal pro-brain natriuretic peptide (NT-proBNP; normal [<125 pg/mL] or high [≥125 pg/mL]) levels. Patients with a non-dipper HR profile and high NT-proBNP levels had a significantly worse prognosis compared to patients with a dipper HR profile and high NT-proBNP levels ($p = 0.002$). Prognosis did not differ significantly between dipping status subgroups in patients with normal NT-proBNP levels ($p = 0.232$). *Source*: Ogoyama et al. Am J Hypertens. 2020; 33: 430–438 [23]. Reprinted by permission of Oxford University Press.

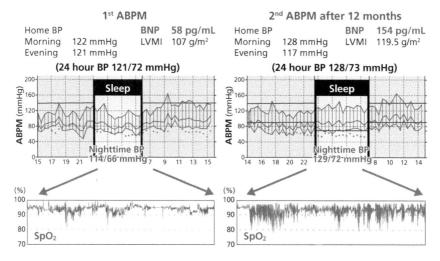

Figure 1.18 How to use brain natriuretic peptide (BNP) as a biomarker to achieve perfect 24-hour blood pressure (BP) control. A 68-year-old woman treated with amlodipine 2.5 mg/day and candesartan 12 mg/day had well-controlled home and 24-hour ambulatory BP (first ambulatory blood pressure monitoring [ABPM]). However, her BNP level increased (from 58 to 154 pg/mL) even when office and home BP remained well controlled. The second ABPM and nocturnal pulse oximetry detected uncontrolled nocturnal hypertension with sleep apnea. LVMI, left ventricular mass index. *Source*: Kario. Essential Manual on Perfect 24-hour Blood Pressure Management from Morning to Nocturnal Hypertension: up-to-date for Anticipation Medicine. Wiley, 2018: 1–309 [24].

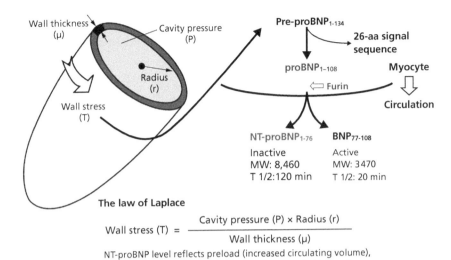

The law of Laplace

$$\text{Wall stress (T)} = \frac{\text{Cavity pressure (P)} \times \text{Radius (r)}}{\text{Wall thickness (}\mu\text{)}}$$

NT-proBNP level reflects preload (increased circulating volume), afterload (systolic blood pressure), and myocardial ischemia

Figure 1.19 Systolic left ventricular wall stress is a major determinant of N-terminal pro-brain natriuretic peptide (NT-proBNP) levels. *Source*: Kario. Essential Manual on Perfect 24-hour Blood Pressure Management from Morning to Nocturnal Hypertension: up-to-date for Anticipation Medicine. Wiley, 2018: 1–309 [24].

pressure and left ventricular cavity radius, an increase in serum NT-proBNP level reflects an increase in preload (increased circulating volume) and afterload (SBP), and myocardial ischemia.

Riser pattern and brain damage

Elderly patients with hypertension, a non-dipper or riser pattern, and high night-time BP have been shown to have atrophy of the brain and insular cortex (Figures 1.20 and 1.21) [26, 27]. In addition, a non-dipper pattern and nocturnal

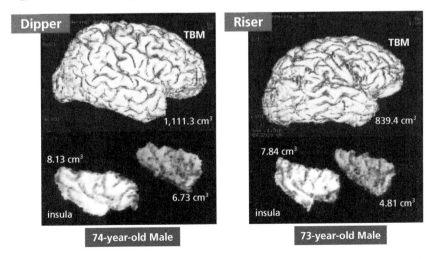

Figure 1.20 Brain volume in individual patients with a riser versus dipper pattern (JMS ABPM study, wave 2 core). TBM, total brain matter. *Source*: Nagai et al. J Hypertens. 2008; 26: 1636–1641 [26].

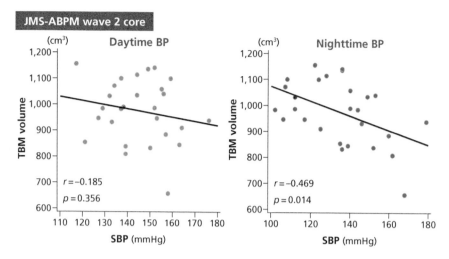

Figure 1.21 Ambulatory blood pressure (BP) and brain volume in elderly patients with hypertension (JMS ABPM study, wave 2 core). SBP, systolic BP; TBM, total brain matter. *Source*: Nagai et al. J Hypertens. 2008; 26: 1636–1641 [26].

hypertension are significantly associated with cognitive dysfunction and slow walking speed in elderly subjects (Figure 1.22) [28].

In patients with HF, a riser pattern was significantly associated with mild cognitive impairments [29]. A quantitative brain MRI study in patients with HF demonstrated that deep white matter lesions are in the presence of a riser pattern of nighttime BP (Figure 1.23) [30].

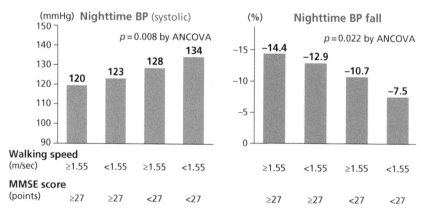

Figure 1.22 Non-dipping pattern of nighttime blood pressure (BP) in elderly patients with heart failure (*n* = 148, mean age 75 years). The four groups are divided based on median values for walking speed and MMSE score. ANCOVA, analysis of covariance; HDL, high-density lipoprotein; MMSE, mini-mental state examination. Data are shown as mean values after adjustment for age, sex, blood glucose and HDL cholesterol. *Source*: Yano et al. Am J Hypertens. 2011; 24: 285–291 [28].

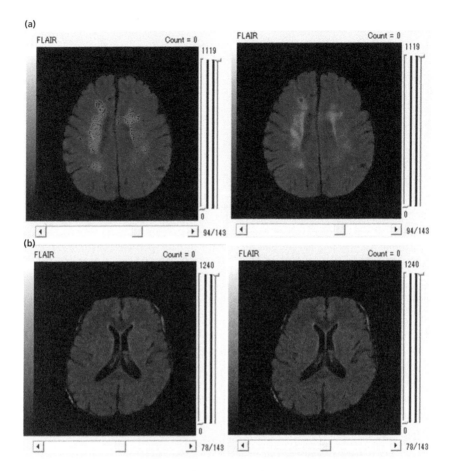

Figure 1.23 Quantitative evaluation of white matter hyperintensity (WMH). (a) Brain imaging scan of a patient with a non-dipper nighttime blood pressure pattern, showing detection of a large amount of WMH (left); image before software analysis (right). (b) Brain imaging scan of a patient with a dipper nighttime blood pressure pattern, showing only a small amount of WMH (left); image before software analysis (right). *Source*: Komori et al. J Clin Hypertens (Greenwich). 2021; 23: 1089–1092 [30].

Nocturnal hypertension

Nocturnal hypertension is diagnosed when the average of nighttime BP measurements is ≥120/70 mmHg. Patients with a non-dipper or riser BP pattern are likely to have nocturnal hypertension.

In prospective studies, nocturnal hypertension was associated with an increased risk of cardiovascular events, both stroke and coronary artery disease. This risk increased in parallel with increasing daytime and nighttime BP readings, but only the increase in nighttime BP was significantly associated with elevated ten-year risk of cardiovascular events, particularly in medicated patients (Figure 1.24) [6]. However, these findings were based only on baseline BP meaning that any change in medication would be based on office BP, which relates more closely to daytime BP

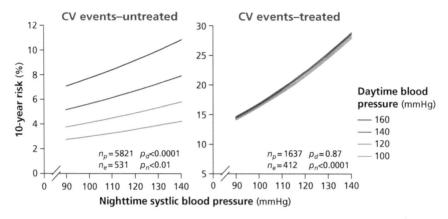

Figure 1.24 Nighttime systolic blood pressure and the risk of cardiovascular (CV) events based on data from the International Database on Ambulatory blood pressure monitoring in relation to Cardiovascular Outcomes (IDACO); n = 7458, 9.6-year follow-up. np and ne indicate the number of participants at risk and the number of events, respectively. pd and pn denote the significance of the independent contributions of daytime and nighttime blood pressures. *Source*: Boggia et al. Lancet. 2007; 370(9594):1219–29 [6].

rather than nighttime BP. Therefore, elevated nighttime BP is likely to persist during long-term follow-up. This highlights the fact that antihypertensive therapy guided by office BP measurements may not reduce the risk of nocturnal hypertension.

The risk of cardiovascular events in the ABP-International registry showed a synergistic relationship between nighttime SBP and nighttime pulse rate (Figure 1.25) [31]. Another study in well-medicated patients with congestive HF

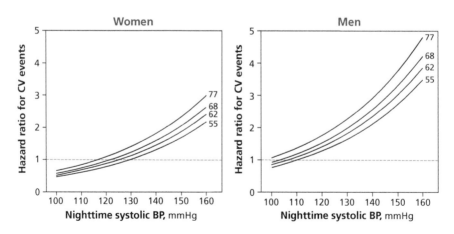

Figure 1.25 Synergistic increase in cardiovascular (CV) risk based on nighttime blood pressure (BP) and pulse rate based on data from the ABP-International registry; n = 7600 from Italy, USA, Australia and Japan). Nighttime pulse rate groups were defined based on midpoints within each pulse rate quartile (55, 62, 68, and 77 beats/min). Risk estimates were adjusted to 52 years of age, non-smoking, no diabetes, total cholesterol level 206 mg/dL, and serum creatinine 0.9 mg/dL. *Source*: Palatini et al. Int J Cardiol. 2013;168:1490–5 [31].

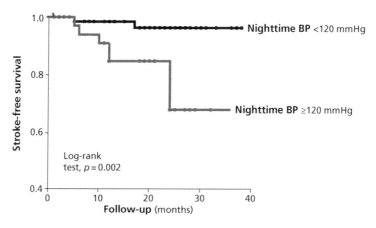

Figure 1.26 Nighttime systolic blood pressure (SBP) on ambulatory blood pressure monitoring and stroke prognosis in patients with ischemic/hypertensive heart failure (Jichi Medical University Cardiovascular Center, n = 111). *Source*: Komori et al. Hypertens Res. 2008; 31: 289–294 [32].

and uncontrolled nocturnal hypertension showed that a nighttime/sleep SBP >120 mmHg) was associated with a significant increase in stroke risk during follow-up (Figure 1.26) [32]. Nighttime SBP in particular appeared to be an important risk factor for HF compared with other cardiovascular events (Figure 1.27) [16].

The negative impact of nocturnal hypertension is greater in patients with hypertension and diabetes than in those with hypertension without diabetes. In a

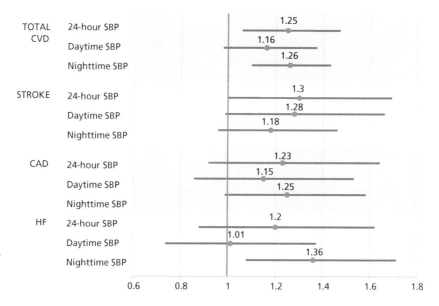

Figure 1.27 Risk of cardiovascular disease by different ambulatory BP measures (per 20-mmHg increase in systolic blood pressure [SBP]). JAMP study (n = 6359, 4.5 years' follow-up). CAD, coronary artery disease; CVD, cardiovascular disease; HF, heart failure. *Source*: Kario et al. Circulation. 2020; 142: 1810–1820 [16].

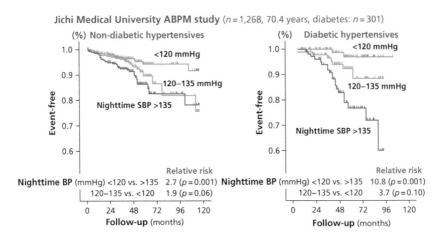

Figure 1.28 Interaction between hypertension and diabetes with respect to the association between nighttime systolic blood pressure (SBP) and cardiovascular prognosis. RR, relative risk. *Source*: Eguchi et al. Am J Hypertens. 2008; 21: 443–450 [33].

prospective study, the increase in cardiovascular risk associated with nocturnal hypertension (nighttime SBP >135 mmHg) vs. nocturnal normotension (nighttime SBP <120 mmHg) was 10.8 times in patients with diabetes compared with 2.7 times in those without diabetes (Figure 1.28) [33].

In treated patients with hypertension who have well-controlled home BP, the presence of uncontrolled nocturnal hypertension (nighttime SBP ≥120 mmHg on ABPM) attenuated effects of antihypertensive therapy on the urinary albumin-creatinine ratio (UACR) and BNP compared to patients with well-controlled home and nighttime BP (both $p<0.001$) (Figure 1.29) [25]. Isolated and masked nocturnal hypertension are also significant risk factors for target organ damage, which in turn increases cardiovascular risk [34–36]. For example, patients with isolated nocturnal hypertension show greater arterial stiffness than those with ambulatory normotension, as assessed using peripheral and central augmentation index, the ambulatory arterial stiffness index, and brachial-ankle pulse wave velocity (PWV).

Taken together, the above data indicate that controlling nighttime BP during sleep, as well as morning and evening home BP levels, is essential to reduce target organ damage in patients receiving antihypertensive therapy.

Associated Conditions and Mechanisms of Nocturnal Hypertension

Risk factors for nocturnal hypertension include aging, orthostatic hypotension, diabetes, and Asian ethnicity, while nocturnal hypertension is common in patients with conditions such as CKD or obstructive sleep apnea. In addition, secondary hypertension and diseases with an increase in sympathetic nervous activity or renin-angiotensin system activity increase circulating volume, resulting in nocturnal hypertension (Table 1.2) [37].

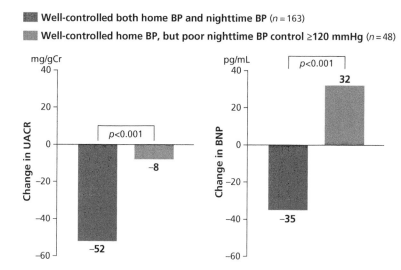

Figure 1.29 Clinical implications of controlling nighttime blood pressure (BP) in hypertension. BNP, B-type natriuretic peptide; SBP, systolic BP; UACR, urinary albumin-creatinine ratio. *Source*: Yano et al. Am J Hypertens. 2012; 25: 306–312 [25].

With respect to circadian BP patterns, increased circulating volume, autonomic nervous dysfunction, poor sleep quality, and structural vascular disease are the major mechanisms of nocturnal hypertension in individuals with a non-dipper or riser pattern of nighttime BP (Figure 1.30) [38]. Increased circulating volume may have a compensatory effect and increase nighttime BP as well as daytime BP by excreting sodium from the kidney based on Guyton's theory of the pressure–natriuresis relationship, resulting in nocturnal hypertension of the non-dipper/

Table 1.2 Determinants of nocturnal hypertension.

Environmental factors	Salt sensitivity
Summer (hot temperature)	
Behavioral factors	**Secondary hypertension**
High salt intake	Endocrine disease (primary aldosteronism,
Reduced physical activity	renovascular hypertension, Cushing syndrome,
Poor sleep quality	pheochromocytoma)
Nocturia	Chronic kidney disease (CKD)
Shift-working	Obstructive sleep apnoea syndrome (OSAS)
Risk factors	
Aging	
Hypertension	**Disease**
Orthostatic hypotension	Heart failure
Diabetes	Stroke
Asian ethnicity	Cognitive dysfunction

Source: Kario. Essential Manual of 24-hour Blood Pressure Management from Morning to Nocturnal Hypertension, Wiley–Blackwell, 2015: 1–138 [37].

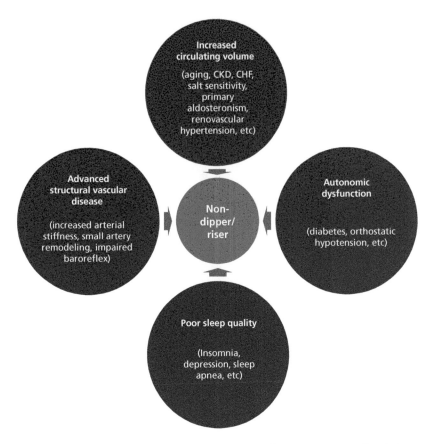

Figure 1.30 Mechanism of non-dipper/riser type nocturnal hypertension. CHF, chronic heart failure; CKD, chronic kidney disease. *Source*: Kario. Clinician's Manual on Early Morning Risk Management in Hypertension. Science Press, London, UK, 2004: 1–68 [38].

riser type [39]. Thus, conditions that increase sympathetic nervous activity, and renin–angiotensin–aldosterone system-associated increases in circulating volume due to reduced sodium excretion, result in a non-dipper/riser pattern of nighttime BP. Activation of neurohumoral factors due to orthostatic hypotension during the daytime may persist during sleep when an individual is in the supine position. Poor sleep quality (such as that associated with obstructive sleep apnea), insomnia, anxiety, and depression (Figure 1.31) [40], and shift work can all contribute to nocturnal hypertension.

Mechanism of cardiovascular risk of nocturnal hypertension

The specific increase in cardiovascular risk associated with nocturnal hypertension can be accounted for by several heterogeneous pathophysiological mechanisms (Figure 1.32). First, nighttime BP surges driven by increased sympathetic activity could trigger nocturnal cardiovascular events and potentiate age-related target organ damage (Figure 1.32). These surges in nighttime BP have a number of potential triggers (including an episode of obstructive sleep apnea, arousals,

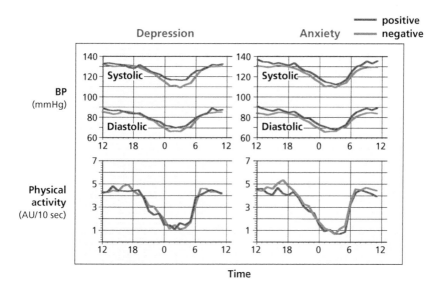

Figure 1.31 Depression and non-dipping profile of nighttime blood pressure (BP) (New York work site study). *Source*: Kario et al. Hypertension. 2001; 38: 997–1002 [40].

rapid-eye-movement sleep, and nocturia) and are augmented by an impaired baroreflex secondary to increased sympathetic tone and vascular stiffness.

Second, nocturnal hypertension may represent the final stage of hypertension in individuals with target organ damage and other comorbidities (Figure 1.32). Sympathetic activity during sleep is lower than that in the morning and daytime

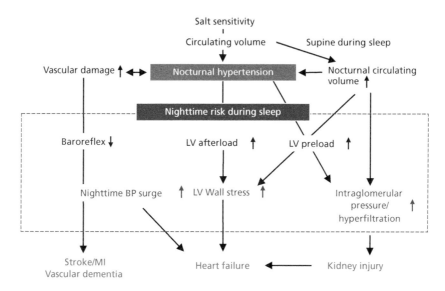

Figure 1.32 Mechanisms underlying the reilationship between nocturnal hypertension and cardiovascular risk. BP, blood pressure; LV, left ventricular; MI, myocardial infarction. *Source*: Kario. Hypertension. 2018; 71: 997–1009 [1].

periods, meaning that nighttime BP is less likely to increase than BP at other times of the day. In general, BP increases with age; morning BP increases first due to the higher level of sympathetic activity in the morning, while nighttime BP is the last to increase because sympathetic tone is lower at night. This means that increases in night-time BP probably indicate advanced structural changes in the large and small arteries (i.e. increased arterial stiffness and vascular resistance) and increased circulating volume because the ability of the kidneys to excrete sodium is reduced.

Third, the supine position during sleep results in increased venous return from the lower body to the heart, which increases left ventricular (LV) preload (Figure 1.32). LV wall stress secondary to the increase in afterload associated with nocturnal hypertension is augmented by the nighttime increase in LV preload (Law of Laplace). Increased LV wall stress is a risk factor for nocturnal-onset HF. Furthermore, LV preload is also increased by a shift of interstitial fluid from the soft tissue of the lower body into the circulating volume. The simultaneous increase in nighttime circulating volume and nighttime BP could combine to worsen renal function by increasing intraglomerular pressure and hyperfiltration (Figure 1.32).

Finally, morning dosing of existing antihypertensive agents may not provide sufficient BP-lowering coverage through the nighttime period, despite reductions in daytime BP. This means that nocturnal hypertension could go undetected if not specifically assessed.

Extreme dipping

Extreme dippers with nighttime BP fall of ≥ 20% also show increased cardiovascular risk, including advanced silent cerebral disease detected by brain MRI (Figure 1.33) [7]. A typical case of extreme dipping is shown in (Figure 1.34) [41]. In addition, the prospective JMS-ABPM study wave 1 showed that elderly patients with hypertension who had an extreme dipper pattern were at increased risk of future clinical stroke events (Figure 1.6) [8]. Results from the JAMP study are consistent, showing that patients with an extreme dipper pattern were at high risk of experiencing a stroke event (Figure 1.35) [16]. This relationship was due to an increase in stroke risk in extreme dipper patients with well-controlled 24-hour BP, whereas the risk of stroke was not significantly increased in extreme dipper patients for whom 24-hour BP was uncontrolled (Figure 1.36) [16]. In a meta-analysis of data from 17 312 hypertensive patients from three continents, the Ambulatory Blood pressure Collaboration in patients with hypertension (ABC-H) study found that an extreme dipper pattern was only significantly associated with cardiovascular events in patients with hypertension not receiving antihypertensive medication (Figure 1.37) [42]. Furthermore, the relationship between extreme dipping and cardiovascular events appears to be modified by patient age, being greatest in those aged 70–79 and, especially, ≥80 years (Figure 1.38) [43].

The increase in cardiovascular risk associated with extreme dipping can be predicted by the target organ damage documented in these patients. In the CARDIA study of young normotensive subjects, extreme dippers, non-dippers, and risers (based on baseline ABPM) went on to develop more advanced coronary calcification over the next ≥10 years. Even after controlling for baseline

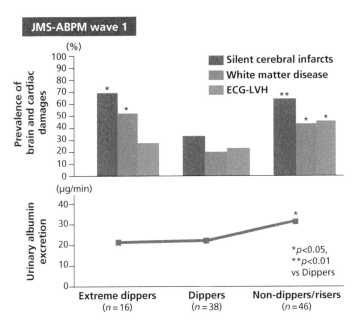

Figure 1.33 Nighttime blood pressure dipping status and organ damage in older patients with sustained hypertension. LVH, left ventricular hypertrophy. *Source*: Kario. Hypertension. 1996; 27: 130–135 [7].

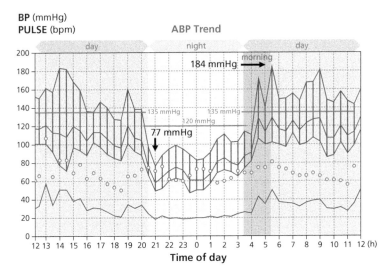

Figure 1.34 Example of 24-hour ambulatory blood pressure (ABP) monitoring from a patient showing an extreme dipper profile of nighttime blood pressure (BP) (37.7% nocturnal BP fall). The patient is a 70-year-old male with a 6-year history of hypertension, treated with amlodipine 5 mg/day and losartan 25 mg/day. 24-hour BP = 135/85 mmHg, daytime BP = 154/96 mmHg, nighttime BP = 96/62 mmHg, sleep-trough morning surge = 68 mmHg, pre-wakening morning surge = 44 mmHg. *Source*: Kario J Hum Hypertens. 2017; 31: 231–243 [41].

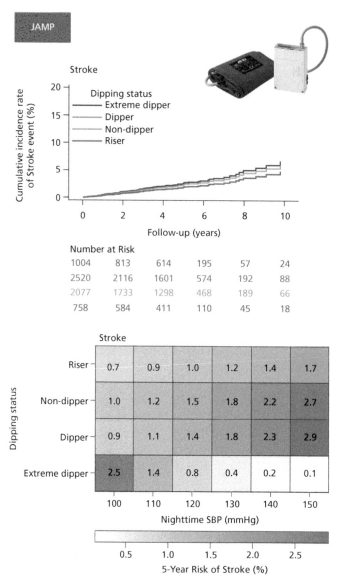

Figure 1.35 Stroke risk associated with nighttime systolic blood pressure (SBP) and nocturnal dipping status. JAMP Study (*n* = 6359, 4.5 years' follow-up, 119 stroke events). Upper: Cumulative incidence of stroke events by dipping status (adjusted for age, sex, body mass index, smoking, alcohol use, diabetes, dyslipidemia, history of cardiovascular disease, use of antihypertensive drugs, bedtime antihypertensive dosing, office SBP, and 24-hour SBP, with dipper status as the reference). Lower: Heat map showing 5-year risk of stroke events by nighttime SBP and dipping status (adjusted for age, sex, body mass index, smoking, alcohol use, diabetes, dyslipidemia, history of cardiovascular disease, use of antihypertensive drugs, bedtime antihypertensive dosing, and office SBP). CHF, chronic heart failure; HR, hazard ratio. *Source*: Kario et al. Circulation. 2020; 142: 1810–1820 [16].

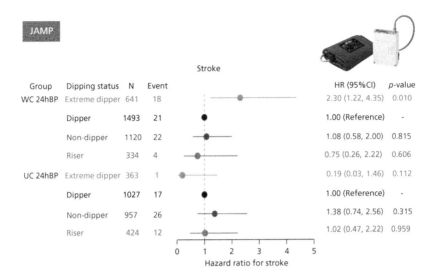

Figure 1.36 Risk of stroke by nocturnal blood pressure (BP) dipping status and 24-hour systolic blood pressure control status. JAMP Study (n = 6359, 4.5 years' follow-up, 119 stroke events). CI, confidence interval; HR, hazard ratio; UC 24hBP, uncontrolled 24-hour BP (24-hour systolic BP >130 mmHg); WC 24hBP, well-controlled 24-hour BP (24-hour systolic BP ≤130 mmHg). Values are adjusted for age, sex, body mass index, smoking, alcohol intake, diabetes, dyslipidemia, prevalent cardiovascular disease, use of antihypertensive drugs, bedtime antihypertensive drug dosing, and office and 24-hour systolic BP. *Source*: Kario et al. Circulation. 2020; 142: 1810–1820 [16].

covariates, the risk of having coronary calcium was at least four times greater in both extreme dippers and non-dippers/risers compared with normal dippers (Figure 1.39) [44]. Extreme dippers have also been shown to have deep white matter lesions on brain MRI [45], reduced cerebral blood flow [46], and increased PWV [47].

The pathophysiology of extreme dipping not well understood. Baroreflex failure caused by increased daytime sympathetic activity in patients with increased arterial stiffness is one possible pathophysiological mechanism (Figure 1.40) [41]. Furthermore, increases in the plasma vasopressin level following head-up tilting have been shown to be significantly greater in extreme dippers than in dippers, which might counteract lower circulating blood volume in extreme dippers [48]. Extreme dipping is also associated with other phenotypes of BP variability, increasing the risk of organ damage and cardiovascular events.

Morning surge in BP

There is significant diurnal variation in the time of onset of cardiovascular events. Morning is the most important period for cardiovascular diseases [38, 49], with cardiovascular events occurring most frequently in the morning just after awakening, at the time of peak ambulatory BP (Figure 1.41) [49]. Exaggerated MBPS and morning hypertension are risk factors for cardiovascular events (Figure 1.42),

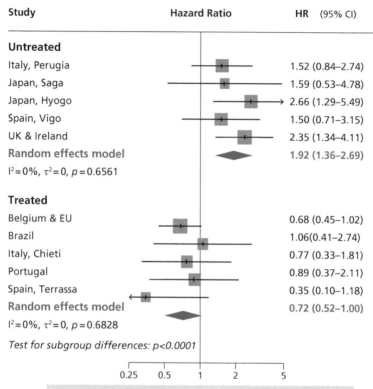

Study	Hazard Ratio	HR (95% CI)
Untreated		
Italy, Perugia		1.52 (0.84–2.74)
Japan, Saga		1.59 (0.53–4.78)
Japan, Hyogo		2.66 (1.29–5.49)
Spain, Vigo		1.50 (0.71–3.15)
UK & Ireland		2.35 (1.34–4.11)
Random effects model		1.92 (1.36–2.69)
$I^2=0\%$, $\tau^2=0$, $p=0.6561$		
Treated		
Belgium & EU		0.68 (0.45–1.02)
Brazil		1.06(0.41–2.74)
Italy, Chieti		0.77 (0.33–1.81)
Portugal		0.89 (0.37–2.11)
Spain, Terrassa		0.35 (0.10–1.18)
Random effects model		0.72 (0.52–1.00)
$I^2=0\%$, $\tau^2=0$, $p=0.6828$		
Test for subgroup differences: p<0.0001		

0.25   0.5   1   2   5

The Ambulatory Blood pressure Collaboration in patients with Hypertension (ABC-H) examined this issue in a meta-analysis of 17,312 hypertensives from 3 continents.

Figure 1.37 Forest plot from a meta-analysis evaluating the association between an extreme dipping pattern and total cardiovascular events in 17 312 patients with hypertension from three continents (adjusted for average 24-hour systolic blood pressure). CI, confidence interval; EU, European Union; HR, hazard ratio. *Source*: Salles et al. Hypertension. 2016; 67: 693–700 [42].

and are associated with advanced organ damage (Figure 1.43) [2, 37, 50–53]. The risk of MBPS is independently of the risk of riser pattern of nighttime BP (Table 1.3) [2]. Morning BP level is more closely associated with damage to the

Table 1.3 Relative stroke risk in patients with hypertension.

JMS-ABPM Wave 1 ($n = 519$)		
Covariants	**Relative risk (95% CI)**	**p-value**
Morning BP surge (10 mmHg) (systolic)	1.25 (1.06–1.48)	0.008
Nocturnal BP dipping status (vs. dippers)		0.025
Extreme dippers	1.43 (0.59–3.43)	0.426
Non-dippers	1.76 (0.78–4.01)	0.175
Risers	2.71 (1.02–7.21)	0.047

BP, blood pressure; CI, confidence interval.
Source: Created based on data from Kario et al. Circulation. 2003; 107: 1401–1406 [2].

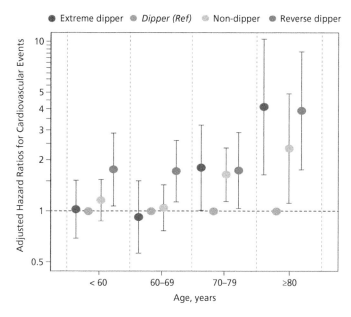

Figure 1.38 Adjusted hazard ratio (HR) values for fatal and nonfatal cardiovascular events based on dipping pattern of nighttime blood pressure and stratified by age group. Data are adjusted for age, sex, smoking, diabetes mellitus, total cholesterol, estimated glomerular filtration rate, and 24-hour systolic blood pressure. Alcohol intake was not accepted in the final parsimonious model. The dipper category was considered as the reference. *Source*: Palatini et al. Hypertension. 2020; 75: 324–330 [43].

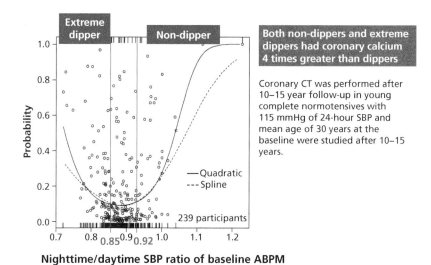

Figure 1.39 U-shaped association between nighttime blood pressure dipping status and coronary calcium (CARDIA study). ABPM, ambulatory blood pressure monitoring; CT, computed tomography; SBP, systolic blood pressure. *Source*: Viera et al. Hypertension. 2012; 59: 1157–63 [44].

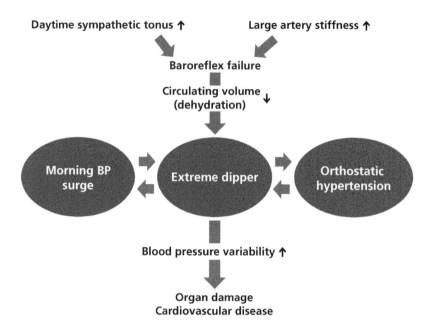

Figure 1.40 Mechanism of an extreme dipper pattern of nighttime blood pressure (BP), and related phenotypes of blood pressure variability. *Source*: Kario J Hum Hypertens. 2017; 31: 231–243 [41].

brain, heart, and kidney, as well as the risk of cardiovascular and cerebrovascular events (Table 1.4) [51] and disability in the elderly, than office BP, both in patients with hypertension and community-based normotensive populations [54, 55].

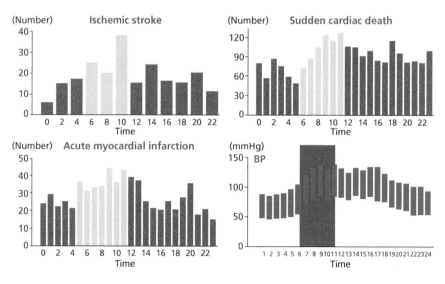

Figure 1.41 Onset time of cardiovascular events. BP, blood pressure. *Source*: Muller et al. Circulation. 1989; 79: 733–43 [49].

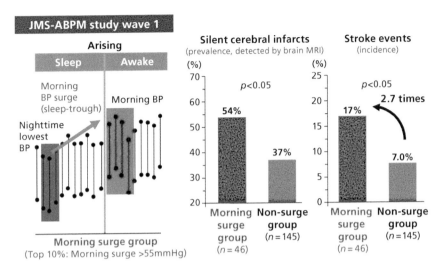

Figure 1.42 Morning blood pressure (BP) surge and stroke risk in patients with hypertension (matching for age and 24-hour systolic BP). ABPM, ambulatory blood pressure monitoring; MRI, magnetic resonance imaging. *Source*: Left: Kario. Hypertension. 2010; 56: 765–773 [53]. Right: Created based on data from Kario et al. Circulation. 2003; 107: 1401–1406 [2].

Recent evidence also shows that uncontrolled morning hypertension is a strong predictor of cardiovascular events in medicated hypertensive patients [56].

MBPS is one component of diurnal BP variability [3, 38, 53, 57–59], and normal MBPS is a physiological phenomenon. However, we first demonstrated that "exaggerated" MBPS is a pathological form of BP variability, which is significantly associated with other phenotypes of BP variability. In addition to the 24-hour

Table 1.4 Morning blood pressure (calculated as the 2-hour average of systolic blood pressure values after rising determined using ambulatory blood pressure monitoring). JMS-ABPM study wave 1.

Covariates	Relative risk (95% CI)	*p*-value
Clinic SBP (10 mmHg)	–	
24-hour SBP (10 mmHg)	–	
Daytime SBP (10 mmHg)	–	
Evening SBP (10 mmHg)	–	
Nighttime SBP (10 mmHg)	–	
Pre-awake SBP (10 mmHg)	–	
Morning SBP (10 mmHg)	**1.44 (1.25–1.67)**	**<0.0001**

Findings are adjusted for age, sex, body mass index, smoking status, diabetes, hyperlipidemia, silent cerebral infarct, and antihypertensive medication status). All systolic blood pressure variables were added into the model, and analyzed using stepwise Cox regression analysis.

CI, confidence interval; SBP, systolic blood pressure.

Source: Created based on data from Hypertens Res. 2006; 29: 581–587 [51].

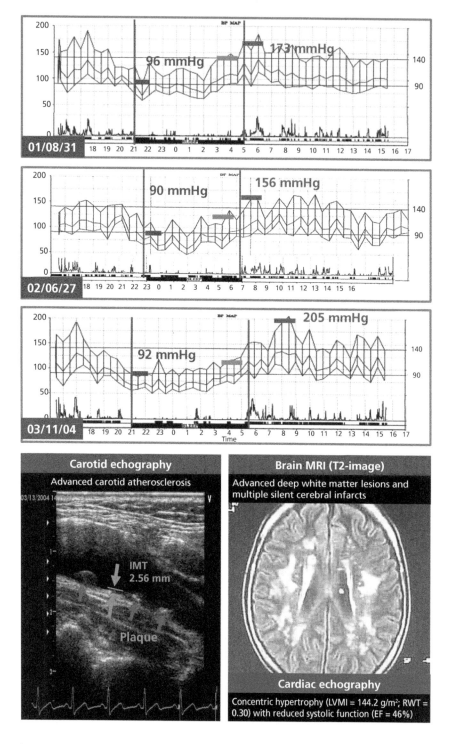

Figure 1.43 A 69-year-old man with morning hypertension, showing advanced organ damage. Echocardiography shows concentric hypertrophy (left ventricular mass index [LVMI] 144.2 g/m², relative wall thickness [RWT] 0.30, with reduced systolic function (left ventricular ejection fraction [EF] 46%). IMT, intima media thickness. *Source*: Kario. Essential Manual of 24-hour Blood Pressure Management from Morning to Nocturnal Hypertension. Blackwell, 2015: 1–138 [37].

persistent pressure overload, dynamic BP variability from the nadir during sleep to peak early in the morning could contribute to the cardiovascular event continuum, from the early stage of subclinical vascular disease to the final trigger of cardiovascular events [3, 38, 53, 57–59].

Definition of MBPS

There is no consensus on the definition and threshold of pathological MBPS. Use of different definitions and studies of different populations may contribute to the lack of consistency in current findings. MBPS is usually assessed using ABPM; however, there are several definitions of MBPS, such as sleep-trough surge, pre-wakening surge, and rising BP surge (Figure 1.44) [2, 38, 53]. Sleep-trough surge is one of the dynamic diurnal surges during the specific period from sleep to early morning [2], when cardiovascular risk is exaggerated. Thus, it is important to exclude the effects of overall diurnal BP variation, such as the dipping status of nighttime BP, in order to establish the clinical implications of sleep-trough morning surge (STMS). As expected, STMS is likely to be most common in extreme dippers with a marked nighttime BP fall, and will be less common in non-dippers (who show a smaller or nonexistent dipping of nighttime BP) or risers (who have

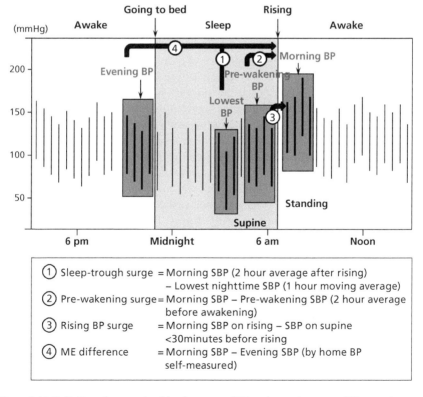

Figure 1.44 Definitions for morning blood pressure (BP) and morning surge. ME, morning-evening; SBP, systolic BP. *Source*: Kario et al. Circulation. 2003; 107: 1401–1406 [2] and Kario. Hypertension. 2010; 56: 765–773 [53].

higher nighttime vs. daytime BP [2]. Even after controlling for nighttime BP dipping status or mean nighttime BP level, the risk associated with STMS remains significant [2]. Prewakening surge refers to the BP change occurring from four hours before to after rising [2]. Although STMS and prewakening surges are defined based on the BP difference, theoretically, the speed of the surge (the slope of the increase in morning BP against time) may be a better indicator of the risk of morning surge [60]. A recently proposed measure of MBPS, calculated as the product of the rate of morning surge and the amplitude (day–night difference), providing information on the "power" of the MBPS, may better clarify morning cardiovascular risk [61]. Given that the rising BP surge may detect morning risk just after rising [62], it may highlight the BP surge that is subsequently augmented by physical activity in the morning.

Morning BP surge and cardiovascular disease

There are numerous studies indicating that MBPS is a strong predictor for the risk of cardiovascular diseases (stroke, coronary artery disease, total mortality) in both outpatients with hypertension and community-dwelling subjects. Although some studies have shown that this predictive ability is independent of average of 24-hour BP, others did not.

The Jichi Medical School (JMS)-ABPM study wave 1 enrolled 519 unmedicated elderly Japanese patients with hypertension (mean age 72 years) [2]. Two measure of MBPS were determined: STMS (defined as morning BP [2-hour average of four 30-minute BP readings just after waking up] minus the lowest nighttime BP); and prewakening surge (defined as morning BP minus prewakening BP [2-hour average of four BP readings just before waking up]). The exaggerated morning surge group was defined as the top tenth percentile of patients with STMS (>55 mmHg), and these patients had a higher incidence of stroke than the non-surge group (19% vs. 7.3%, $p = 0.004$). After matching for age and 24-hour BP, the relative risk of stroke in the surge vs. the nonsurge group was 2.7 ($p = 0.04$) (Figure 1.42) [2]. This association remained significant after adjusting for nighttime BP dipping status. The prewakening surge tended to be associated with stroke risk, although the association was not statistically significant ($p = 0.07$). In another Japanese population study, MBPS was associated with cerebral hemorrhage [63].

The International Database on Ambulatory Blood Pressure in Relation to Cardiovascular Outcome (IDACO), including 5645 subjects, provided definitive data showing that both morning surges (STMS and pre-wakening surges) are independent risk factors for total mortality and cardiovascular events [52]. Similar to the JMS-ABPM study, the IDACO study also found that only individuals with MBPS values in the top tenth percentile were at risk of mortality or cardiovascular events (Figure 1.45) [52], even after controlling for covariates including age and 24-hour BP. For the risk of patients with HF, an another follow-up study of patients hospitalized with HF showed that STMS was a significant predictor of the composite outcome of all-cause mortality and worsening HF (hazard ratio 2.84, 95% confidence interval 1.58–5.10, $P < 0.01$) in the HFrEF but not HFpEF patients (Figure 1.46) [64].

A meta-analysis demonstrated that a 10 mmHg increase in MBPS was associated with an 11% increase in the risk of stroke [65]. In the JAMP study, MBPS

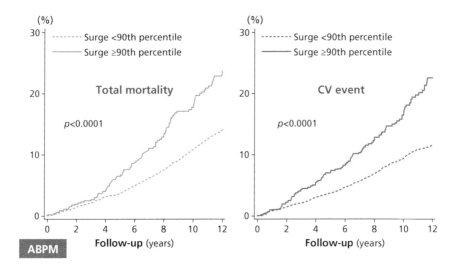

Figure 1.45 Prognostic value of the morning blood pressure surge (sleep-trough surge) in 5645 subjects from eight populations. CV, cardiovascular. *Source*: Li et al. Hypertension. 2010; 55: 1040–8 [52].

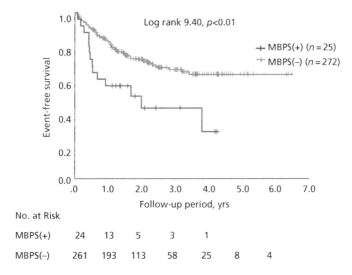

Figure 1.46 Kaplan-Meier curves for the composite endpoint according to the presence or absence of the morning blood pressure surge (MBPS)* in patients with heart failure (HF) with reduced ejection fraction (HFrEF; n = 297). The composite outcome were occurred 90 events (all-cause mortality 33, worsening HF 66 [9 patients are duplicate]; 16.3 per 100 person-years) in the HFrEF group. There was a significantly higher incidence of endpoints in MBPS than non-MBPS patients in the HFrEF group. *MBPS was defined as >40 mmHg increase in average morning systolic blood pressure (2 hours after waking) from the lowest sleep blood pressure. *Source*: Komori et al. Circ J. 2021, 85: 1535–1542 [64].

was significantly associated with a risk of stroke incidence in the dipper group, whereas it was not found in the non-dipper group. After adjusting covariates, this association between MBPS and stroke still remained in the dipper group (HR, 1.14; 95% CI, 1.00–1.30; p = 0.050) (Figure 1.47).

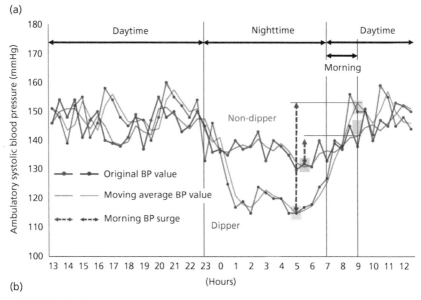

(a)

(b)

Morning blood pressure surge and stroke incidence according to dipping status				
	Dipper, n = 3490		Non-dipper, n = 2804	
ABPM characteristics				
24-hour SBP, mmHg	131.7±13.5		135.0±16.2*	
Daytime SBP, mmHg	139.5±14.2		136.2±16.1*	
Nighttime SBP, mmHg	115.1±13.1		132.4±17.5*	
Morning BP surge, mmHg	49.2±18.9		34.6±17.2*	
Outcome				
Events, number	57		62	
Model	HR (95%CI) for morning BP surge, +10 mmHg	P	HR (95%CI) for morning BP surge, +10 mmHg	P
Adjusted	1.19 (1.05, 1.35)	0.006	1.06 (0.92, 1.22)	0.423
Fully adjusted	1.14 (1.00, 1.30)	0.050	1.03 (0.90, 1.19)	0.635

The adjusted model included 24-h SBP. The fully adjusted model included age, sex, body mass index, smoking, diabetes, hyperlipidemia, prevalent cardiovascular disease, antihypertensive treatment, and 24h SBP. BP indicates blood pressure: HR, hazard ratio;CI, confidence interval; SBP, systolic blood pressure. *P<0.001 vs. dipper group.

Figure 1.47 Morning blood pressure (BP) surge separated for dipper and non-dipper and its association with stroke events (a) Illustration of the definition of morning BP surge in patients with dipper and non-dipper status. (b) Results of the hazard ratio of morning BP surge for stroke events in the dipper and non-dipper groups. Source: Hoshide S and Kario K. Morning Surge in Blood Pressure and Stroke Events in a Large Modern ABPM Cohort: Results of the JAMP study. Hypertension. 2021; 78: 894–896.

In addition, a population-based prospective study demonstrated that STMS was positively associated with the risk of cardiovascular and all-cause death and was directly related to indices of 24-hour SBP variability [59]. In a prospective study of patients with hypertension, blunted MBPS was an independent predictor of cardiovascular events [66]. Similarly, a study of patients referred for ABPM showed that an increased MBPS was significantly associated with decreased mortality, especially in non-dippers [67]. Thus, both extremes, that is, the absence (or a negative value) of MBPS and exaggerated MBPS, may be pathological, resulting in nonlinear J-shaped (or U-shaped) associations between MBPS and cardiovascular events with specific thresholds [53]. Thus, the identification of pathological thresholds of MBPS is clinically important. In the JMS-ABPM study, the top tenth percentile of SBP was 55 mmHg in elderly patients with hypertension [2], and in IDACO was 37 mmHg for community-dwelling individuals [52]. Thus, the threshold of pathological MBPS should be identified for clinical practice in the future. Recent prospective studies in elderly patients with treated hypertension demonstrated that high morning surge (MS) of SBP predicted coronary events in dippers but not non-dippers [68]. In the same group of patients, even those who achieved normal ambulatory BP during antihypertensive therapy were at increased cardiovascular risk when they had a dipper profile and high MS or a non-dipper profile [69].

In a meta-analysis of seven prospective studies, evaluating MS in a total of 14 133 patients with a mean follow-up period of 7.1 years, excess STMS was a strong predictor for future all-cause mortality (relative risk 1.29; $p = 0.001$ [four studies]) [70]. Another meta-analysis of 17 studies did not find any clear evidence for the impact of prewakening MBPS on prognosis. However, using a continuous scale, which has more power to detect an association, there was evidence that a 10-mmHg increase in MBPS was related to an increased risk of stroke (three studies; hazard ratio 1.11, 95% CI 1.03–1.20) [65].

In a recent long-term prospective study of 2020 participants with 24-hour ambulatory BP data and a median 20-year follow-up, STMS rate was an independent predictor of cardiovascular death. The amplitude of STMS was derived from the difference between morning SBP and lowest nighttime SBP. The rate of STMS was derived as the slope of linear regression of sequential SBP measures on time intervals within the STMS period. Thresholds for high STMS amplitude and rate were determined by the 95th percentiles (43.7 and 11.3 mmHg/h, respectively). A high STMS rate (HR 2.61), but not STMS amplitude, was significantly associated with the risk of cardiovascular mortality [71].

Morning BP surge and organ damage

MBPS is positively correlated with inflammatory biomarkers and other types of BP variability, such as orthostatic hypertension (orthostatic increase in BP) and increased daytime ambulatory BP variability [53]. MBPS is associated with target organ damage, including left ventricular hypertrophy (LVH), albuminuria, and large and small artery diseases such as carotid atherosclerosis, arterial stiffness, and silent cerebrovascular disease, independent of the 24-hour BP level (Figure 1.48) [53].

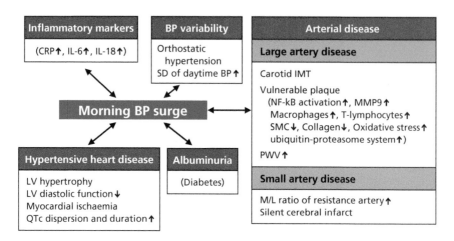

Figure 1.48 Morning blood pressure (BP) surge and target organ damage. CRP, C-reactive protein; IL-6, interleukin 6; IL-18, interleukin 18; IMT, intima-media thickness; LV, left ventricular; M/L ratio, media thickness to lumen diameter ratio; MMP-9, matrix metallopro-teinase-9; NF-κB, nuclear factor kappa B; PWV, pulse wave velocity; SD, standard deviation; SMC, smooth muscle cell. *Source*: Kario. Hypertension. 2010; 56: 765–773 [53].

Hypertensive heart disease

Many previous studies have demonstrated that an exaggerated MBPS is associated with echocardiographic measures of hypertensive heart disease. MBPS increases cardiac afterload and arterial stiffness, contributing to the progression of LVH.

In elderly hypertensive patients, Kuwajima et al. first reported that the rising surge (change in SBP after rising from bed) was significantly correlated with LV mass index (LVMI) and the A/E ratio (a measure of diastolic function) [72]. In the Bordeaux study on unmedicated patients with hypertension, rising surge was a significant determinant of LVMI [62]. In addition, patients with hypertension who had an exaggerated MBPS had a prolonged QTc duration and QTc dispersion in the morning period (detected by Holter ECG recording) compared to those without MBPS [73]. Given that increased QTc dispersion has been reported to be associated with LVH and cardiac arrhythmia, an exaggerated MBPS could increase the risk of cardiac arrhythmia and sudden death in the morning in patients with hypertension.

The association between MBPS and LVH has also been documented in normotensive individuals and patients with well-controlled hypertension. In a community-dwelling sample, exaggerated morning BP reactivity (highest quartile of the slope of MBPS against morning physical activity) was associated with LVH [74]. In patients with well-controlled hypertension who had 24-hour BP values <130/80 mmHg, MBPS (sleep-trough surge) was significantly associated with increases in LVMI and carotid intima-media thickness (IMT) (Figure 1.49) [75]. The associations found in both studies were not linear, but appeared to be nonlinear with a threshold of morning surge. Even in normotensive individuals with office BP <140/90 mmHg and 24-hour BP <130/80 mmHg, sleep-trough MBPS

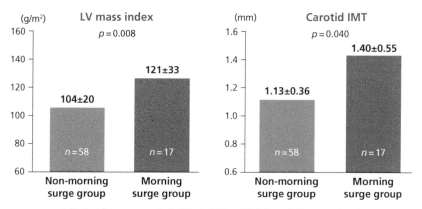

Adjusted for awake systolic BP, nighttime BP fall, and LDL-cholesterol

Figure 1.49 Morning blood pressure (BP) surge and cardiovascular remodeling in treated patients with well-controlled hypertension (24-hour BP <130/80mmHg; n = 75). LV, left ventricular; IMT, intima-media thickness. *Source*: Yano et al. Am J Hypertens. 2009; 22: 1177–1182 [75].

was significantly correlated with LVMI [76]. In a study on coronary flow reserve in patients with prehypertension or Stage 1 hypertension, increased change in MBPS was associated with microvascular dysfunction in the absence of obstructive coronary artery disease [77].

Vascular disease and inflammation

The morning surge in BP and increased time rate of BP variation in the morning have been associated with carotid atherosclerosis in untreated patients with hypertension [78–81]. This association may be accompanied by increased vascular inflammation that can induce plaque instability.

Hypertensive patients with MBPS (n = 128) had greater carotid IMT and higher urinary catecholamine excretion ($p<0.001$), and higher levels of inflammatory markers such as C-reactive protein (CRP), interleukin-6, and interleukin-18 ($p<0.001$) vs. those without MBPS (n = 196) [79]. In our JMS-ABPM study of patients with hypertension, MBPS was significantly correlated with the high-sensitivity CRP (hsCRP) level in patients with the highest quartile of MBPS (sleep-trough surge), but not in the other quartiles [81]. In addition, a histological study on carotid endarterectomy specimens demonstrated that carotid plaques in those with exaggerated MBPS had characteristics of vulnerable plaques (higher numbers of macrophages and T-lymphocytes, increased expression of HLA-DR antigen, reduced numbers of smooth muscle cells, and lower collagen content), increased levels of markers of oxidative stress, and activation of the ubiquitin–proteasome system [80]. In that study, the finding that subjects with exaggerated MBPS had higher levels of activated subunits (p50, p65) of nuclear factor kappa B (NF-κB: a central transcription factor regulating inflammatory genes), and matrix metalloproteinase-9 (MMP-9: an important enzyme in plaque rupture) suggests that exaggerated MBPS is associated with vascular inflammation and plaque instability. Together, these findings suggest that exaggerated MBPS accelerates both atherosclerotic plaque formation and plaque instability in relation to vascular inflammation. Clinically, patients with hypertension who have carotid plaques, which are likely to be vulnerable, may benefit from anti-inflammatory treatment using statins, renin–angiotensin system (RAS) inhibitors, and thiazolidinediones, as well as from treatment to suppress the MBPS [82].

In Asian patients with hypertension, consecutive three-hourly mean SBP readings during the day were significantly associated with intracranial arterial stenosis (ICAS) (odds ratio [OR] 1.28–1.38 for each 10 mmHg increase; $p \leq 0.001$). However, only mean SBP obtained between 5:00 AM and 7:59 AM was significantly associated with ICAS after adjusting for all consecutive three-hourly mean SBP readings (OR 1.30; $p = 0.019$). This highlights a significant association between early morning SBP and asymptomatic intracranial stenosis (Figure 1.50) [83].

In 743 patients with hypertension or diabetes and healthy normotensives, STMS were significantly correlated with PWV ($r = 0.126$, $p < 0.001$ in patients with hypertension; $r = 0.434$, $p < 0.0001$ in patients with diabetes) and LVMI ($r = 0.307$, $p < 0.001$ [hypertension]; $r = 0.447$, $p < 0.0001$ [diabetes]) [84]. In 602 consecutive patients with untreated hypertension (mean age 48 years), STMS ($r = 0.16$, $p < 0.001$) and rising MBPS ($r = 0.12$, $p = 0.003$) showed a direct correlation with the carotid-femoral PWV (cf-PWV), and only STMS was independently associated with cf-PWV ($p = 0.04$) after adjustment for age, sex, height, clinic mean arterial pressure, heart rate, and renal function. Average real variability (ARV), a measure of BP variability, was a significant mediator of the relationship between STMS and cf-PWV ($p = 0.003$). In untreated patients with hypertension, STMS showed a direct relationship with aortic stiffness, which is mediated by increased ARV [85].

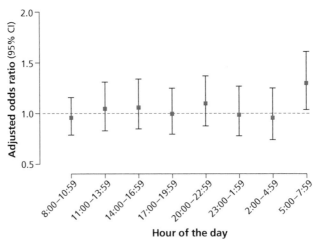

*Computed for a 10 mmHg increase in the consecutive 3-hourly means of SBP during the day.

Figure 1.50 Association between ambulatory systolic blood pressure (SBP) during the day and asymptomatic intracranial arterial stenosis. *Source*: Chen et al. Hypertension. 2014; 63: 61–7 [83].

In 241 younger adult patients (mean age 36.6 years), those with higher STMS were older ($p = 0.003$), had higher carotid IMT ($p = 0.05$) and lower E/A ratio ($p = 0.01$) than those with lower STMS. A relationship between MBPS and cardiovascular alterations was observed both in dippers and non-dippers, although this was less pronounced in non-dippers [86]. A recent study in 170 patients with prehypertension showed that independent predictors of greater carotid IMT were greater MBPS (OR 8.47; $p < 0.001$), male sex, and elevated mean platelet volume levels [87]. Thus, even in relatively young adults who have not yet developed hypertension, MBPS seems partly to be associated with vascular disease.

Silent cerebrovascular disease

Silent cerebral infarcts (SCIs) are the strongest surrogate markers of clinical stroke, particularly in those with an increased CRP level [88]. In the JMS-ABPM study, SCIs (particularly multiple SCIs) were detected more frequently by brain MRI in the morning surge group than in the nonsurge group. The OR for SCI was significantly higher only for patients with MBPS in the highest quartile and higher (above median) hsCRP levels compared with other MBPS quartiles and with lower hsCRP (below median) (Figure 1.51) [81]. This indicates that the relationship between exaggerated MBPS and the presence of SCI is slightly modified by the presence of low-grade inflammation. Although it is well known that sympathetic activity, particularly alpha-adrenergic activity, is increased in the morning, SCI has been shown to be more closely associated with the exaggerated MBPS related to alpha-adrenergic activity (defined as the reduction of MBPS by an alpha-adrenergic blocker [doxazosin]) than the overall MBPS (Figure 1.52) [89].

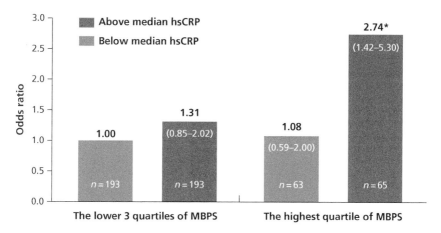

Figure 1.51 Association between the morning blood pressure surge (MBPS) and silent cerebral infarcts in relation to inflammation in elderly patients with hypertension (Jichi Medical University ABPM study wave 1, logistic regression analysis adjusted for age, sex, body mass index, smoking status, abnormal glycemic control, dipping status, and 24-hour systolic blood pressure). *$p<0.01$ vs. patients with MBPS in the lower 3 quartiles of MBPS and a high-sensitivity C-reactive protein (hsCRP) level below the median. Values are odds ratio with 95% confidence interval. *Source*: Shimizu et al. Atherosclerosis. 2011; 219: 316–321 [81].

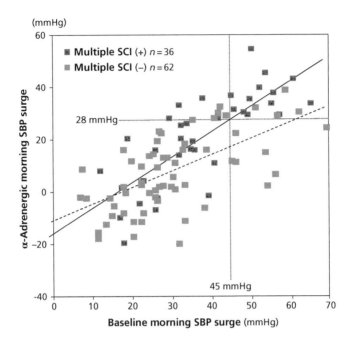

Figure 1.52 Association between the alpha-adrenergic morning systolic blood pressure (SBP) surge and the presence of silent cerebral infarcts (SCI) on brain magnetic resonance imaging in elderly patients with hypertension. *Source*: Kario et al. Am J Hypertens. 2004; 17: 668–675 [89].

Chronic kidney disease

Despite the aforementioned associations between MBPS and cardiac and vascular complications, there have been few studies demonstrating positive associations between MBPS and renal disease. Patients with CKD are likely to have a non-dipping pattern of nighttime BP fall [39, 90], and this non-dipping pattern might precede microalbuminuria [91]. One cross-sectional study in newly diagnosed normotensive patients with type 2 diabetes demonstrated that morning BP and MBPS were significantly higher in patients with vs. without microalbuminuria [92]. This indicates that a systemic BP surge might directly induce a morning surge in intraglomerular pressure in the presence of diabetes-associated disrupted autoregulation of the afferent arteriole of the glomerulus. Another study of normotensive subjects and patients with hypertension or diabetes demonstrated only a weak correlation between rising BP surge and albuminuria ($r = 0.126$, $p < 0.05$) [84].

The resistive index (RI) in renal Doppler ultrasonography is thought to be a good indicator of renal vascular resistance caused by atherosclerosis. It has been shown that MBPS (sleep-trough surge) was significantly associated with higher RI in patients with risks of atherosclerosis [93]. Furthermore, a prospective study of 622 hypertensive patients (mean age: 57.6 years) with a median of 3.33 years' follow-up, showed that higher MBPS (analyzed both as a continuous and categorical variable), was associated with incident CKD in all models [94].

Determinants of MBPS

Table 1.5 shows the factors associated with MBPS and morning hypertension [37]. MBPS is increased by various factors, including aging, hypertension, high-normal normotension, inflammation, alcohol intake [95], smoking, physical stress, psychological stress, and poor sleep quality [53, 96, 97]. In addition, higher fasting glucose was associated with greater MBPS in elderly patients with hypertension [96], suggesting that the dawn phenomenon may activate sympathetic activity to augment MBPS, especially in those with increased arterial stiffness.

As the underlying mechanism of diurnal BP variation and MBPS, diurnal variation and activation of neurohumoral factors that regulate vascular tone and cardiac output, such as the renin-angiotensin-aldosterone system (RAAS) and sympathetic nervous activity, potentially in relation to central and peripheral clock genes, may be involved. Orthostatic hypertension, which is associated with an extreme dipper pattern, was also associated with an increase in morning BP level, suggesting that orthostatic hypertension partly contributes to MBPS.

There are weekly and seasonal variations in the MBPS. MBPS is augmented on Mondays (Figure 1.53) [98] and over the winter, particularly in elderly subjects [99]. Prewakening MBPS was significantly associated with lower outdoor temperature [100]. These BP variations may partly account for the Monday peak and winter peak of cardiovascular events in the elderly [101]. In addition, nocturnal hypoxia or poor sleep quality may augment MBPS, probably through an increase in sympathetic activation and endothelial dysfunction. MBPS has also been shown to be augmented in children with sleep apnea without any early vascular damage [102]. MBPS is also augmented in the winter (Figure 1.54) [99], especially in the elderly (Figure 1.55) [103]. Patients with "thermosensitive hypertension" may exhibit "winter morning surge in BP," which may contribute to the increase in cardiovascular events seen during winter. In addition, colder temperature and less availability of well-insulated housing may partly account for regional differences in the winter increase in cardiovascular events.

Table 1.5 Determinants of morning hypertension and morning blood pressure surge.

Environmental factors	Risk factor
Winter (cold temperature)	Aging
Monday	Hypertension (high-normal normotension)
Behavioural factors	Diabetes
Alcohol	Orthostatic hypertension
Smoking	Inflammation
Physical stress	
Psychological stress	**Vascular disease**
Poor sleep quality	
Insomnia	**Short-acting antihypertensive drug**
Obstructive sleep apnoea	

Source: Kario. Essential Manual of 24-hour Blood Pressure Management from Morning to Nocturnal Hypertension. Wiley Blackwell, 2015: 1–138 [37].

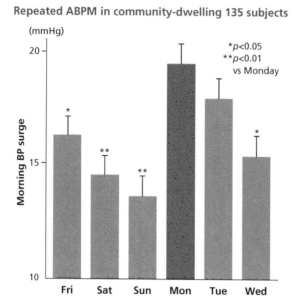

Figure 1.53 Weekly variation in morning blood pressure (BP) surge based on ambulatory BP monitoring in community-dwelling subjects ($n = 135$). *Source*: Murakami et al. Am J Hypertens. 2004; 17(12 Pt 1): 1179–83 [98].

Mechanism of morning risk

Factors related to an increase in cardiovascular risk in the morning include MBPS, imbalance between thrombotic and fibrinolytic activities, and endothelial dysfunction (Figures 1.56 and 1.57) [104, 105]. Neurohumoral factors show circadian rhythm. For example, sympathetic nervous activity gradually increases

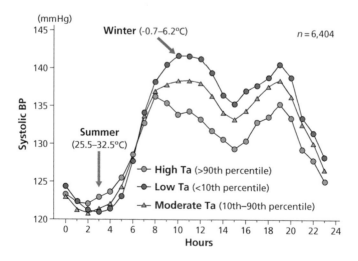

Figure 1.54 Daily variation in systolic (BP) based on daily mean outdoor air temperature (Ta). *Source*: Modesti et al. Hypertension. 2006; 47: 155–61 [99].

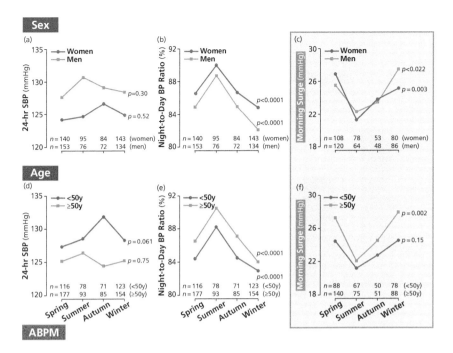

Figure 1.55 Seasonal variation in 24-hour systolic blood pressure (SBP) (A and D), night-to-day SBP ratio (B and E), and morning surge in SBP (C and F), stratified by sex and age group. Spring was from March 1 to May 31, summer from June 1 to August 31, autumn from September 1 to November 30, and winter from December 1 to the last day of the following February. Plotted values are means. Analysis of variance (ANOVA) p-values indicate the significance of the overall differences across seasons. The season-by-sex ($p \geq 0.35$) and season-by-age group ($p \geq 0.13$) interactions were all nonsignificant. ABPM, ambulatory BP monitoring. Source: Sheng et al. Hypertension. 2017; 69: 128–135 [103].

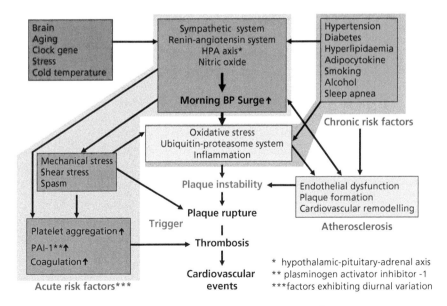

Figure 1.56 Morning blood pressure (BP) surge-related cardiovascular risk. Source: Kario. Hypertension. 2007; 49: 771–772 [104].

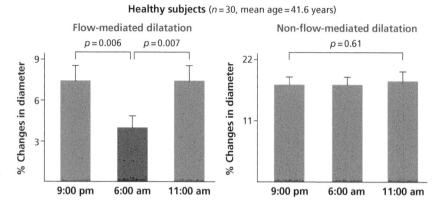

Figure 1.57 Morning endothelial dysfunction in healthy subjects (*n* = 30, mean age 41.6 years). *Source*: Otto et al. Circulation. 2004; 109: 2507–10 [105].

before awakening, and overshooting is found after rising, and plasma norepinephrine levels have been shown to surge just after awakening (Figure 1.58-upper) [106]. In a study of muscle sympathetic nerve activity in younger subjects, the ability of the baroreflex to buffer increases in BP via reflexive changes in muscle sympathetic nerve activity and may play a role in determining the magnitude of the MBPS [107]. Similar circadian variations are seen in the RAS, with the surge beginning earlier than the sympathetic nervous system. The RAS is activated from midnight to early in the morning, resulting in a peak early in the morning (Figure 1.58-lower) [108].

Circadian variation in these factors is related partly to circadian variation in hemodynamics, including BP, pulse rate, and circulating volume. The risk of MBPS triggering a cardiovascular event is partly due to increased hemodynamic stress, such as vertical pressor stress and increased shear stress, generated by exaggerated blood flow at plaques of the vessel wall. In addition, plaque instability may be caused by exaggerated hemodynamic stress, as described previously [80].

Morning BP surge and hemostatic abnormalities

Thrombotic tendency augments the morning risk of cardiovascular events. Thrombus formation results in acute thrombosis at the site of plaque rupture, hemostatic imbalance in the morning is due to hypercoagulability and hypofibrinolytic activity (increase in plasma levels of tissue-type plasminogen activator inhibitor-1 [PAI-1]), and increased platelet aggregation contributes to accelerating thrombus formation at the site of plaque rupture.

In the JMS-ABPM study, an additive increase in stroke risk was found for MBPS and increased plasma level of prothrombin fragment 1+2 (F1+2) and PAI-1 in patients with hypertension (Figure 1.59) [109]. F1+2 is a biomarker for activated coagulation factor Xa, and PAI-1 is a well-known inhibitor of fibrinolysis. These biomarkers are known to show circadian variation, with increases in the morning. However, the degree of MBPS per se was not significantly

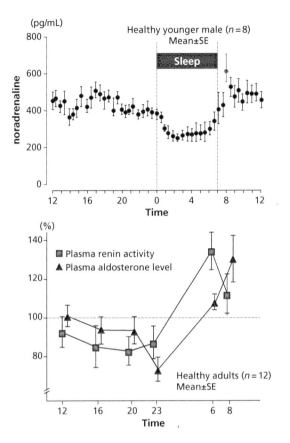

Figure 1.58 Diurnal variation of plasma noradrenaline level, plasma renin activity and aldosterone levels. Lower panel: Time-qualified levels of plasma renin activity and plasma aldosterone concentration, expressed as percent change of the mean, determined 6 times over a 24-hour span in 12 clinically healthy young subjects. SE, standard error. *Source*: Upper panel, Linsell et al. J Clin Endocrinol Metab. 1985; 60: 1210–5 [106]. Reprinted by permission of Oxford University Press; lower panel, Kawasaki et al. Horm Metab Res. 1990; 22: 636–9 [108].

correlated with morning plasma levels of these biomarkers in our study. These results indicate that exaggerated MBPS additively increases the cardiovascular risk when accompanied by hemostatic abnormalities. In addition, MBPS has been shown to be significantly associated with increased platelet aggregation, assessed using the newly developed laser scattering intensity method to assess platelet aggregation in different size particles [110]. Spontaneous platelet aggregation in small size particles was significantly correlated with the degree of MBPS (Figure 1.60) [110]. The association between morning surge and platelet aggregation was found both in the morning and in the afternoon, but was stronger in the morning. This indicates a very important aspect of BP variability. High shear-stress-induced platelet activation per se due to increased BP variability in the morning may partly account for this result. Practically, this is important because when patients with hypertension and cardiovascular disease

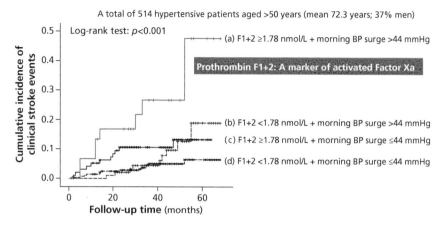

Figure 1.59 Additive impact of morning hemostatic risk factors and morning blood pressure (BP) surge on stroke risk in older Japanese patients with hypertension (n = 514; mean age 72.3 years; 37% male). F1+2, prothrombin fragment 1+2. *Source*: Kario et al. Eur Heart J. 2011; 32: 574–580 [109].

or paroxysmal atrial fibrillation are treated with antithrombotic therapy, they are at risk for both thrombotic and hemorrhagic episodes. The Ohasama study demonstrated that MBPS is also a risk for cerebral hemorrhage [63]. Antiplatelet and/or anticoagulation therapy without sufficient reduction of exaggerated MBPS may increase the risk of hemorrhagic events. Therefore, strict reduction of exaggerated MBPS in patients with hypertension receiving antithrombotic therapy is essential to maximize the clinical benefits of treatment [111].

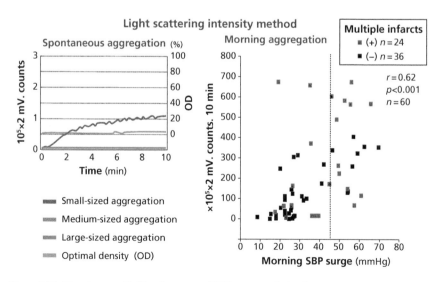

Figure 1.60 Morning systolic blood pressure (SBP) surge and platelet aggregation in patients with hypertension. *Source*: Kario et al. J Hypertens. 2011; 29: 2433–2439 [110].

Vascular mechanism of exaggerated morning BP surge

Vascular diseases of both the small and large arteries are not only a consequence of MBPS, but are also one of the leading causes, resulting in a vicious cycle of cardiovascular risk [53, 104, 112].

An interesting study that directly assessed small artery remodeling by examining biopsy specimens demonstrated that the sleep-trough surge was significantly and positively correlated with increased media thickness to lumen diameter ratio (M/L ratio, a measure of remodeling) of the subcutaneous small arteries in patients with essential hypertension (Figure 1.61) [113]. The association between contraction of the resistance arteries and vascular resistance is not linear but rather curvilinear in keeping with Folkow's principle [114], which explains the acceleration of hypertension (Figure 1.62).

Narrowing of the small arterioles has been hypothesized to contribute to the pathogenesis of hypertension [115], but there is little prospective clinical data on this association. Structural narrowing of the small resistance arteries shifts this association curve to the left, compared to the curve for normal arteries. Compared with during sleep, when vascular tonus is decreased, the difference in vascular resistance between small arteries with remodeling, and those without remodeling is augmented in the morning when vascular tonus is increased.

Activation of various pressor neurohumoral factors, including the sympathetic nervous system and the RAS, occurs early in the morning. Increased sympathetic activity, particularly of the alpha-adrenergic component [116], increases vascular tone in the small resistance arteries and may contribute to MBPS. In fact, bedtime dosing of an alpha-adrenergic blocker was shown to preferentially reduce morning BP levels and MBPS, particularly in those with small artery diseases [89]. The RAS is activated in the morning and could contribute to the MBPS and morning increase in cardiovascular risk. Plasma renin activity, angiotensin II,

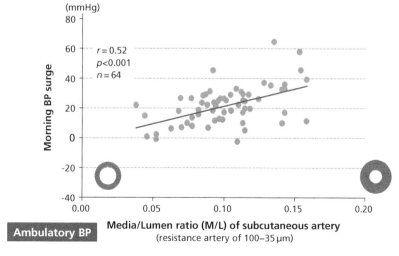

Figure 1.61 Morning blood pressre (BP) surge and small resistance artery remodelng in hypertension. *Source*: Rizzoni et al. J Hypertens. 2007; 25: 1698–703 [113].

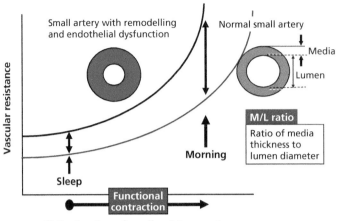

% Contraction of small resistance artery

Figure 1.62 Folkow's principle-based mechanism of exaggerated morning blood pressure surge in patients with small artery disease. M/L, media/lumen. *Source*: Kario. Morning surge in blood pressure in hypertension: clinical relevance, prognostic significance and therapeutic approach. In: Special Issues in Hypertension (A. E. Berbari, G. Manccia, eds). Springer Inc., pp. 71–89, 2012 [3].

and aldosterone levels are all increased before awakening and then further increase after awakening [117]. In addition, a previous experimental study demonstrated that mRNA levels for RAS components at the tissue level of the cardiovascular system exhibit diurnal variation, particularly in models of hypertension, with increases during the awakening period [118]. A vaccine-targeting angiotensin II significantly reduced ambulatory BP throughout the 24-hour period [119]. However, the reduction in BP was most prominent in the morning hours. The fact that the BP reduction by complete 24-hour RAS inhibition was most prominent in the morning period indicates that both the RAS and the related pressor effect are highly activated in the morning. In addition, endothelial dysfunction is found in the morning, even in healthy subjects, and reduces the capacity for vasodilatation [105]. Thus, the threshold of augmentation of BP surge by pressor stimulation may be lowest in the morning. In other words, the morning is a sensitive period for detecting pathological surge and variability in BP, which reflects vascular status. Using BP surge, the morning may be the best time window to detect the early stage of vascular damage, such as small artery remodeling and endothelial dysfunction. Considering these data, even when mean office BP is within the normal range, masked (isolated) morning hypertension could be considered as "prehypertension" in patients in the early stage of vascular disease (the morning hypertension–prehypertension hypothesis) (Figure 1.63) [112]. Other ambulatory BP surges such as sleep apnea-related nighttime BP surge, orthostatic hypertension, and stress hypertension at the workplace, all of which reflect ambulatory BP variability, could also be considered as forms of "prehypertension." When the duration of pressor conditions persists longer and increases mean 24-hour ambulatory BP to ≥130/80 mmHg, this could be considered as masked hypertension before office BP level increases.

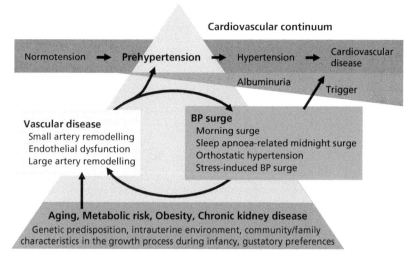

Figure 1.63 Clinical relevance of blood pressure (BP) surge on the cardiovascular continuum. *Source*: Kario et al. J Hypertens. 2007; 25: 1573–1575 [112].

In addition to being a consequence of morning surge, increased stiffness in large arteries is important as a leading cause of exaggerated BP variability, and MBPS is correlated with vascular disease [84–87]. Baroreceptor sensitivity (BRS) decreases as large arterial stiffness increases and shows diurnal variation with a decrease early in the morning [120]. Thus, reduced BRS in patients with large artery disease may be insufficient to suppress BP surges [112], especially in the morning. In fact, in patients with hypertension, impaired dynamic Valsalva-BRS has been significantly correlated with an increase in morning BP [121].

The MBPS can be characterized into two types (Table 1.6) [122]: cardiac reactive type and vascular stiffness type. Clinical implications of the former may be the phenotypes of prehypertension before an increase in average BP in younger adults, while the latter may be a direct trigger for cardiovascular events in individuals with advanced vascular disease, which seems difficult to treat.

Table 1.6 Age-related characteristics of the morning blood pressure (BP) surge.

Type	Cardiac reactive type	Vascular stiffness type
Age	Younger adult	Elderly
Clinical implication	Prehypertension	Advanced vascular disease
BP characteristics hypertension	Increased heart rate	Systolic
Response to treatment	Easy to treat	Difficult to treat
Day-by-day variability	Stable	Variable
Morning BP surge reactivity	Lower	Higher

Source: Kario. Hypertension. 2015; 65: 1163–1169 [122].

BP Variability and systemic hemodynamic atherothrombotic syndrome (SHATS)

BP variability combines with a number of other factors to cause asymptomatic organ damage, which eventually manifests as clinical cardiovascular disease (Figure 1.64) [122–137].

There are various types of BP variability with different time phases, from short-term to long-term [122, 123]. These include beat-by-beat, orthostatic, physical, or psychological stress-induced, diurnal, day-by-day, visit-to-visit, seasonal, and yearly BP variability, and clinically, these are detected by different office, home, and ABPM methods (Figure 1.65) [122, 123].

BP variability is considered the master biomarker of human healthcare because it is not only a modifiable risk factor for organ damage and cardiovascular disease but also a marker of cardiovascular dysregulation that is affected by individual characteristics and stressors related to daily psychobehavioral factors and environmental conditions, as well as medication status [138–142]. Almost all BP variability phenotypes are at least partly related and are reported to increase cardiovascular risk [58, 143–145].

Different components of BP variability may have different clinical impacts on cardiovascular disease. A long-term increase in average BP would be considered a chronic risk factor for advancing endothelial dysfunction and subsequent atherosclerosis, whereas relatively short-term exaggerated BP variability (e.g. MBPS) is a more acute risk factor, which triggers an atherothrombotic cardiovascular disease event by a mechanical stress-induced plaque rupture (Figure 1.1). These different roles for BP

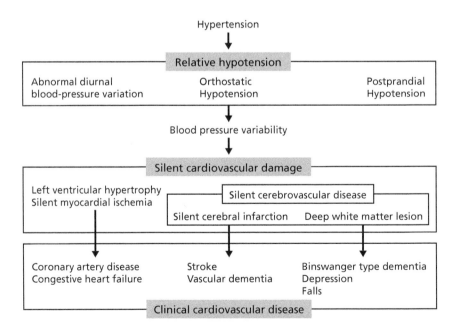

Figure 1.64 Blood pressure variability combined with other factors to cause asymptomatic organ damage, resulting in clinical cardiovascular disease. *Source*: Reprinted from the Kario and Pickering Lancet. 2000; 355: 1645–1646 [124]. Copyright (2000), with permission from Elsevier.

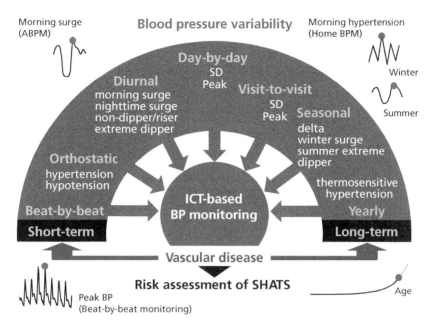

Figure 1.65 Information and communication technology (ICT)-based assessment of different blood pressure (BP) variability parameters and vascular damage in systemic hemodynamic atherothrombotic syndrome (SHATS). ABPM, ambulatory blood pressure monitoring; BPM, blood pressure monitoring; SD, standard deviation. *Source*: Modified from Kario. Hypertension. 2015; 65: 1163–1169 [122].

variability in cardiovascular risk are similar to those seen in HF, where chronically advancing left ventricular hypertrophy eventually results in clinical HF, while acute HF might be triggered by afterload mismatch due to an abrupt increase in SBP.

The resonance hypothesis of BP surge

The "resonance hypothesis" of BP surge has been proposed [138, 146]. On the basis of reduced baroreceptor sensitivity and small artery remodeling associated with aging, each type of BP variability has different time phase increases. The magnitude of increase in each type of BP variability may be different in different individuals. There are a number of triggers of BP surge in the real world, such as physical and mental stress, and environmental factors (especially cold temperature), diet, and sleep (Figure 1.66) [146]. When the timing of each type of BP surge wave does not coincide, the summation of BP surge is small. However, when the timing of many BP surge waves with different time phases is synchronized and resonance of the pulse wave occurs, this might generate a critically large dynamic BP surge (defined as "dynamic surge BP") that would trigger a cardiovascular disease event (Figure 1.66).

For example, MBPS is one of the typical surges [122] that can be synergistically potentiated by a resonance of various components of BP surges, resulting in morning-onset cardiovascular disease [146]. In ABPM studies, the MBPS was exaggerated in the winter, especially in elderly patients [101]. Added to the underlying MBPS,

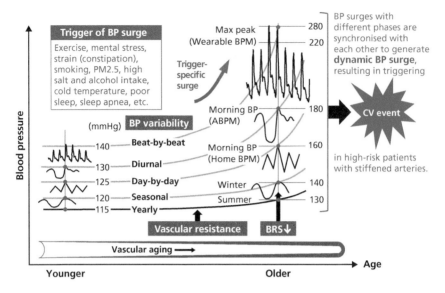

Figure 1.66 Synergistic resonance hypothesis of blood pressure (BP) variability. ABPM, ambulatory blood pressure monitoring; BPM, blood pressure monitoring; BRS, baroreceptor sensitivity; CV, cardiovascular; PM2.5, particulate matter of <2.5 microns. *Source*: Modified from Kario. Am J Hypertens. 2016; 29: 14–16 [146]. Reprinted by permission of Oxford University Press.

coincident exposure to airborne particulate matter of <2.5 microns (PM2.5) [142] and smoking, with high salt and alcohol intake at the evening meal and poor sleep the previous night, could occur in the morning in the cold winter (Figure 1.66). This cluster of triggers results in a marked dynamic morning BP surge and could precipitate a cardiovascular event, especially in high-risk patients with vascular disease.

The age-related increase in dynamic surge BP generated by resonance with synchronization of each BP surge with a different time-phase exceeds the average of BP (Figure 1.67). Given that the risk associated with surge BP increases more rapidly than that of average BP-based diagnosis of hypertension, earlier intervention is especially important to protect against the age-related cardiovascular burden associated with exaggerated (dynamic) surge BP.

Orthostatic hypertension

We first demonstrated that orthostatic BP increase was not transient, but persistent, in elderly patients with hypertension who have an extreme dipper pattern of nighttime BP (Figure 1.68) [143]. This phenomenon was unexpectedly found in a previous study of ABPM and head-up tilting test looking at the association between disrupted circadian rhythm of BP and orthostatic BP change. In addition, this orthostatic hypertension was also associated with MBPS evaluated by ABPM (Figure 1.69) [144]. Along with orthostatic hypotension, orthostatic hypertension is now one of the phenotypes of positional BP variability, and is a new risk factor for cardiovascular disease [58, 148, 149].

In our brain MRI study, there was U-shaped relationship between the change in orthostatic BP and SCIs, especially multiple SCIs (Figure 1.70) [144]. The 241

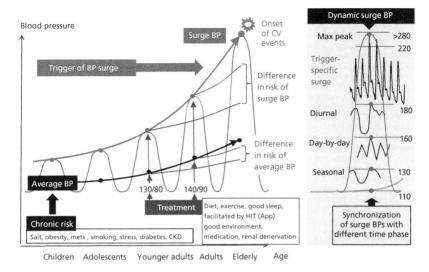

Figure 1.67 Lifelong increase in surge blood pressure (BP) and risk of cardiovascular (CV) disease. The impact of age-related risk reduction of surge blood pressure by the shift of the average blood pressure from 140/90 to 130/80 mmHg as the diagnostic threshold and treatment goal of hypertension. App, application; CKD; chronic kidney disease; HIT, health information technology (e.g. application for remote monitoring and self-monitoring of BP); mets, metabolic disease. *Source*: Kario and Wang Hypertension. 2018; 71: 979–984 [148].

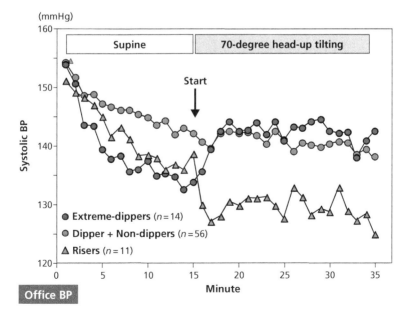

Figure 1.68 Persistent orthostatic hypertension evaluated by head-up tilting test (70 degrees), detected in subjects with an extreme dipping pattern of nighttime blood pressure (BP) by the head-up tilting test. *Source*: Kario et al. Hypertension. 1998; 31: 77–82 [143].

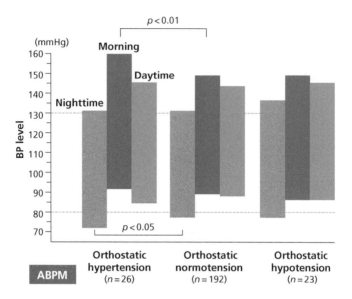

Figure 1.69 Orthostatic hypertension and 24-hour ambulatory blood pressure (BP) profile in elderly patients with hypertension. ABPM, ambulatory blood pressure monitoring. *Source*: Created based on data from Kario et al. J Am Coll Cardiol. 2002; 40: 133–141 [144].

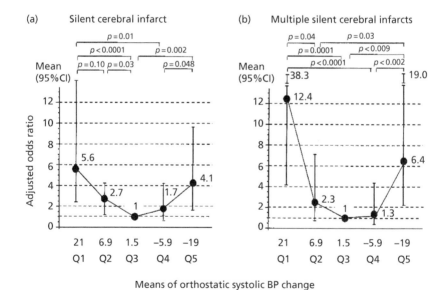

Figure 1.70 U-shaped relationship between orthostatic systolic blood pressure (BP) change and silent cerebral infarcts in elderly subjects with sustained hypertension. Odds ratio (95% confidence interval [CI]) values are shown and were adjusted for age, gender, body mass index, smoking status, presence/absence of hyperlipidemia, and 24-hour systolic BP using multiple logistic regression analysis, with quintile (Q) 3 the reference group. *Source*: Kario et al. J Am Coll Cardiol. 2002; 40: 133–141 [144].

patients were classified into an orthostatic hypertension (OHT) group (orthostatic SBP increase ≥20 mmHg; n =26), an orthostatic hypotension (OHYPO) group (orthostatic SBP decrease ≥20 mmHg; n = 23), and a normal group (with neither of the other two patterns; n = 192). SCIs were significantly more common in the OHT (3.4/person, p < 0.0001) and OHYPO groups (2.7/person, p = 0.04) than in the normal group (1.4/person). Morning SBP was higher in the OHT group than in the normal group (159 vs. 149 mmHg, p = 0.007), while there were no significant between-group differences in ambulatory BPs during other periods. The OHT and OHYPO groups had higher BP variability than the normal group (standard deviation [SD] of awake SBP of 21 and 20 mmHg vs. 17 mmHg, respectively; both p ≤ 0.01).

In a recent post hoc analyses of Systolic Blood Pressure Intervention Trial (SPRINT), orthostatic hypertension (defined as ≥20 mmHg increase in SBP or ≥10 mmHg increase in DBP on standing) was associated with a higher risk of cardiovascular events in the intensive treatment group but not the standard treatment group; intensive treatment of BP did not reduce the risk of cardiovascular events compared with standard treatment in patients with orthostatic hypertension [150].

Three phenotypes of BP variability—the morning BP surge, nighttime BP dipping, and orthostatic BP change—are partly associated with each other. Exaggerated morning surge, extreme dipper, and orthostatic hypertension all show hyper-reactive BP variability, while blunted or inverse morning surge, riser, and orthostatic hypotension are all indicative of disrupted BP variability (Figure 1.71) [122]. Thus, increased BP variability might be a residual risk factor even when average BP is well controlled.

Ambulatory BP variability

There is also significant evidence for an association between ambulatory BP variability and organ damage/cardiovascular events. An increase in ambulatory BP variability (SD of daytime ambulatory SBP values) has been shown to be signifi-

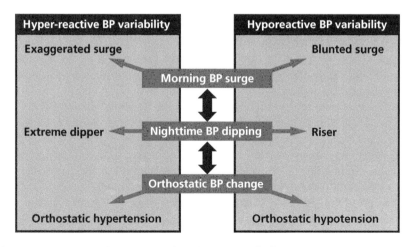

Figure 1.71 Associations between pathological extremes of differences in blood pressure (BP) variability. *Source*: Kario. Hypertension. 2015; 65: 1163–1169 [122].

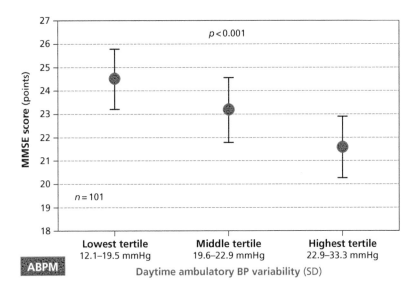

Figure 1.72 Ambulatory blood pressure (BP) variability and cognitive function in the very elderly (age >80 years; mean 84 years). ABPM, ambulatory blood pressure monitoring; MMSE, mini mental state examination; SD, standard deviation. *Source*: Created based on data from Sakakura et al. Am J Hypertens. 2007; 20: 720–727 [151].

cantly associated with cognitive dysfunction assessed by the Mini Mental State Examination (MMSE) in the very elderly (age >80 [mean 84] years) (Figure 1.72) [151]. In addition, even those with well-controlled ambulatory BP, increased ambulatory BP variability (weighted SD of ambulatory SBP), but not average ambulatory BP level, was significantly associated with cognitive dysfunction (based on the Japanese version of the Montreal Cognitive Assessment [MoCA-J] score) (Figure 1.73) [152].

Visit-to-visit variability in office BP
There is a lot of evidence for the association between visit-to-visit variability of office BP and organ damage and cardiovascular events. Rothwell et al. demonstrated the prognostic importance of visit-to-visit variability of office BP and maximum SBP for stroke and coronary events in the ASCOT-BPLA database [127]. We have previously shown that delta SBP (peak minus the lowest reading of office BP over 12 months, a measure of visit-to-visit variability of office BP readings) was significantly correlated with measures of vascular disease (IMT and stiffness of the common carotid artery) in 201 elderly patients at high risk of cardiovascular disease (mean age 80 years) [153]. This relationship is augmented by insomnia [154]. In addition, delta SBP was a significant determinant of cognitive dysfunction (MMSE score <24 points), independent of average office BP readings over a 12-month period (Figure 1.74) [129]. The impact of increased delta SBP on cognitive impairment was increased in the presence of advanced vascular disease (Figure 1.75) [134].

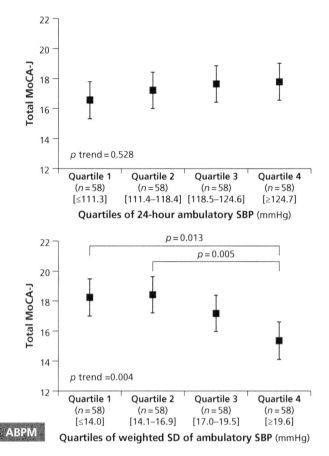

Figure 1.73 Association between the Japanese version of the Montreal Cognitive Assessment (MoCA-J) score and quartiles of 24-hour systolic blood pressure (SBP) or weighted standard deviation (SD) of SBP in patients with well-controlled blood pressure (n = 232, mean age 77.7 years, antihypertensive treatment 85%, 24-hour blood pressure 118/68 mmHg). ABPM, ambulatory blood pressure monitoring. *Source*: Cho et al. Am J Hypertens. 2018; 31: 293–298 [152]. Reprinted by permission of Oxford University Press.

Vicious cycle between BP variability and vascular disease—SHATS

Clinically, the pathogenesis and impact of BP variability should be considered in the context of vascular disease. In 2013, we first proposed a novel disease entity, called systemic hemodynamic atherothrombotic syndrome (SHATS), which is characterized by a vicious cycle between hemodynamic stress and vascular disease and is a risk factor for cardiovascular events and organ damage (Figure 1.76) [57, 58, 155].

The novel contribution of SHATS is its synergistic consideration of various types of BP variability and hemodynamic stress in relation to vascular disease [57, 58, 157]. That is, SHATS is defined by both vascular (one or more clinical/subclinical

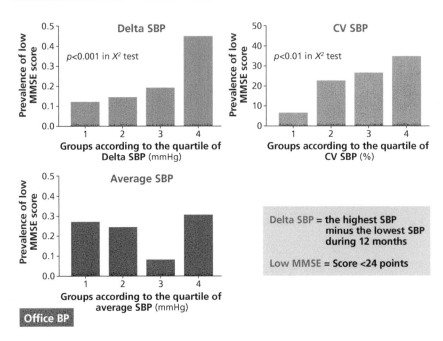

Figure 1.74 The relationships between visit-to-visit systolic blood pressure (SBP) variation and cognitive function. BP, blood pressure; CV, coefficient of variation; MMSE, Mini Mental State Examination. *Source*: Created based on data from Nagai et al. J Hypertens. 2012; 30: 1556–1563 [129].

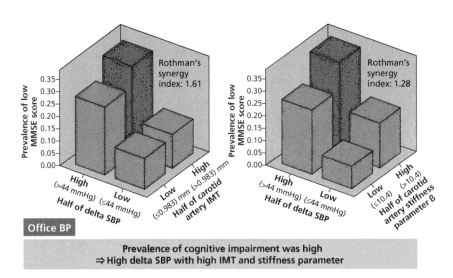

Figure 1.75 Visit-to-visit systolic blood pressure (SBP) variability and cognitive impairment, with influencer from carotid artery remodelling (*n* = 205). BP, blood pressure; IMT, intima media thickness; MMSE, Mini Mental State Examination. *Source*: Nagai et al. Atherosclerosis. 2014; 233: 19–26 [134].

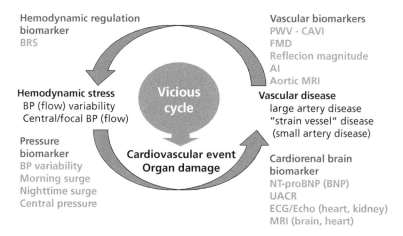

Figure 1.76 Concept and biomarkers of the systemic hemodynamic atherothrombotic syndrome (SHATS). AI, augmentation index; BNP, B-type natriuretic peptide; BRS, baroreceptor sensitivity; BPV, blood pressure variability; CAVI, cardio-ankle vascular index; ECG, electrocardiography; Echo, echography; FMD, flow-mediated dilation; MRI, magnetic resonance imaging; NT-proBNP; N-terminal pro-brain natriuretic peptide; PWV, pulse wave velocity; UACR, urinary albumin/creatinine ratio. *Source*: Kario. Nat Rev Nephrol. 2013; 9: 726–738 [58] and Kario. Prog Cardiovasc Dis. 2016; 59: 262–281 [156].

vascular diseases) and BP components (one or more phenotypes of BP variability) [158, 159]. The concept underscores the fact that clinicians should recognize the synergistic risk posed by exaggerated BP variability and vascular damage in clinical practice.

There are four domains of SHATS biomarkers: pressure; hemodynamic; vascular; and cardiorenal/brain (Figure 1.76). Pressure biomarkers of SHATS could be detected using HBPM, ABPM, and the active standing test.

The clinical relevance of SHATS is different for younger and older subjects. SHATS is clinically important for predicting future sustained hypertension in younger subjects. Early detection of SHATS may facilitate prevention of organ damage in this early stage. In older subjects, SHATS is important as a direct risk for triggering cardiovascular events. The suppression of SHATS should be directly related to a reduction in cardiovascular events.

A typical case of SHATS

A 72-year-old woman who had been registered and was being followed in the Japan Morning Surge Home Blood Pressure (J-HOP) study [160] developed acute stroke just after rising in the morning to take a walk (Figure 1.77) [155]. Neurological deficits were dizziness and conjugate deviation. The responsible lesion (shown in diffusion MRI) was located in a small artery, the paramedian branch (the perforating artery supplying the posterior circulation) of the posterior cerebral artery. The patient had a 36-year history of hypertension, a 15-year history of hyperlipidemia, and had experienced an acute myocardial infarction 14 years previously. Before the onset of stroke, she had achieved good control of

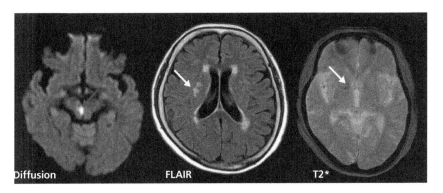

Figure 1.77 A 72-year-old woman who developed morning-onset stroke. The paramedian branch of the posterior cerebral artery showed signs of branch atheromatous disease and this anatomical location corresponded to the site of high intensity on diffusion magnetic resonance imaging (MRI) and the neurological deficit. The red arrow shows the acute infarction in diffusion MRI and the white arrows show old deep white matter infarcts (FLAIR) and microbleed (T2*). *Source*: Kario. J Clin Hypertens (Greenwich). 2015; 17: 328–331 [155].

office BP (<130/80 mmHg), home BP self-measured in the sitting position (125/70 mmHg), average 24-hour BP (<120/75 mmHg) (Figures 1.78 and 1.79), and other metabolic risk factors using a treatment regimen consisting of aspirin, candesartan, hydrochlorothiazide (HTCZ), bisoprolol, and a statin. However, prior to the stroke, vascular evaluation tests revealed advanced systemic vascular disease (flow-mediated dilatation of the brachial artery 2.4%; normal range >5%; high IMT of the common carotid artery [right 2.2 mm, left 2.2 mm; normal range

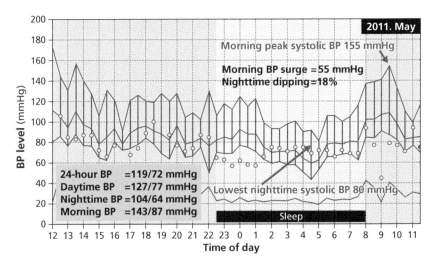

Figure 1.78 Ambulatory blood pressure monitoring (ABPM) performed 13 months before the onset of stroke event, showing an exaggerated morning blood pressure (BP) surge with marked daytime BP variability, even when average 24-hour BP was well controlled (<130/80 mmHg). *Source*: Kario. J Clin Hypertens (Greenwich). 2015; 17: 328–331 [155].

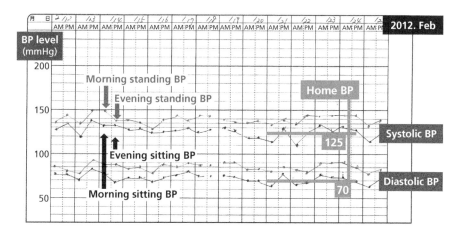

Figure 1.79 Self-measured home active standing blood pressure (BP) monitored in the morning and evening for 14 days at four months before the onset of stroke. The recordings clearly demonstrate persistent orthostatic hypertension (systolic BP increase >15 mmHg). Black dots and lines represent the second sitting BP measurements and red dots/lines represent standing BP readings measured just after standing. *Source*: Kario. J Clin Hypertens (Greenwich). 2015; 17: 328–331 [155].

<1.0 mm], a brachial-ankle PWV (baPWV) of 1935 cm/sec [corresponding to the healthy reference value for a 93-year-old], and carotid augmentation index of 26%) (Figure 1.80). The patient also had advanced hemodynamic risk factors, including an exaggerated MBPS (SBP >55 mmHg) (Figure 1.78) and orthostatic hypertension detected by orthostatic HBPM before the stroke (Figure 1.79). This case indicates that even if conventional risk factors are well controlled, cardiovascular

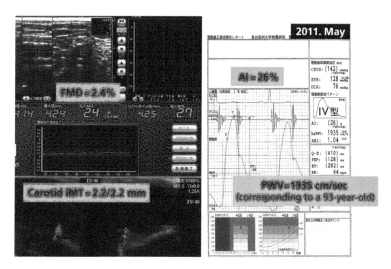

Figure 1.80 Vascular evaluation tests performed prior to stroke onset. AI, augmentation index; FMD, flow-mediated dilation; IMT, intima-media thickness; PWV, pulse wave velocity. *Source*: Kario. Essential Manual of 24-hour Blood Pressure Management from Morning to Nocturnal Hypertension. Wiley Blackwell, 2015: 1–138 [37].

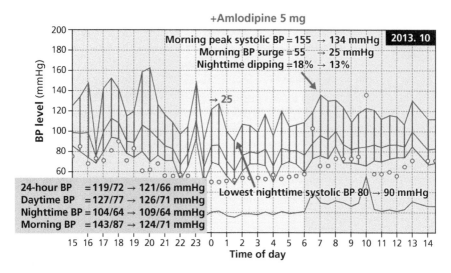

Figure 1.81 Data showing the change in ambulatory blood pressure (BP) during treatment with amlodipine 5 mg/day after the stroke event. *Source*: Kario. Essential Manual of 24-hour Blood Pressure Management from Morning to Nocturnal Hypertension. Wiley Blackwell, 2015: 1–138 [37].

risk can remain significant. The patient recovered from the poststroke neurological deficit and had amlodipine added to her cardiovascular therapy, which markedly reduced the peak of morning BP without altering the lowest BP during sleep, resulting in specific suppression of MBPS (Figure 1.81).

Pathological targets in SHATS

Different-sized arteries and organ-related microcirculation interaction are the target of SHATS (Figure 1.82) [58]. In high-risk patients, an advanced vulnerable

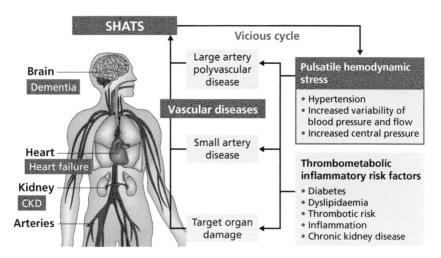

Figure 1.82 Clinical phenotypes of the systemic hemodynamic atherothrombotic syndrome (SHATS). CKD, chronic kidney disease. *Source*: modified from Kario. Nat Rev Nephrol. 2013; 9: 726–738 [58].

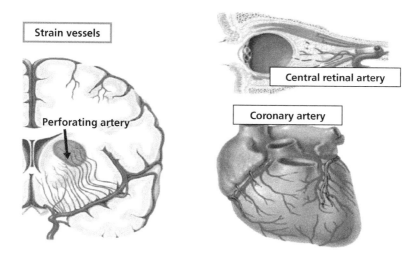

Figure 1.83 Strain vessel hypothesis: a viewpoint for the association between albuminuria and cerebrocardiovascular risk. *Source*: Ito et al. Hypertens Res. 2009; 32: 115–21 [161].

plaque may be the first target. MBPS triggers plaque rupture due to BP-related mechanical stress and shear stress from exaggerated variability of blood flow, resulting in the onset of cardiovascular events. Small arteries branching rectangularly from large arteries may be an appropriate second target [57, 58, 157]. These vessels are the so-called "strain vessels" that are anatomically exposed to high pressure and that must maintain strong vascular tone in order to provide large pressure gradients from the parent vessels to the capillaries [161]. These vascular structures are found in the cerebral perforating arteries, renal juxtamedullary afferent arterioles, and retinal and coronary arteries (Figure 1.83) [161].

Large artery disease augments the impact of exaggerated BP variability on atherosclerotic and small artery-related cardiovascular events. Increasing large artery stiffness decreases attenuation of the pulse transmitted to the peripheral arteries (Figure 1.84) [162]. As shown in Figure 1.84, the soft ascending aorta dilate (11.562% dilatation) to absorb the power of the pulse (Figure 1.85 left). However, dilation of a stiffened aorta is limited (2.675% dilatation) (Figure 1.85 right). Thus, the pulse is transmitted to the brain without being absorbed in the ascending aorta (Figure 1.86). When plaque exists in the major artery, pulse reaching a disrupted plaque could trigger cerebral infarction (Figure 1.86). Even when such a plaque does not exist, pulse transmission to small perforating arteries could result in silent cerebrovascular disease (cerebral infarcts and/or white matter disease)((Figure 1.86), which predispose elderly patients to dementia, depression, apathy, and falls. These small artery cerebrovascular diseases progress with small artery remodeling and disrupted autoregulation of small arteries (Figure 1.87) [163].

Cerebral hemorrhage and infarction occur most frequently in the regions of the small perforating arteries. In fact, in elderly hypertensive patients, SCIs, particularly when occurring as multiple SCIs, are more frequently detected by brain

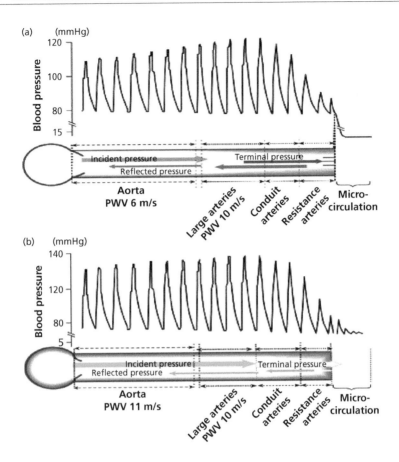

Figure 1.84 Attenuation of transmission of pulsatile pressure energy to the microcirculation by arterial stiffness gradient. (a) When an arterial stiffness gradient is present (aortic pulse wave velocity [PWV] < peripheral PWV), partial reflections occur far from the microcirculation and return to the aorta at low PWV in diastole, thereby maintaining central-to-peripheral amplification. Partial reflections limit the transmission of pulsatile pressure energy to the periphery and protect the microcirculation. (b) When the stiffness gradient disappears or is inverted (aortic PWV > peripheral PWV), pulsatile pressure is not sufficiently dampened and is transmitted, damaging the microcirculation; in parallel, the central-to-peripheral pressure amplification is attenuated. *Source*: Briet et al. Kidney Int. 2012; 82: 388–400 [162].

MRI in individuals with an exaggerated MBPS than in those with a normal MBPS (Figures 1.42 and 1.43) [2]. In addition, cerebral hemorrhage has been reported to occur more frequently when MBPS is exaggerated versus normal [63].

In the kidney, the nearer the large artery (arcuate artery), the greater the pressure overload in the afferent arterioles of the glomeruli (Figure 1.88) [161]. The source of microalbuminuria is first the glomeruli in the cortex near the arcuate arteries of the outer medulla with increased intraglomerular hypertension (Figure 1.89).

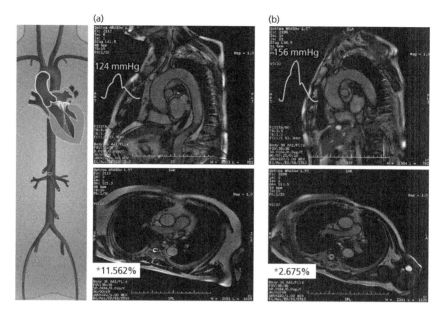

Figure 1.85 Assessment of aortic stiffness using dynamic magnetic resonance imaging. (a) soft aorta. (b) stiffened aorta. *% dilation of ascending aorta during systolic phase. *Source*: Kario. Essential Manual on Perfect 24-hour Blood Pressure Management from Morning to Nocturnal Hypertension: Up-to-date for Anticipation Medicine. Wiley, 2018: 1–309 [24].

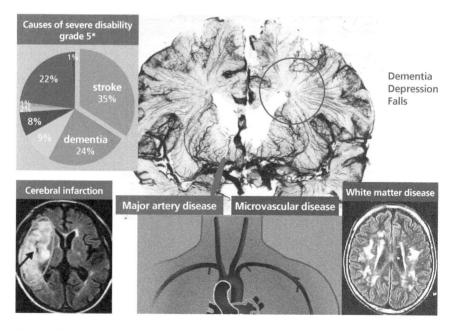

Figure 1.86 Hypertension influences two causes of severe disability (stroke and dementia). *Source*: Created based on Dr. Vladimir Hachinski's slide, with his permission. *Created based on data from 2013 Comprehensive Survey of Living Conditions (Ministry of Health, Labour and Welfare; http://www.mhlw.go.jp/toukei/saikin/hw/k-tyosa/k-tyosa13/; accessed on December 23, 2017)

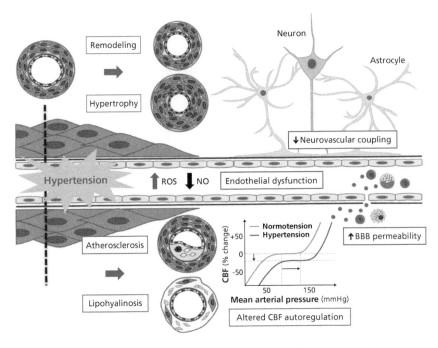

Figure 1.87 Hypertension and cerebral blood vessels. BBB, blood–brain barrier; CBF, cerebral blood flow; ROS, reactive oxygen species. *Source*: Faraco and Iadecola Hypertension. 2013; 62: 810–7 [163].

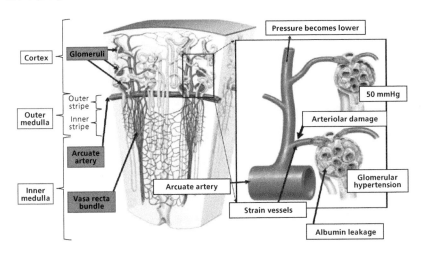

Figure 1.88 Strain vessel hypothesis: a viewpoint for linkage of albuminuria and cerebro-cardiovascular risk. *Source*: Ito et al. Hypertens Res. 2009; 32: 115–21 [161].

Mechanisms underlying the vicious cycle of BP variability and vascular disease

Exaggerated MBPS, specifically potentiated by neurohumoral activation in the morning, is the BP variability phenotype of SHATS. SHATS is characterized by an increase in BP variability. This is detected clinically as one of the specific BP surges,

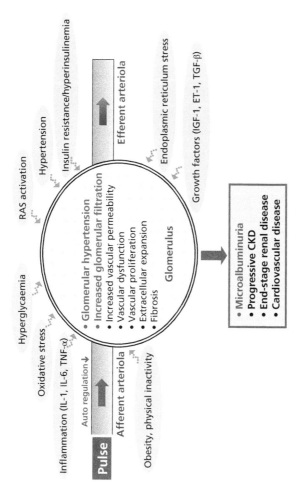

Figure 1.89 Cardiometabolic syndrome and chronic kidney disease (CKD). ET-1, endothelin-1; IGF-1, insulin-like growth factor-1; IL-1, interleukin-1; IL-6, interleukin-6; RAS, renin–angiotensin system; TGF-β, transforming growth factor-β; TNF-α, tumor necrosis factor-α. *Source:* Kario. Essential Manual on Perfect 24-hour Blood Pressure Management from Morning to Nocturnal Hypertension: Up-to-date for Anticipation Medicine. Wiley, 2018: 1–309 [24].

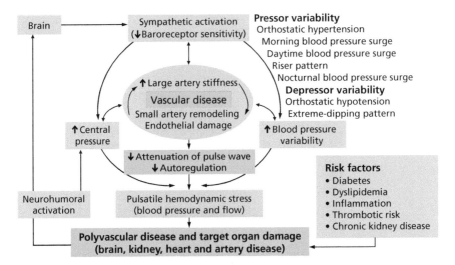

Figure 1.90 Mechanism of the systemic hemodynamic atherothromotic syndrome. *Source*: Kario. Nat Rev Nephrol. 2013; 9: 726–738 [58].

which may partly be associated with each other. MBPS is associated with other BP variability phenotypes such as orthostatic hypertension, increased SD of daytime ambulatory BP readings, and circadian BP variation (especially extreme dipping of nighttime BP [nighttime SBP fall ≥20%]) [57, 58, 143, 144, 157].

Increases in BP variability, central pressure, and impaired baroreceptor sensitivity are the three BP measures of SHATS, and are closely related (Figure 1.90) [58]. Baroreflex is a negative feedback loop in the autonomic nervous system (Figure 1.91) [164]. The overall underlying mechanism of SHATS may include

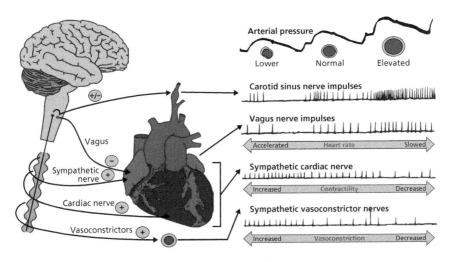

Figure 1.91 Carotid sinus reflexes. *Source*: Amerena and Julius. Role of the nervous system in human hypertension. In: Hollenberg NJ, Braunwald E, eds. Atlas of Hypertension. 5th ed. Current Medicine, Philadelphia, PA, LLC, 2005. Reprinted with permission of Springer Nature [164].

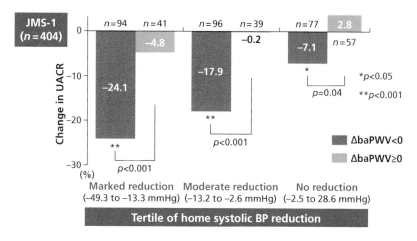

Figure 1.92 Reduction of brachial-ankle pulse wave velocity (baPWV) is important for reduction of the urinary albumin-creatinine ratio (UACR) in patients with hypertension. BP, blood pressure. *Source*: Matsui et al. J Hypertens. 2010; 28: 1752–1760 [165].

impaired neural and vascular components of baroreflex due to increased central sympathetic activity and decreased carotid dispensability, respectively. In addition, small artery remodeling and large artery disease may contribute to increases in BP variability [58, 157]. Arterial stiffness and pressure wave reflections are two important components of pulsatile hemodynamics. Measurements provided by ABPM, including MBPS, can reflect pulsatile hemodynamics through the influences of arterial stiffness and wave reflections. The degree of central and peripheral neurohumoral activation and their related cardiovascular reactivity in each specific condition may determine the different phenotypes of BP variability.

Improvement in BP and vascular disease could provide synergistic end-organ protection. Titrating doxazosin therapy to a target home BP of <135/85 mmHg reduced not only home BP but also PWV, both of which are important for reducing microalbuminuria (Figure 1.92) [165].

Even when conventional risk factors are well controlled, patients with hypertension may be at risk of advanced organ damage and cardiovascular events. The detection of phenotypes of BP variability to assess SHATS, especially in high-risk patients with cardiovascular disease and during antihypertensive treatment, can be achieved by considering the time of medication dosing targeting BP peaks, by measures to confer vascular protection, and/or by neuromodulation with renal denervation or baroreceptor sensitization therapy, resulting in more effective organ protection.

White-coat and masked hypertension

The terms "white-coat hypertension" and "masked hypertension" were defined by Thomas G Pickering [166, 167]. While white-coat hypertension is defined as normotension when assessed using out-of-office BP measurement and hypertension when office BP is assessed, whereas masked hypertension is diagnosed when office BP is

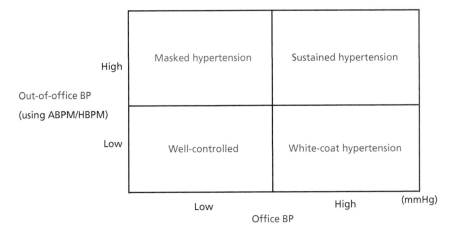

Figure 1.93 Hypertension Classification using office and out-of-office blood pressures. ABPM, ambulatory blood pressure monitoring; HBPM, home BPM; SBP, systolic BP. *Source*: Kario. Essential Manual of 24-hour Blood Pressure Management from Morning to Nocturnal Hypertension. UK: Wiley Blackwell; 2015:1–138 [37].

normal, and hypertension is detected using out-of-office BP monitoring (Figure 1.93) [37]. All four different subtypes of hypertension (white-coat, masked, sustained, and well controlled) are determined based on the average of multiple measurements of office BP and out-of-office BP. Out-of-office BP is measured using ABPM and/or HBPM. The clinical characteristics of and treatment strategies for white-coat hypertension and masked hypertension are summarized in Table 1.7 [168].

Table 1.7 Clinical characteristics and treatment strategies for white-coat and masked hypertension.

White-coat hypertension (WCH)	Masked hypertension (MH)
• Prevalence is dependent on the definition used • Detect using out-of-office BP monitoring • Target use of out-of-office BP monitoring based on co-existing risk factors • Isolated WCH is relatively benign, but may indicate higher risk of developing sustained hypertension • WCH with other CV risk factors increases cardiovascular morbidity and mortality • Lifestyle modifications may be sufficient to manage WCH in most patients • Antihypertensive treatment should be considered for patients with WCH and evidence of target organ damage or high CV risk • Recommendations for ongoing monitoring and follow-up of WCH vary between major guidelines	• Prevalence is dependent on the definition used • Detect using out-of-office BP monitoring (ABPM preferred) • Consider screening for MH in patients with normal clinic BP and target organ damage or other CV risk factors • MH is not a benign condition • MH is associated with a significantly increased risk of target organ damage, CVD and death • Lifestyle modifications and antihypertensive treatment of MH are justified based on the CV risk profile • There is an urgent need for robust data to support recommendations about the diagnosis, treatment and monitoring of MH • Long-term monitoring with out-of-office BP techniques is recommended

ABPM, ambulatory BP monitoring; BP, blood pressure; CV, cardiovascular.
Source: Kario et al. Circ Res. 2019; 124: 990–1008 [168].

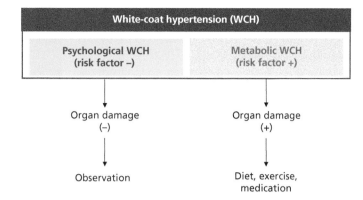

Figure 1.94 White-coat hypertension phenotypes. *Source*: Reproduced with permission from Kario and Pickering Arch Intern Med. 2000;160: 3497–8 [169]. Copyright©2000. American Medical Association. All rights reserved.

White-coat hypertension

White-coat hypertension is generally a benign condition, but it could increase the risk of developing sustained hypertension in the future. The white-coat hypertension phenotype is psychological when it is present without other risk factors or organ damage, and metabolic when there are coexisting risk factors and/or target organ damage (Figure 1.94) [168, 169]. The former does not increase cardiovascular risk, while follow-up is necessary for the latter, which could increase the risk of cardiovascular disease and may therefore require intervention [168].

In our JMS-ABPM Wave 1 study of elderly patients with hypertension, the risk of future clinical stroke events in those with white-coat hypertension was comparable to that in the normotension group and one-quarter of that in the group with sustained (Figure 1.95) [88]. In addition, brain MRI detected a similar

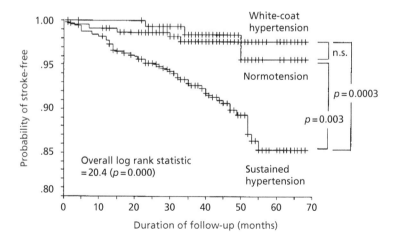

Figure 1.95 Stroke-free survival curves for normotensive individuals, and patients with white-coat or sustained hypertension. n.s., not statistically significant. *Source*: Reprinted from Kario et al. J Am Coll Cardiol. 2001; 38: 238–45 [88], Copyright (2001), with permission from Elsevier.

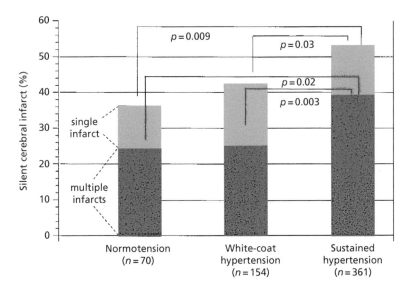

Figure 1.96 Prevalence of silent cerebral infarcts (SCI) detected by brain magnetic resonance imaging. Multiple infarcts are defined as ≥2 infarcts per person. Overall p-values for three-group comparisons are 0.006 for SCIs and 0.002 for multiple SCIs. *Source*: Kario et al. J Am Coll Cardiol. 2001; 38: 238–45 [88].

prevalence of SCI in the white-coat hypertension and normotension groups, both of which were significantly lower than the that in patients with sustained hypertension (Figure 1.96) [88]. However, the prevalence of SCI in patients with diabetes and white-coat hypertension was comparable to that in nondiabetic patients with sustained hypertension, while the prevalence of SCI (especially multiple SCI) was highest in patients with both diabetes and sustained hypertension (Figure 1.97) [170].

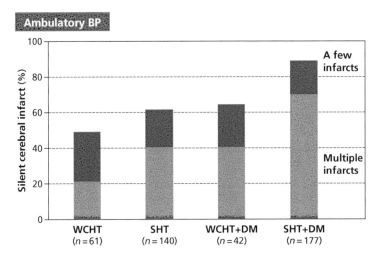

Figure 1.97 Prevalence of silent cerebral infarcts in patients with hypertension and diabetes mellitus (DM). SHT, sustained hypertension; WCHT, white-coat hypertension. *Source*: Eguchi et al. Stroke. 2003; 34: 2471–2474 [170].

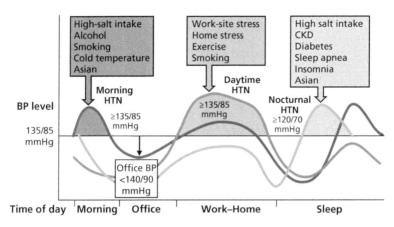

Figure 1.98 Three forms of masked hypertension (HTN) and influencing factors. BP, blood pressure; CKD, chronic kidney disease. *Source*: Kario. Circulation. 2018; 137: 543–545 [171].

Masked hypertension

There are three subtypes of masked hypertension, namely morning hypertension, daytime (stress-induced) hypertension, and nocturnal hypertension (Figure 1.98) [171]. Factors influencing the pressor effect on BP values are different between these subtypes. Of the masked hypertension subtypes, only morning hypertension could be definitively detected by the routine measurement of home BP. Use of ABPM can detect isolated stress-induced daytime, BP surge during a stressful event even when home BP and ambulatory BP during other periods are well-controlled (Figure 1.99).

Advances in ABPM

Development of information and communication technology-based multi-sensor (IMS)-ABPM

We developed a new multisensor IMS HBPM and ABPM (TM2441; A&D Company, Tokyo), which is equipped with a high-sensitivity actigraph that can detect the wearer's fine-scale physical movements in three directions, a thermometer, and a barometer (Figure 1.100). This device could be used for both ABPM and HBPM. Using these data obtained using the new device, we can examine three hemodynamic properties under resting-home and active-ambulatory conditions: BP variability; central hemodynamics; and trigger-specific BP sensitivity (Figure 1.100) [172]. Figure 1.101 [172] shows a 24-hour ambulatory BP profile measured with this device (in a seventy-seven-year-old female with hypertension) [172]. The device could also store intracuff pressure waves during oscillometric measurement of BP and use this information to detect various types of arrhythmia (Figure 1.102) [173], including atrial fibrillation using an algorithm based on pulse wave intervals (Figure 1.103 and Table 1.8) [174].

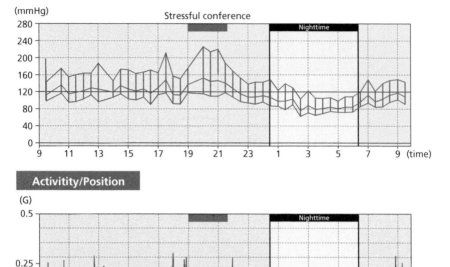

Ambulatory blood pressure (24-hour blood pressure =151/94 mmHg)

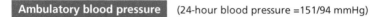

Figure 1.99 Uncontrolled hypertension triggered by worksite stress. Ambulatory blood pressure (even when physical activity is almost zero) is markedly increased during a very important 2-hour stressful conference for a 47-year-old woman taking losartan 50 mg/day. Home morning blood pressure was 132/87 mmHg. *Source*: Kario. Essential Manual on Perfect 24-hour Blood Pressure Management from Morning to Nocturnal Hypertension: Up-to-date for Anticipation Medicine. Wiley, 2018: 1–309 [24].

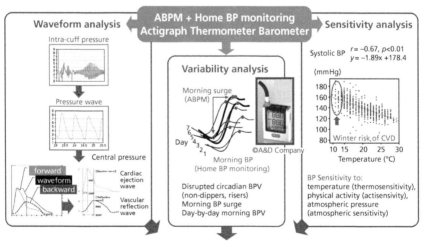

New hemodynamic biomarker-initiated anticipation medicine

Figure 1.100 Development information and communication technology-based multi-sensor (IMS) blood pressure (BP) monitoring to determine three hemodynamic properties of BP variability. ABPM, ambulatory BP monitoring; BPV, BP variability. *Source*: Kario. Am J Hypertens. 2017; 30: 226–228 [175]; Reproduced by permission of Oxford University Press.

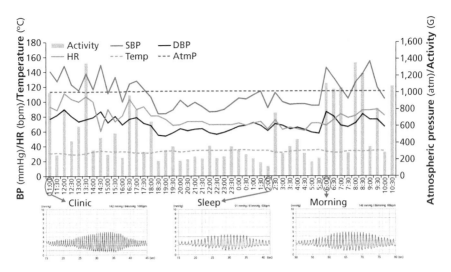

Figure 1.101 The 24-hour ambulatory blood pressure (BP) profile measured using information and communication technology-based multi-sensor (IMS) ambulatory BP monitoring in a 77-year-old woman with hypertension. Upper figure: 24-hour trend of ambulatory BP and trigger parameters measured by sensors within the ABPM device. Lower figures: envelopes of intra-cuff pressures during oscillometric BP measurement at three time points, i.e., at the clinic, during sleep (when physical activity is at a minimum), and in the morning just after arising (when activity is high). All these envelopes and waveforms are stored in the device. Act, activity (summation of the physical activity detected by 3-direction, high-sensitivity actigraphy sensors); SBP, systolic BP; DBP, diastolic BP; HR, heart rate; Temp, temperature; AtmP, atmospheric pressure. *Source*: Reprinted from Kario et al. Prog Cardiovasc Dis. 2017;60:435–449 [172]. Copyright (2017), with permission from Elsevier.

New ABPM indices
BP variability
The IMS-ABPM device can be used for both ABPM and HBPM [175]. For example, the device can be initially used in 24-hour ABPM mode, and then the mode is automatically changed to HBPM. Thus, the IMS-ABPM can evaluate ambulatory and home BP variability simultaneously using the same device and the same oscillometric BP measurement algorithm. For example, the combination of exaggerated ambulatory MBPS and increased day-by-day home morning BP variability may be associated with a higher risk of triggering cardiovascular disease events than either of these factors alone [53].

In addition to the reproducible exaggerated MBPS (Figure 1.104, Patient B), exaggerated MBPS with poor reproducibility increases cardiovascular risk (Patient C; Figure 1.104) [53]. Given that the degree of MBPS in high-reactive patients is very dependent on morning physical activity [53, 176], high-reactive patients would exhibit poorly reproducible exaggerated MBPS with increased day-by-day variability of morning BP (Patient C; Figure 1.104). Exaggerated MBPS reactivity may be associated with the greatest risk when physical activity is high. Thus, an unstable MBPS with increased day-by-day variability might reflect a phenotype with a worse prognosis (Figure 1.104) [53].

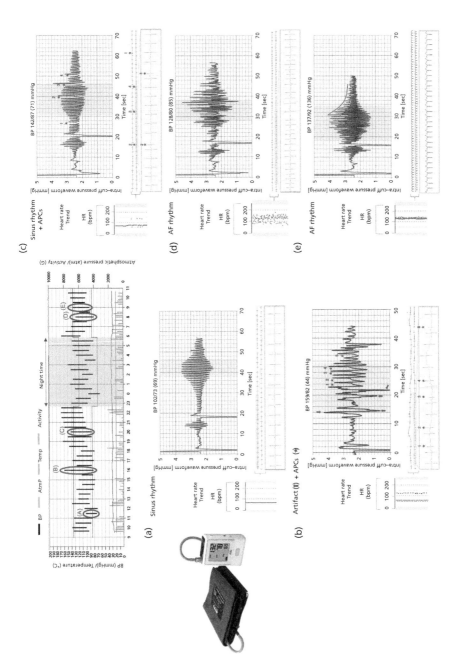

Figure 1.102 Multisensor ambulatory blood pressure (BP) monitoring technology for pulse waveform analysis to detect arrhythmias. AF, atrial fibrillation; AFL, atrial flutter; APC, atrial premature contraction; AtmP, atmospheric pressure; bpm, beats per minute; HR, heart rate; Temp, temperature. *Source:* Watanabe et al. J Clin Hypertens (Greenwich). 2020; 22: 1525–1529 [173].

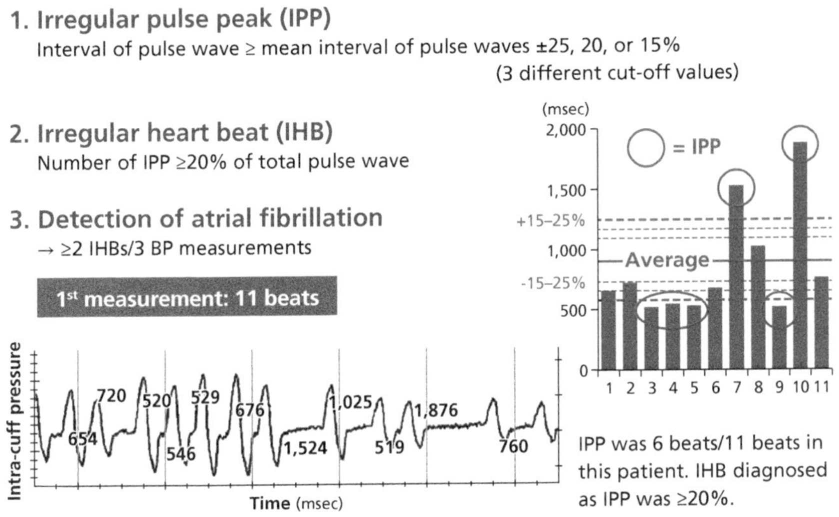

1. Irregular pulse peak (IPP)
Interval of pulse wave ≥ mean interval of pulse waves ±25, 20, or 15%
(3 different cut-off values)
2. Irregular heart beat (IHB)
Number of IPP ≥20% of total pulse wave
3. Detection of atrial fibrillation
→ ≥2 IHBs/3 BP measurements
1st measurement: 11 beats
Intra-cuff pressure
720
520
529
676
1,025
1,876
654
546
1,524
519
760
Time (msec)
(msec)
2,000
1,500
+15–25%
1,000
-15–25%
500
0
= IPP
Average
1 2 3 4 5 6 7 8 9 10 11
IPP was 6 beats/11 beats in this patient. IHB diagnosed as IPP was ≥20%.

Figure 1.103 Atrial fibrillation detection algorithm. *Source*: Kabutoya et al. J Clin Hypertens (Greenwich). 2017; 19: 1143–1147 [174].

Systolic BP
135
7
6
5
4
3
2
1
Day
Patient A
Patient B
Good reproducibility
Patient C
Poor reproducibility

Figure 1.104 Poor reproducibility does not decrease the importance of morning blood pressure (BP) surge as an important cardiovascular risk factor. *Source*: Kario. Hypertension. 2010; 56: 765–773 [53].

Table 1.8 Diagnostic accuracy of a new algorithm to detect atrial fibrillation (AF).

Accuracy of the monitor for diagnosing AF				
Monitor detection AF +/–		Sensitivity	Specificity	κ
IPP 25%	14/22	0.88	1.00	0.89
IPP 20%	15/21	0.94	1.00	0.94
IPP 15%	16/20	1.00	1.00	1.00

BP, blood pressure; bpm, beats/min; IPP, irregular pulse peak.

Source: Kabutoya et al. J Clin Hypertens (Greenwich). 2017; 19: 1143–1147 [174].

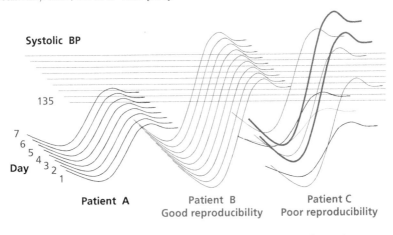

Central hemodynamics

Using intra-cuff pressure data and each of the waveforms obtained by time-series oscillometric BP measurement, we are currently analyzing the shape of the envelope of intra-cuff pressure and the waveform of estimated central BP.

Trigger-specific BP sensitivity

Change in ambulatory BP is closely related to the level of physical activity and may reflect the characteristics of individual cardiovascular properties (Figure 1.105) [53, 176]. Trigger-specific BP sensitivities based on ambulatory BP reactivity as defined by the slope of BP change in response to triggers are as follows: (1) actisensitivity—the slope of BP change versus physical activity before BP measurement; (2) thermosensitivity—the slope of BP change versus temperature; and (3) atmospheric sensitivity—the slope of BP change versus atmospheric pressure [53, 172, 175]. Negative (inverse), absent or exaggerated trigger-specific sensitivity is likely to be pathological. Using pathological thresholds defined using these hemodynamic biomarkers, it is possible to identify specific high-risk patients, such as those with thermosensitive, actisensitive, or atmospheric condition-sensitive hypertension or hypotension, who may have increased cardiovascular risk in that specific situation (Figure 1.100) [175].

Actisensitivity. As shown in Figure 1.106, actisensitivity differs between patients [172]. One regression line is calculated from six or more ambulatory BP readings with a corresponding 5-minute average of physical activity just before each BP measurement. The individual differences were large, indicating that actisensitivity would be a very useful marker for identifying high-risk patients with different BP sensitivities to physical activity. Actisensitivity is significantly steeper in winter than in summer (Figure 1.106) [172]. Our hypothesis is that hyperactisensitive patients are likely to have increased daytime BP variability, resulting in exertional onset of cardiovascular disease, while negative actisensitive (inverse slope) patients may have severe cardiac dysfunction or severe coronary artery disease (Figure 1.107 left) [172]. Figure 1.108 shows IMS-ABPM data from a 38-year-old patient with obesity and obstructive sleep apnea (apnea-hypopnea index 42.9/h) and HF with reduced ejection fraction (left ventricular ejection fraction [LVEF] 27%) before (Figure 1.108 left) and after (Figure 1.108 right) treatment [177]. After treatment, the LVEF increased to 56%, and a normal actisensitivity pattern was restored (Figure 1.109).

Thermosensitivity. Exaggerated cold thermosensitivity is thought to identify patients at risk of cardiovascular events in cold locations in winter, while exaggerated summer thermosensitivity may be associated with hypotensive episodes at hot locations in summer (Figure 1.107 right) [172]. In summer, negative thermosensitivity (i.e. a significant increase in BP in hot temperatures) may be at least partially responsible for poor sleep quality. In addition, negative thermosensitivity may be associated with autonomic nervous dysfunction. The clinical implications and pathological threshold of these trigger-specific BP sensitivity indices should be investigated in a prospective clinical study.

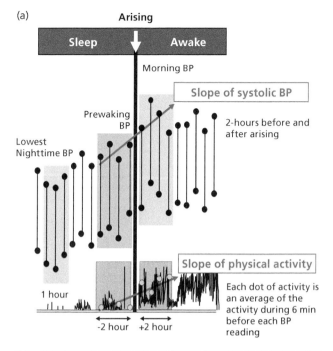

(a) Arising

Sleep | Awake

Morning BP

Slope of systolic BP

Prewaking BP

2-hours before and after arising

Lowest Nighttime BP

Slope of physical activity

1 hour

Each dot of activity is an average of the activity during 6 min before each BP reading

-2 hour   +2 hour

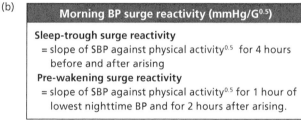

(b)

Morning BP surge reactivity (mmHg/G^0.5)

Sleep-trough surge reactivity
= slope of SBP against physical activity^0.5 for 4 hours before and after arising

Pre-wakening surge reactivity
= slope of SBP against physical activity^0.5 for 1 hour of lowest nighttime BP and for 2 hours after arising.

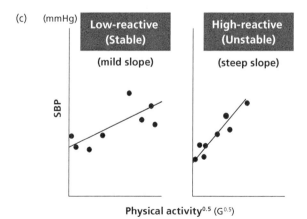

(c) (mmHg)

Low-reactive (Stable)

(mild slope)

High-reactive (Unstable)

(steep slope)

SBP

Physical activity^0.5 (G^0.5)

Figure 1.105 Morning blood pressure (BP) surge reactivity detected by ambulatory BP monitoring (ABPM). SBP, systolic BP. *Source*: Kario et al. Hypertension. 1999; 34: 685–691 [176] and Kario. Hypertension. 2010; 56: 765–773 [53].

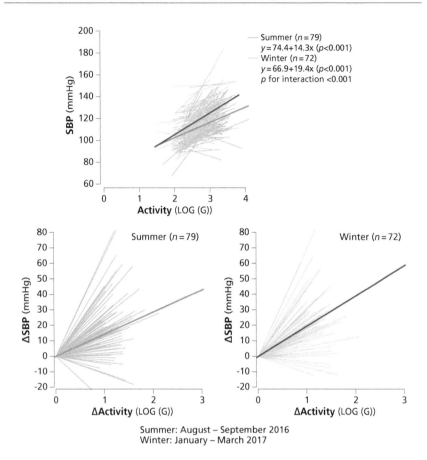

Summer: August – September 2016
Winter: January – March 2017

Figure 1.106 Differential actisensitivity between winter and summer in the same patients with hypertension. Actisensitivity is defined as the slope of blood pressure (BP) change against physical activity. Each regression line was calculated from six or more ambulatory BP readings with the corresponding 5-minute average of physical activity just before each BP measurement. The thin line represents a regression line calculated from the daytime ambulatory BP measurements in a single patient. The thick line shows the average of all regression lines for each patient (thin lines). SBP, systolic BP. *Source*: Reprinted from Kario et al. Prog Cardiovasc Dis. 2017; 60: 435–449 [172]. Copyright (2017), with permission from Elsevier.

HI-JAMP registry

The national general practitioner-based cohort, Home-Activity ICT-based Japan Ambulatory Blood Pressure Monitoring Prospective (HI-JAMP) of patients treated with antihypertensive agents was started in 2017. The aim of the registry is to clarify seasonal and regional differences in trigger-specific sensitivities and their impact on cardiovascular events (Figure 1.110).

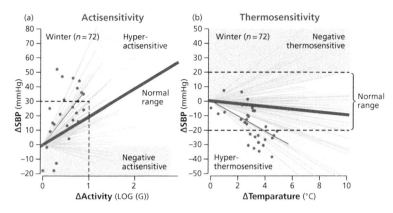

Figure 1.107 Classification of high-risk groups based on actisensitivity and thermosensitivity. The blue thick line shows the average of all regression lines from each patient (thin blue lines). (a) Actisensitivity is defined as the slope of blood pressure (BP) change against physical activity. For example, actisensitive hypertension with hyperactisensitivity may be defined as a ≥30 mmHg increase in systolic BP (SBP) when there is an increase in physical activity from 100 G (resting level) to 1000 G (walking level). The red plots and the regression line represent 24-hour information and communication technology-based multi-sensor ambulatory BP monitoring (IMS-ABPM) data from a 77-year-old woman with hypertension, chronic kidney disease (CKD), and hyperuricemia; brachial-ankle pulse wave velocity (baPWV) was high (right: 2168 cm/s; left: 2090 cm/s, corresponding to the reference value [vascular age] for an individual aged >90 years). (b) Thermosensitivity is defined as the slope of BP change against change in temperature. For example, cold thermosensitive hypertension with hyperthermosensitivity may be defined as a ≥20 mmHg increase in SBP triggered by a 10°C decrease in temperature. The red plots and the regression line represent 24-hour IMS-ABPM data from a 69-year-old woman with hypertension, hyperlipidemia, and insomnia; baPWV was high (right: 1701 cm/s; left: 1719 cm/s; vascular age: 75 years). *Source*: Kario et al. Prog Cardiovasc Dis. 2017; 60: 435–449 [172]. Copyright (2017), with permission from Elsevier.

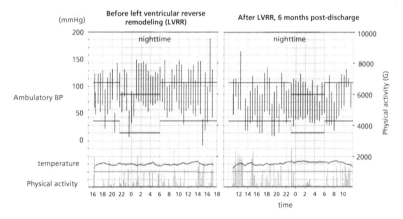

Figure 1.108 Change in ambulatory blood pressure (BP) levels from before to after the improvement of cardiac systolic function (left ventricular reverse remodeling [LVRR]). Information and communication technology-based multi-sensor ambulatory BP monitoring (IMS-ABPM) data from before and after LVRR are shown. Changes in ambulatory BP vs. physical activity are evident. Daytime ambulatory BP variability measured as the coefficient of variation for systolic BP did not increase from before to after LVRR (baseline, 0.14; follow-up, 0.12). *Source*: Narita et al. Am J Hypertens. 2020; 33: 161–164 [177]. Reprinted by permission of Oxford University Press.

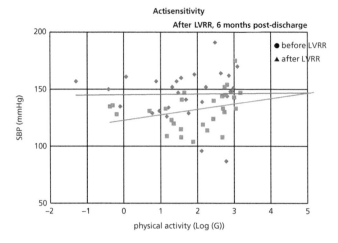

Figure 1.109 Change in actisensitivity from before to after left ventricular reverse remodeling (LVRR). Actisensitivity improved after LVRR (before, $\beta = 0.34$; after, $\beta = 4.79$). Actisensitivity of ambulatory blood pressure (BP) is defined as the slope of the regression line which is calculated from daytime ambulatory systolic BP values with the log-transformed corresponding 5-minute average of physical activity just before each BP measurement. The dotted line and solid line indicate the regression line of the actisensitivity before and after LVRR, respectively. *Source*: Narita et al. Am J Hypertens. 2020; 33: 161–164 [177]. Reprinted by permission of Oxford University Press.

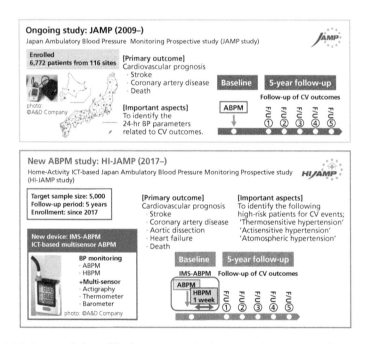

Figure 1.110 Japan ambulatory blood pressure monitoring prospective (JAMP) study. Since 2009, the JAMP study has investigated the impact of ambulatory blood pressure (BP) control status on cardiovascular (CV) prognosis in patients with a history of and/or risk factors for cardiovascular disease. ABPM, ambulatory BP monitoring; HBPM, home BP monitoring; IMS-ABPM, information and communication technology-based multi-sensor ABPM. *Source*: Kario. Essential Manual on Perfect 24-hour Blood Pressure Management from Morning to Nocturnal Hypertension: Up-to-date for Anticipation Medicine. Wiley, 2018: 1–309 [24].

CHAPTER 2

Scientific rationale for HBPM

The term "home blood pressure-monitoring (HBPM)" commonly refers to the self-measurement of blood pressure (BP) at home, although in some studies, HBPM describes a provider or research assistant measuring an individual's BP in his/her home. Both ambulatory blood pressure monitoring (ABPM) and HBPM can identify white-coat hypertension (diagnostic disagreement between office and out-of-office BP in untreated subjects) and white-coat uncontrolled hypertension (diagnostic disagreement in treated subjects) [41, 111, 156, 178–182]. Although ABPM has been the preferred out-of-office measurement tool, the 2017 American Heart Association/American College of Cardiology (AHA/ACC) hypertension guidelines suggest that HBPM may be a more practical approach in clinical practice, particularly during antihypertensive therapy.

Five prospective, general practitioner-based, home BP studies

A commonly recommended HBPM monitoring schedule consists of performing morning and evening BP measurements twice on each occasion over a minimum of three days with a preferred period of seven days (Figure 2.1) [183–185]. Several clinic-based prospective studies have investigated the prognostic importance of home BP measurements in treated patients with hypertension (Table 2.1) [56, 186–190]. All studies demonstrated that home BP is superior to office BP for the prediction of cardiovascular events. In the J-HOP study, patients with masked hypertension had a worse prognosis with respect to stroke than those with well-controlled or white-coat hypertension, and the risk of stroke associated with masked hypertension was comparable to that of patients with sustained hypertension (Figure 2.2) [191].

Morning hypertension

Morning hypertension is the most important and effective clinical target in the management of hypertension. In particular, for medicated patients with hypertension, once daily dosing of antihypertensives means that BP-lowering effects

Essential Manual of 24-Hour Blood Pressure Management: From Morning to Nocturnal Hypertension,
Second Edition. Kazuomi Kario.
© 2022 John Wiley & Sons Ltd. Published 2022 by John Wiley & Sons Ltd.

Morning, within 1 h of waking, after urination,
before breakfast and drug intake

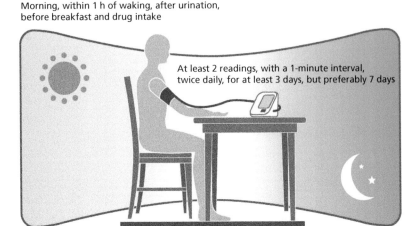

At least 2 readings, with a 1-minute interval,
twice daily, for at least 3 days, but preferably 7 days

Evening before going to bed

Figure 2.1 Recommendations for home blood pressure measurements. *Source*: Kario et al. J Clin Hypertens (Greenwich). 2018; 20: 456–461 [184]; Kario et al. J Clin Hypertens. 2020; 22: 351–362 [185]; Park et al. J Hum Hypertens. 2018; 32: 249–258 [183].

are weakest first thing in the morning, immediately prior to the next dose. Thus, morning BP control is the "blind spot" for current hypertensive medication.

Morning BP can easily be self-measured using a HBPM device. Two types of morning hypertension are detected by HBPM [156, 178]. One is the "morning surge" type, characterized by an exaggerated morning blood pressure surge (MBPS), and the other is the "sustained nocturnal hypertension" type with continuous hypertension from nocturnal hypertension (non-dipper/riser type) (Figure 2.3).

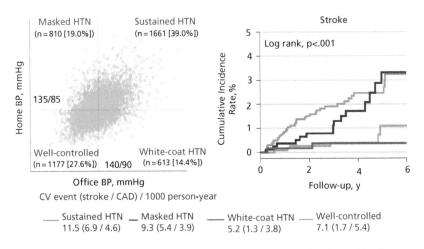

Figure 2.2 Prevalence of different forms of hypertension (HTN) based on home blood-pressure monitoring (left, and risk of stroke in different hypertension groups (right). *Source*: Reproduced with permission from Fujiwara et al. JAMA Cardiology. 2018; 3: 583–590 [191]. Copyright©(2018) American Medical Association. All rights reserved.

Table 2.1 Prospective, general practitioner-based, home BP studies.

Name of study	Study subjects and follow-up	BP measurement schedule	Outcomes
1. SHEAF study[†] Bobrie G, et al. (JAMA. 2004)	France (4939 treated hypertensive patients; mean age, 70 years; mean follow-up, 3.2 years)	4-day HBPM (baseline HBP) (24 readings)	Adjusted HR of fatal or non-fatal cardiovascular events with a BP increase of 1 mmHg was 1.02 (95% CI, 1.01 to 1.02; $P < 0.001$)
2. Fagard RH, et al. (J Hum Hypertens. 2005)	Belgium (391 older outpatients; mean age, 71 years; follow-up, 10.9 years)	1-day HBPM (baseline HBP) (3 readings) (not by self-measurement, by a physician or assist physician with mercury device)	Adjusted relative HR of cardiovascular events with a HBP increase of 1 SD. (22.9 mmHg) was 1.32 (95%CI, 1.06–1.64; $P = 0.01$)
3. HOMED BP[‡] Asayama K, et al. (Hypertens Res. 2012)	Japan (3,518 hypertensive patients; mean age, 59.6 years; median follow-up, 5.3 years)	5-day HBPM (follow-up HBP) (5 readings)	Adjusted HR of fatal or non-fatal cardiovascular events with a HBP increase of 1 s.d. (13.2 mmHg) was 1.47 (95% CI 1.23–1.75, $P < 0.0001$)
4. HONEST[§] Kario K, et al. (Hypertension. 2014)	Japan (21,591 hypertensive patients, mean age, 64.9 years, mean follow-up, 2.02 years)	2-day HBPM (follow-up HBP) (8 readings)	HR of incidence of cardiovascular events for morning HSBP>=145 mHg and CSBP >=150 mmHg compared to morning HSBP 125 mmHg and CSBP <130 mmHg was 3.92, 95% CI 2.22–6.92)
5. JHOP[‖] Hoshide S, et al. (Hypertension. 2016)	Japan (4310 patients with a history of and/or risk factors for cardiovascular disease; mean age, 65 years, mean follow-up, 4 years)	14-day HBPM (baseline HBP) (84 readings)	Adjusted HR of stroke events with a home SBP increase of 10 mmHg was 1.36 (95%CI, 1.19 to 1.56; $P < 0.001$)
6. JHOP Nocturnal BP study Kario K, et al. (Hypertension 2019)	Japan (2547 patients with a history of and/or risk factors for cardiovascular disease; mean age, 63 years, mean follow-up, 7.1 years)	14-day HBPM (baseline HBP) (morning and evening 84 readings + nighttime 42 readings)	A 10-mm Hg increase of nighttime home SBP was associated with an increased risk of CVD events (hazard ratios [95% CIs]: 1.201 [1.046–1.378]), after adjustments for covariates including office and morning home SBPs.

BP, blood pressure; CI, confidence interval; CSBP, clinic systolic BP; CVD, cardiovascular disease; HBPM, home BP monitoring; HR, hazard ratio; SBP, systolic BP; SD, standard deviation.

[†]Self-Measurement of Blood Pressure at Home in the Elderly: Assessment and Follow-up (SHEAF) study
[‡]Hypertension Objective Treatment Based on Measurement by Electrical Devices of Blood Pressure (HOMED-BP)
[§]Home Blood Pressure Measurement With Olmesartan Naive Patients to Establish Standard Target Blood Pressure (HONEST) study
[‖]Japan Morning Surge-Home Blood Pressure (J-HOP) study.
Source: Modified from Kario et al. Hypertension. 2019; 74: 229–236 [192].

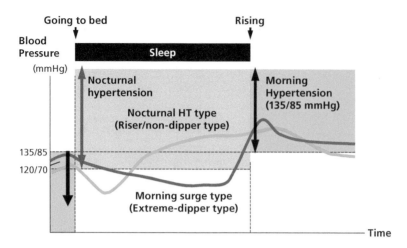

Figure 2.3 Two types of morning hypertension (HT). *Source*: Modified from Kario. Am J Hypertens. 2005;18:149–151 [50].

These two forms of morning hypertension both increase the risk of cardiovascular and renal diseases, but this occurs via different pathogenic mechanisms and each are associated with different conditions. The only way to reliably differentiate between "morning surge" and "sustained nocturnal hypertension" is to measure home BP during sleep, either using ABPM or newer automated HBPM devices.

Control status of morning home BP in the J-HOP study

Figure 2.4 [171] shows the morning systolic blood pressure (SBP) control status and changes associated with application of new cut-off values based on the AHA/ACC 2017 guidelines [178] compared with those classified by the previous Seventh Report of the Joint National Committee on Prevention, Detection, Evaluation, and Treatment of High Blood Pressure (JNC7) guidelines [193] using data from the Japan Morning Surge-Home Blood Pressure (J-HOP) study, a general practice-based national registry of home BP (4310 patients with treated hypertension, mean age 64.9 years, 47% male). Prevalence rates for normotension, white-coat hypertension, masked morning hypertension, and sustained morning hypertension changed from 31%, 15%, 19%, and 36%, respectively, using JNC7 definitions (140/90 mmHg for office BP and 135/85 mmHg for home BP) [193] to 14%, 17%, 10%, and 58%, respectively, based on the AHA/ACC 2017 definitions (130/80 mmHg for both office and home BP) (Figure 2.4) [171, 178]. The lower single BP threshold of 130/80 mmHg for both office and home BP values could be acceptable for two reasons. First, in general, the difference between office and out-of-office BP values decreases to reach a similar level to that shown in Figure 2.4 [171]. Second, clinically, the decrease in masked morning hypertension and the increase in sustained morning hypertension provides physicians with the opportunity to strictly treat hypertension without underestimation of cardiovascular risk due to undetected masked morning hypertension. A lower morning BP (SBP <125 mmHg) target may be ideal for minimization of cardiovascular risk, regardless of office BP level [56].

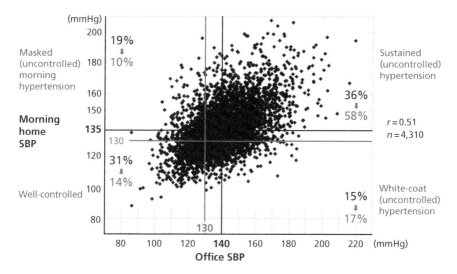

Figure 2.4 Shift in the prevalence of different patterns of hypertension classified by the new American Heart Association/American College of Cardiology 2017 guidelines (shown in red) vs. those classified based on the previous Seventh Report of the Joint National Committee on Prevention, Detection, Evaluation and Treatment of High Blood Pressure guidelines (shown in black) in subjects from the Japan Morning Surge-Home Blood Pressure Study (4310 patients with treated hypertension: mean age 64.9 years, 47% male). SBP, systolic blood pressure. *Source*: Kario. Circulation. 2018;137:543–545 [171].

Evidence for morning hypertension control

The Ohasama study of a general population-based cohort first demonstrated that morning home BP is a better predictor of cardiovascular prognosis than office BP [194].

J-HOP study

The J-HOP study, one of the nationwide, general practitioner-based cohorts of cardiovascular risk patients (Table 2.1) showed that morning home BP was a better predictor of stroke than evening home BP (Figure 2.5) [189]. An analysis of 349 patients aged ≥80 years from this trial found that higher morning SBP was a significant risk factor for composite cardiovascular events (hazard ratio [HR] per 10 mmHg increase in morning SBP, 1.23; 95% confidence interval [CI] 1.01–1.50) and stroke events (HR per 10 mmHg increase in SBP, 1.47; 95% CI 1.08–2.00) after adjustment for four-year cardiovascular risk scores and office SBP (Figure 2.6) [195]. This association was not observed for office BP or evening home BP.

In J-HOP study, participants with nonelevated high-sensitive cardiac troponin T level (hs-cTnT; <0.014 ng/mL, $n = 3307$), an adjusted Cox hazard model showed that home SBP was associated with stroke risk (HR per 1 standard deviation [SD] increase, 1.62). In the group with elevated hs-cTnT, lower home diastolic blood pressure (DBP) was associated with the risk of coronary artery disease (CAD; HR per 1 SD increase, 0.54). These findings suggest that excessive lowering of home

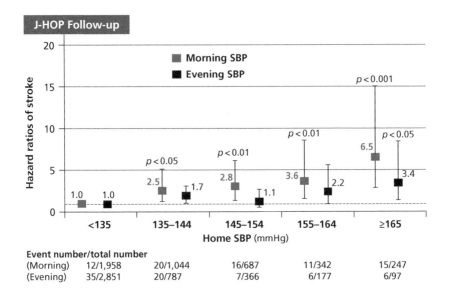

Figure 2.5 Home BP and stroke risk based on data from the Japan Morning Surge-Home Blood Pressure (J-HOP) study. SBP, systolic blood pressure. *Source*: Hoshide et al. Hypertension. 2016; 68: 54–61 [189].

DBP in patients with subclinical myocardial ischemia may be associated with a risk of incident CAD (Figure 2.7) [196].

HONEST study

On-treatment morning home BP was also a stronger predictor of cardiovascular events than office BP in the Hypertension Objective treatment based on Measurement by Electrical Devices of Blood Pressure (HOMED-BP) study [188] and the Home blood pressure measurement with Olmesartan Naïve patients to Establish Standard Target blood pressure (HONEST) study [56]. The HONEST trial is the largest real-world prospective study in the field and included >21 000 patients with hypertension. The results showed that morning SBP of 145 mmHg was the threshold for a statistically significant increase in cardiovascular risk in medicated patients with hypertension. In addition, the morning SBP associated with minimum risk was 124 mmHg (Figure 2.8) [56]. Furthermore, the ability of morning home BP to detect the risk of CAD and stroke was similar, whereas office BP underestimated the risk of CAD (Figure 2.9) [197]. There was no significant J-shaped curve for the association between morning home SBP and both stroke and coronary events until home SBP reached 110 mmHg (Figure 2.10) [197]. When on-treatment morning home SBP was well controlled (<125 mmHg) during two-year follow-up, there was no increase in cardiovascular events even when office SBP remained ≥150 mmHg (Figure 2.11) [56].

Diabetes. In a subanalysis of patients with diabetes, those with morning home SBP 125–134 or 135–144 mmHg showed a tendency for, or a significant increase in, the risk of cardiovascular events compared to patients with well-controlled

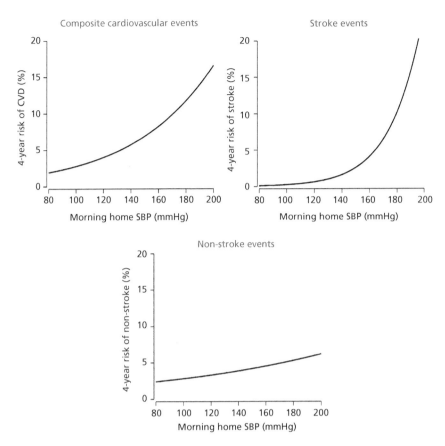

Figure 2.6 Relationship between the occurrence of cardiovascular disease (CVD) events and morning home systolic blood pressure (SBP) levels in very elderly patients (age ≥80 years) from the Japan Morning Surge-Home Blood Pressure (J-HOP) study (*n* = 349; median follow-up 3.0 years). *Source*: Created based on data from Kawauchi et al. Am J Hypertens. 2018; 31: 1190–1196 [195].

hypertension (morning home SBP <125 mmHg) (Figure 2.12) [198]. Morning hypertension in patients with diabetes is associated with the non-dipper/riser pattern of nighttime BP and nocturnal hypertension. In addition, morning hypertension was closely associated with advanced organ damage in patients with diabetes [199].

Elderly. Another subanalysis found that morning home SBP targets during antihypertensive therapy for patients aged <75 years can also be beneficial for reducing cardiovascular risk in those aged ≥75 years if this intensity of therapy is tolerated (Figure 2.13) [200].

High-risk hypertension. In a post hoc analysis, where patients were grouped according to cardiovascular risk level showed that intensive antihypertensive therapy targeting a home SBP of <125 mmHg would be beneficial for high-risk hypertensive patients (Figure 2.14) [201].

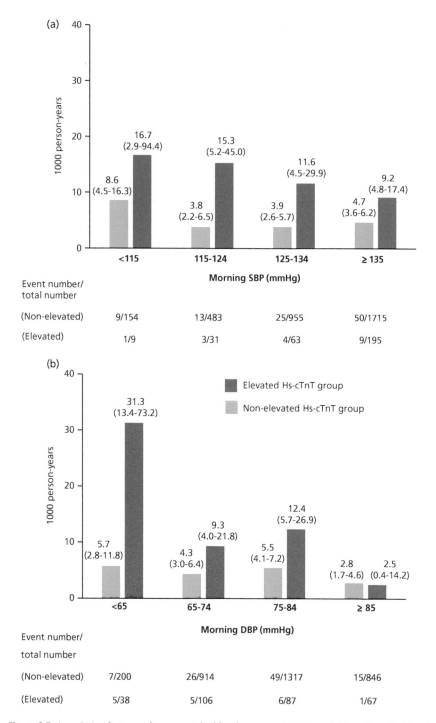

Figure 2.7 Association between home systolic blood pressure (SBP; panel A) or diastolic blood pressure (DBP; panel B) and coronary artery disease incidence in patients with elevated or nonelevated levels of high-sensitive cardiac troponin (Hs-cTnT). Values are the incidence per 1000 person-years (95% confidence interval). *$p < 0.05$, †$p < 0.01$ vs. nonelevated Hs-cTnT group in each blood pressure category. *Source*: Shimizu et al. J Clin Hypertens (Greenwich). 2020; 22 : 2214–2220 [196].

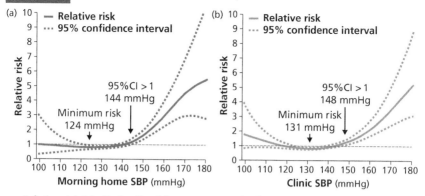

HONEST

Relative risk 1 indicates the risk at mean morning home SBP during the 2-yr follow-up period (a); the risk at mean clinic SBP during the 2-yr follow-up period (b).

Adjusted for sex, age, family history of cardiovascular disease, dyslipidaemia, diabetes mellitus, chronic kidney disease, history of cardiovascular disease, and smoking status. Primary endpoint: stroke event; coronary event; sudden death.

Figure 2.8 Minimum and statistically significant increase in cardiovascular risk associated with different morning home systolic blood pressure (SBP) levels (spline regression analysis). CI, confidence interval. *Source*: Kario et al. Hypertension. 2014; 64: 989–996 [56].

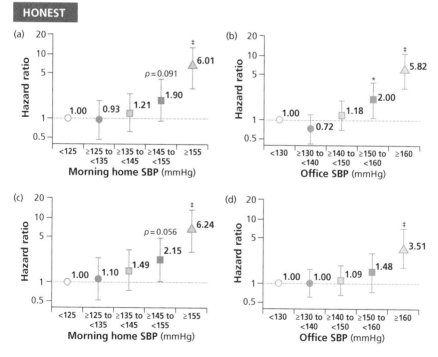

HONEST

Figure 2.9 On-treatment systolic blood pressure (SBP) and the risk of stroke (panels A and B) and coronary artery disease (panels C and D) events. Cox proportional hazards model was adjusted for age, sex, family history of cardiovascular disease, and smoking status. *$p < 0.05$; ‡$p < 0.001$. *Source*: Kario et al. J Am Coll Cardiol. 2016; 67: 1519–1527 [197]. Reproduced with permission from Elsevier.

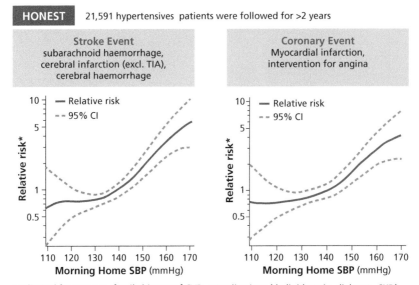

*Adjusted for age, sex, family history of CVD, complications (dyslipidaemia, diabetes, CKD), history of CVD, smoking habit.

Figure 2.10 Relationship between morning home systolic blood pressure (SBP) and stroke/coronary events (spline regression analysis); analysis from 21,591 patients with hypertension who were followed for >2 years. CI, confidence interval; CKD, chronic kidney disease; CVD, cardiovascular disease; TIA, transient ischemic attack. *Source*: Kario et al. J Am Coll Cardiol. 2016; 67: 1519–1527 [197]. Reproduced with permission from Elsevier.

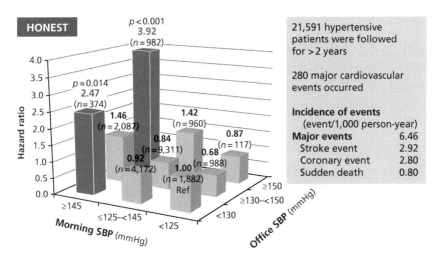

Figure 2.11 On-treatment morning home and office systolic blood pressure (SBP) values and the occurrence of cardiovascular events in medicated patients with hypertension from the Home blood pressure measurement with Olmesartan Naive patients to Establish Standard Target blood pressure (HONEST) study (adjusted for age, sex, family history of cardiovascular disease, dyslipidemia, diabetes mellitus, chronic kidney disease, history of cardiovascular disease, and smoking status). *Source*: Kario et al. Hypertension. 2014: 64: 989–996 [56].

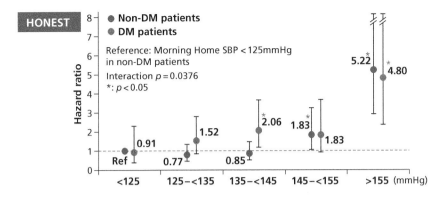

Figure 2.12 Relationship between cardiovascular events and morning home systolic blood pressure (SBP) in patients with and without diabetes mellitus (DM) treated with an angiotensin receptor blocker. CKD, chronic kidney disease; HR, hazard ratio. *Source*: Kushiro et al. Hypertens Res. 2017; 40: 87–95 [198].

Difference between the first and second measurements. In the HONEST study, patients were asked to measure morning home BP twice. There was an interesting V-shape association between the difference between the first and second readings and the rate of cardiovascular events (Figure 2.15) [202]. Risk was higher in those with the greatest variability between the first and second home BP measurements compared with patients whose BP readings were more stable.

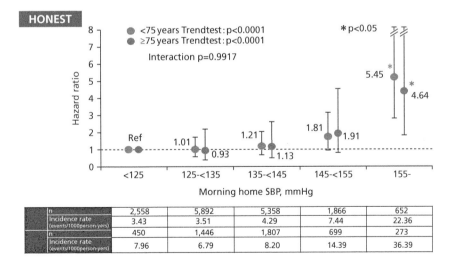

Figure 2.13 Relationship between major cardiovascular events and morning home systolic blood pressure (SBP) during follow-up in patients aged <75 years and ≥75 years from the Home blood pressure measurement with Olmesartan Naive patients to Establish Standard Target blood pressure (HONEST) study (adjusted for sex, family history of cardiovascular disease, dyslipidemia, diabetes mellitus, chronic kidney disease, history of cardiovascular disease, and smoking status). *Source*: Saito et al. Clin Exp Hypertens. 2018; 40: 407–413 [200].

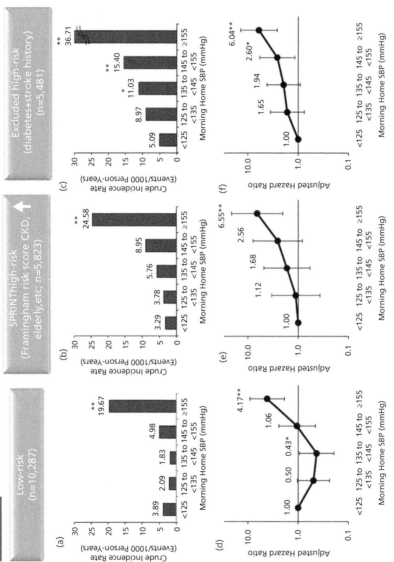

Figure 2.14 Relationship between incidence rates of cardiovascular disease events and morning home systolic blood pressure (SBP) levels (analysis of the Home blood pressure measurement with Olmesartan Naive patients to Establish Standard Target blood pressure (HONEST) study). Crude incidence rate (A–C) and adjusted hazard ratios (D–F) for each morning home SBP category in the non-SPRINT (Systolic Blood Pressure Intervention Trial) low-risk population, SPRINT population, and SPRINT-excluded high-risk population, respectively. Vertical lines indicate the 95% CI. *p<0.05, **p<0.01 (compared with morning home SBP <125 mmHg). *Source:* Kario et al. Hypertension. 2018: 72: 854–861 [201].

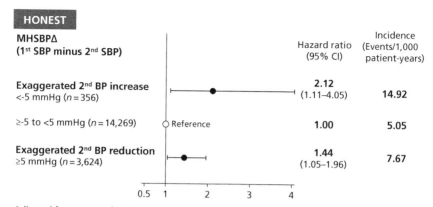

Adjusted for sex, age, family history of cardiovascular disease, dyslipidaemia, diabetes mellitus, chronic kidney disease, history of cardiovascular disease, smoking status, and averaged morning home systolic blood pressure during the follow-up period.

Figure 2.15 Variability in morning home systolic blood pressure (MHSBP) between the first and second measurements taken on the same occasion and the risk of cardiovascular disease (adjusted for sex, age, family history of cardiovascular disease, dyslipidemia, diabetes mellitus, chronic kidney disease, history of cardiovascular disease, smoking status, and averaged MHSBP during follow-up). BP, blood pressure; CI, confidence interval. *Source*: Saito et al. Clin Exp Hypertens. 2018; 40: 407–413 [200].

Target home BP levels. Real-world findings from the HONEST study emphasize the importance of HBPM in clinical practice. This evidence suggests that it is essential to control morning home SBP to <145 mmHg as a first step, even in patients with controlled office BP. The second step is to target morning home SBP to <130 mmHg as per the guidelines, then a target of around 125 mmHg is the ultimate goal of home BP-guided management of hypertension (Figure 2.8) [37, 50].

ANAFIE Study

The All Nippon AF in the Elderly (ANAFIE) Registry home BP subcohort is the first prospective large observational study to investigate the impact of home BP control status on cardiovascular prognosis in elderly patients (age ≥75 years) with nonvalvular atrial fibrillation (NVAF; n = 5204) [203]. It is recommended that patients with NVAF receive anticoagulant therapy and that target BP office and home BP levels are <130/80 and <125/75 mmHg, respectively, to reduce the risk of both embolic and hemorrhagic cardiovascular events. However, early morning hypertension (morning home SBP ≥125 mmHg) was found in 66% of studied patients (Figure 2.16). Although 51.1% of patients had well-controlled office SBP, 52.5% of these still had uncontrolled morning home SBP. In elderly patients with NVAF, morning home BP was poorly controlled, and masked uncontrolled morning hypertension remains significant.

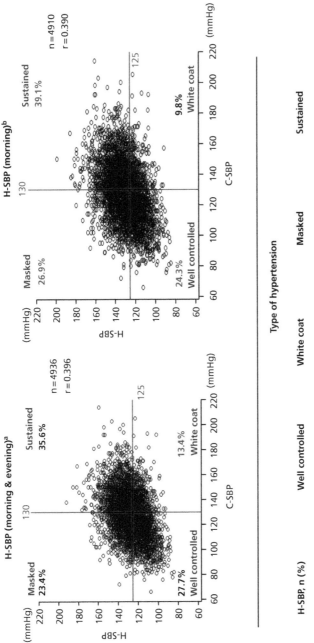

Figure 2.16 High prevalence of masked uncontrolled morning hypertension in elderly nonvalvular atrial fibrillation patients: Home blood pressure substudy of the ANAFIE Registry. *Source: Kario* et al. J Clin Hypertens (Greenwich). 2021; 23: 73–82 [203].

Type of hypertension

H-SBP, n (%)	Well controlled	White coat	Masked	Sustained
Morning & evening[a]	1366 (27.7)	659 (13.4)	1154 (23.4)	1757 (35.6)
Morning[b]	1191 (24.3)	481 (9.8)	1319 (26.9)	1919 (39.1)

Home BP variability

HBPM is the best practical method to detect the wide range of BP variability with different time phases, from relatively short-term (diurnal), intermediate-term (day-by-day), to long-term (seasonal, and yearly) (Figure 2.17) [156]. HBPM could exclude the white-coat effect to detect reproducible pathological BP variability. There are several measures of home BP variability that have clinical relevance in terms of cardiovascular prognosis (Figure 2.18) [3]. These are morning–evening difference (ME-dif), standard deviation (SD), coefficient of variation (CV) average real variability (ARV), and variation independent of mean (VIM), all for home SBP, plus maximum home SBP (max home SBP) and seasonal variation.

Morning–evening difference (ME-dif)
In both medicated and nonmedicated patients with hypertension, the ME difference of self-measured home BP was associated with the left ventricular mass index (LVMI) and the risk of concentric hypertrophy, as well as with increased pulse wave velocity (PWV) [204–206]. ME-dif has also been significantly associated with left ventricular hypertrophy (LVH) and increased brachial-ankle pulse wave velocity (baPWV) (Figure 2.19) [204]. In addition, morning hypertension defined by the ME-dif and the average of morning and evening BP readings (ME-ave) was shown to be a determinant of concentric LVH (Figure 2.20) [199–205]. Even for patients with normal home BP (white-coat hypertension), those with ME-dif ≥15 mmHg had a higher percentage of concentric remodeling than those with ME-dif <15 mmHg (32.5% vs. 14.7%, $p = 0.017$) [205]. Recently, ME-dif assessed using ABPM or HBPM was reported to be associated with cardiovascular risk independently of the ME-ave. [51, 207] The ME-dif from ABPM was an independent predictor of future stroke events in elderly patients with hypertension [51].

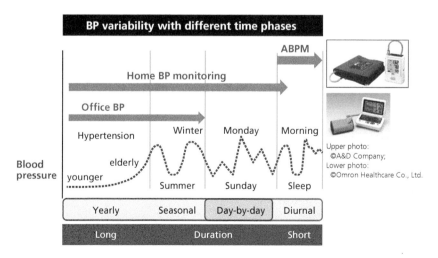

Figure 2.17 Blood pressure (BP) variability with different time phases. *Source*: Kario. Prog Cariovasc Dis 2016; 59: 262–281 [156].

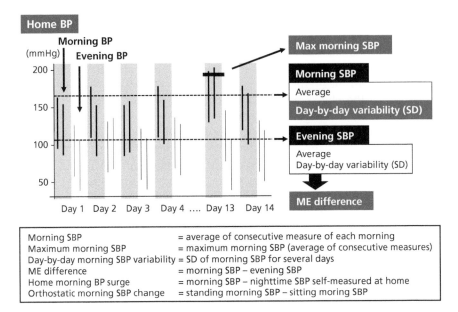

Morning SBP	= average of consecutive measure of each morning
Maximum morning SBP	= maximum morning SBP (average of consecutive measures)
Day-by-day morning SBP variability	= SD of morning SBP for several days
ME difference	= morning SBP – evening SBP
Home morning BP surge	= morning SBP – nighttime SBP self-measured at home
Orthostatic morning SBP change	= standing morning SBP – sitting moring SBP

Figure 2.18 Key indices of home blood pressure (BP) variability. ME, morning-evening; SBP, systolic blood pressure; SD, standard deviation. *Source*: Kario. Morning surge in blood pressure in hypertension: clinical relevance, prognostic significance and therapeutic approach. In: Special Issues in Hypertension (A. E. Berbari, G. Mancia, eds). Springer Inc., pp. 71–89, 2012 [3].

Measurement of evening BP is recommended, in addition to morning BP, especially for patients with both hypertension and diabetes, because reduction of both evening and morning BP is closely correlated with a decrease in the urinary albumin-creatinine ratio (UACR) [208].

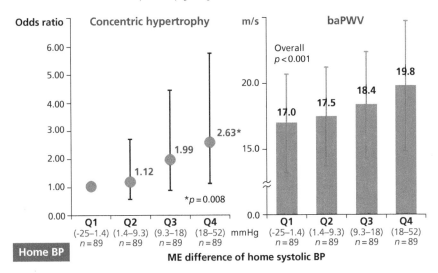

Figure 2.19 Morning-evening (ME) difference of home blood pressure (BP) and cardiovascular disease in unmedicated patients with hypertension (*n* = 356). baPWV, brachial-ankle pulse wave velocity; Q, quartile. *Source*: Matsui et al. J Hypertens 2009; 27: 712–720 [204].

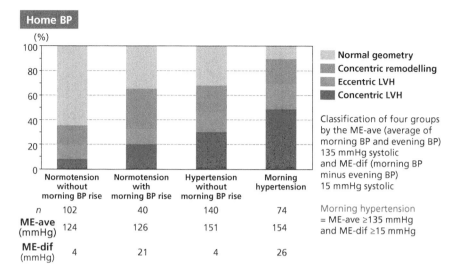

Figure 2.20 Morning hypertension and left ventricular hypertrophy (LVH) in unmedicated patients with hypertension. BP, blood pressure; ME-average, average of morning-evening differences in BP; ME-dif, morning-evening difference in BP. *Source*: Matsui et al. J Clin Hypertens (Greenwich). 2010; 12: 776–783 [205].

SD, CV, ARV, and VIM of home BP

Increased SD of home BP readings is associated with organ damage. In a study of unmedicated patients with hypertension, the SD of home BP readings measured three times at a single time-point in the morning and evening for 14 days was associated with the UACR, LVMI, and carotid intima-media thickness (IMT) (Figure 2.21) [209]. The Ohasama study of a community-dwelling population also demonstrated that an increase in the SD of home BP self-measured in the morning was an independent risk for cardiovascular mortality [125]. In addition, in the recent population-based prospective Finn Home study, the variability of home BP, defined as the SD values of ME-dif, day-by-day, and first minus second measurements, was associated with future cardiovascular events, independent of BP [207]. The association with cardiovascular risk was stronger for BP variability of morning SBP than that for evening SBP. Thus, BP variability assessed by self-measured home BP has clinical relevance independently of average home BP levels.

The impact of three different measures of home BP variability (CV, ARV, and VIM) were evaluated in the J-HOP study (Figure 2.22), and the incidence of cardiovascular events was found to increase significantly as the quartile for all measures of home BP variability increased (Figure 2.23) [210]. In addition, the impact of increased home BP variability (SD, CV, ARV) on cardiac stress (serum amino terminal pro B-type natriuretic peptide [NT-proBNP]) was greater in those with advanced arterial stiffness (baPWV >1800 cm/sec) than in those with less-advanced arterial stiffness (Figure 2.24) [211]. This is indicative of the systemic hemodynamic atherothrombotic syndrome (SHATS), in which BP variability and vascular disease have synergistic effects on cardiovascular overload. Invasive strategies may reduce exaggerated BP variability and pulse wave reflection,

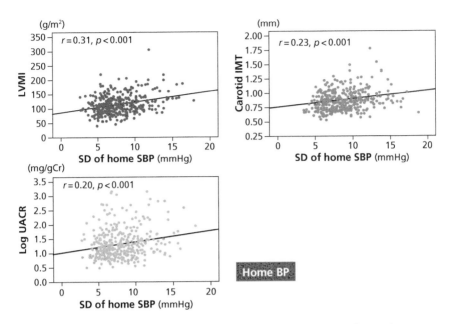

Figure 2.21 Day-by-day variability of home blood pressure (BP) and organ damage in never-treated patients with hyprtension. IMT, intima-media thickness; LVMI, left ventricular mass index; SBP, systolic BP; SD, standard deviation; UACR, urinary albumin-creatinine ratio. *Source*: Matsui et al. Hypertension. 2011; 57: 1087–1093 [209].

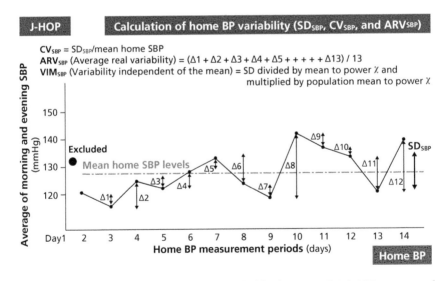

Figure 2.22 Calculation of variability in home systolic blood pressure (SBP). ARV, average real variability; BP, blood pressure; CV, coefficient of variation; SD, standard deviation; VIM, variability independent of the mean. Power X was obtained by fitting a curve through a plot of SD against mean value using the model SD = a times meanX, where X was derived by a nonlinear regression analysis. *Source*. Kario. Essential Manual for Perfect 24-Hour Blood Pressure Management from Morning to Nocturnal Hypertension: Up-to-date for Anticipation Medicine. Wiley, 2018: 1–309 [24].

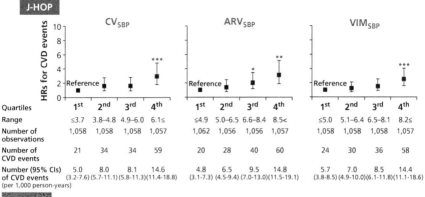

Figure 2.23 Incidence cardiovascular disease (CVD) risk by quartiles of home systolic blood pressure (SBP) measurements (n = 4,231, mean age 65 years, 53% female, 79% taking antihypertensives). Data are presented as hazard ratio (HR) and 95% confidence interval (CI). ARV, average real variability; CV, coefficient of variation; VIM, variability independent of the mean. *Source*: Hoshide et al. Hypertension. 2018; 71: 177–184 [210].

resulting in the suppression of the vicious cycle of SHATS. Carotid artery stenting (CAS) significantly reduces the day-by-day variability of home BP levels in patients with carotid artery disease [212].

Maximum home SBP

Maximum home SBP was significantly associated with increases in LVMI and carotid IMT (evaluated by echocardiography) and microalbuminuria, independent of BP level in unmedicated patients with hypertension (Table 2.2) [209]. In this study, even when home BP was well controlled (<135/85 mmHg), maximum home SBP was significantly correlated with LVMI and carotid IMT. The maximum home SBP was found in the morning BP readings in 67% of all samples. An increase in maximum morning SBP and/or increased SD of morning SBP readings reflects the instability of MBPS. An analysis of the J-HOP study using a Cox regression showed that the hazard ratios of a 1-SD increase in maximum mean home SBP for incident stroke were 1.89 (95%CI, 1.23–2.89) including MEave SBP and 1.68 (1.33–2.14) including the VIM of MEave SBP. The patients in the highest maximum mean home SBP group had a significantly higher incidence rate of stroke compared with the patients in the other groups (Figure 2.25).

Orthostatic Home BP Change

Home BP self-measured conventionally in the morning in a sitting position may underestimate the risk of ambulatory MBPS, which is augmented by standing and morning physical activity. The head-up tilting test is the standard method for assessing orthostatic BP changes. However, the simple home active standing test (HAST) using HBPM (two measurements on active standing after two measurements in the sitting position) is clinically useful to exclude the white-coat effect and to identify reproducible and pathological home orthostatic hypertension or

Table 2.2 Multivariate regression analyses for the association between maximum home systolic blood pressure (SBP) and organ damage parameters in never-treated patients with hypertension (n = 356).

Variable	Total population (n = 356)		Subgroup analysis			
			Mean home BP <135/85 mmHg (n = 135)		Mean home BP ≥135/85 mmHg (n = 221)	
	β (SE)	p	β (SE)	p	β (SE)	p
Dependent variable: LVMI[a] (g/m²)						
Maximum home SBP (mmHg)	0.598 (0.094)	<0.001	0.512 (0.188)	0.007	0.655 (0.145)	<0.001
	Model R^2 = 0.32		Model R^2 = 0.21		Model R^2 = 0.24	
Dependent variable: carotid IMT[b] (mm)						
Maximum home SBP (mmHg)	0.003 (<0.001)	<0.001	0.003 (0.001)	0.006	0.003 (0.001)	<0.001
	Model R^2 = 0.27		Model R^2 = 0.26		Model R^2 = 0.24	
Dependent variable: UACR[c] (mg/gCr)						
Maximum home SBP (mmHg)	0.004 (0.002)	0.02	0.001 (0.003)	0.68	0.003 (0.002)	0.18
	Model R^2 = 0.20		Model R^2 = 0.15		Model R^2 = 0.17	

BP, blood pressure; IMT, intima-media thickness; LVMI, left ventricular mass index; SE, standard error; UACR, urinary albumin-creatinine ratio.

[a] This model was adjusted by age, sex, habitual drinking, and mean office SBP.

[b] This model was adjusted by age, sex, hypertension duration, smoking, diabetes mellitus, and mean office SBP.

[c] This model was adjusted by age, sex, diabetes mellitus, and mean office SBP.

Source: Matsui et al. Hypertension. 2011; 57: 1087–1093 [209].

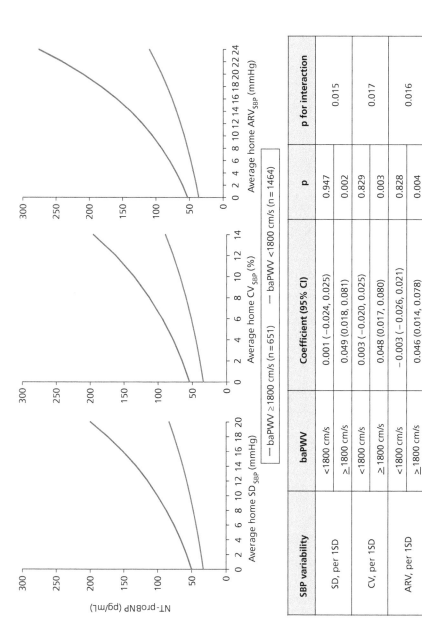

SBP variability	baPWV	Coefficient (95% CI)	p	p for interaction
SD, per 1SD	<1800 cm/s	0.001 (−0.024, 0.025)	0.947	0.015
	≥1800 cm/s	0.049 (0.018, 0.081)	0.002	
CV, per 1SD	<1800 cm/s	0.003 (−0.020, 0.025)	0.829	0.017
	≥1800 cm/s	0.048 (0.017, 0.080)	0.003	
ARV, per 1SD	<1800 cm/s	−0.003 (−0.026, 0.021)	0.828	0.016
	≥1800 cm/s	0.046 (0.014, 0.078)	0.004	

Figure 2.24 Relationship between the average home systolic blood pressure (SBP) and amino terminal pro B-type natriuretic pressure (NT-proBNP) levels in patient subgroups based on brachial artery pulse wave velocity (baPWV). ARV, average real variability; CI, confidence interval; CV, coefficient of variation; SD, standard deviation. *Source:* Ishiyama et al. Hypertension. 2020; 75: 1600–1606 [211].

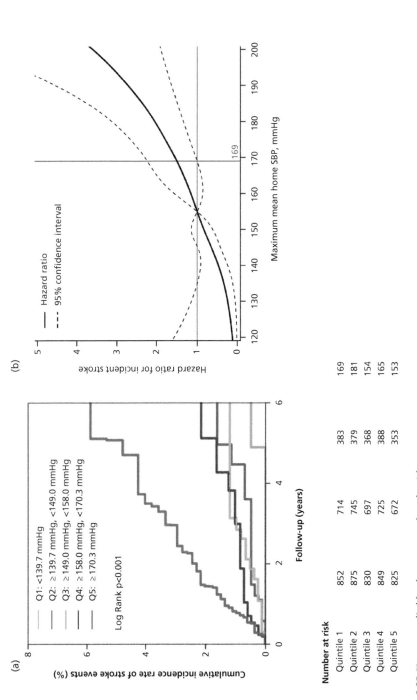

Figure 2.25 Home systolic blood pressure and stroke risk.

a. Cardiovascular disease event risks according to quintiles of the maximum mean home systolic blood pressure (SBP). Kaplan-Meier curves of the cumulative incidence of stroke by the quintiles of maximum mean home SBP are shown. Kaplan-Meier survival curves and the associated log rank test statistic were unadjusted. b. Relationship between maximum mean home SBP and incident stroke risk. The spline curve for incident stroke is shown with adjustment for age, sex, body mass index, smoking status, prevalence of diabetes, pre-existing angina pectoris, myocardial infarction or stroke, total cholesterol to high-density lipoprotein cholesterol ratio, the use of antihypertensive medication drugs, statins and aspirin, and office SBP. The value of maximum mean home SBP was used as a reference. The solid line indicates the hazard ratio for incident stroke event and the dotted line indicates the 95% confidence interval (CI). The maximum mean home SBP value at which the lower limit of 95% CI exceeded a hazard ratio of 1 was 169 mmHg. *Source*: Fujiwara T et al., *Hypertension*, 2021;78:840–850.

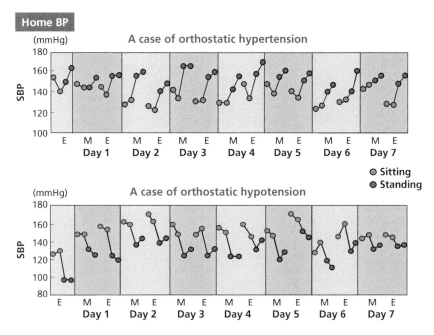

Figure 2.26 Reproducible orthostatic hypertension and hypotension detected by home blood pressure monitoring. E, evening; M, morning; SBP, systolic blood pressure. *Source*: Kario. Circ J. 2009; 73: 1002–1007 [147].

hypotension (Figure 2.26) [148]. Orthostatic stress may also clarify the reactive BP profile, and Table 2.3 shows the different diagnostic methods to detect orthostatic hypertension [58]. Using the HAST, orthostatic hypertension is defined based on an orthostatic BP increase (SBP measured by HBPM in the standing position minus that in the sitting position) of ≥10 mmHg (Table 2.3) [58]. Even in patients classified as normotensive based on sitting home BP, orthostatic hypertension may be a risk factor for future cardiovascular events. In recent studies on orthostatic BP changes evaluated by self-measured BP monitoring at home (four BP measures: two in the sitting position followed by two in the standing position), both orthostatic hypertension and orthostatic hypotension (two standing SBP measures minus two sitting SBP measures) were significantly associated with microalbuminuria (Figure 2.27) and plasma BNP levels in hypertensive patients [145]. After nighttime dosing of doxazosin, a reduction in the orthostatic BP increase in patients with orthostatic hypertension at home was associated with a decrease in the UACR independent of the reduction in sitting home BP (Figure 2.28) [213]. Orthostatic hypertension is closely associated with exaggerated ambulatory MBPS, while orthostatic hypotension is closely associated with nocturnal hypertension. The HAST helps to identify masked hypertension in those with exaggerated MBPS and nocturnal hypertension, and in those for whom masked hypertension could not be detected using conventional sitting HBPM.

Table 2.3 Recommendations for the diagnosis and definition of orthostatic hypertension.

Tests	Method of orthostatic stress	BP measurements	Diagnostic threshold of orthostatic hypertension (orthostatic increase in systolic BP)
Head-up tilting	Supine for 5 minutes or more followed by passive tilting with 60°–70° tilt angle for 20 minutes or more	Every 1 minute	• 20 mmHg (definitive) • 10 mmHg (probable)
Active standing			
Office	Supine for 5 minutes or more followed by active standing for 3 minutes	At least 3 times (one before standing, two during 3-minutes standing)	• 20 mmHg (definitive) • 10 mmHg (probable) • 5 mmHg for predicting masked hypertension and future hypertension
Home	Sitting for 5 minutes or more followed by active standing for 3 minutes	At least 3 times (one before standing, two during 3-minute standing)	• 10 mmHg

BP, blood pressure.
Source: Kario. Nat Rev Nephrol. 2013; 9: 726–738 [58].

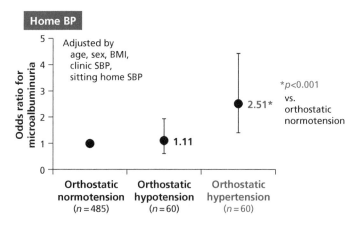

Figure 2.27 Orthostatic hypertension defined by home active standing and microalbuminuria. BMI, body mass index; SBP, systolic blood pressure. *Source*: Hoshide et al. Hypertens Res. 2008; 31: 1509–1516 [145].

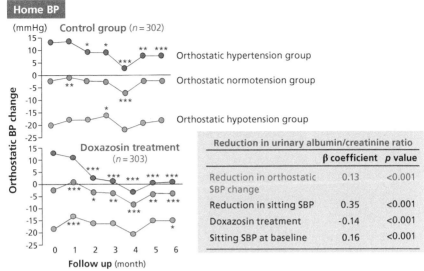

Figure 2.28 Reproducible orthostatic hypertension could be restored by alpha-blockade. SBP, systolic blood pressure. *Source*: Hoshide et al. Hypertens Res. 2012; 35: 100–106 [213].

Seasonal variation of home BP and "thermosensitive hypertension"

There is significant seasonal variation in the occurrence of cardiovascular events, with rates peaking in the winter (Figure 2.29). However, this winter peak could be decreased by improving housing conditions. In Hokkaido, in the north of Japan, the temperature is very cold, but the prevalence of well-insulated housing is higher than other regions, resulting in smaller winter-related increase in cardiovascular

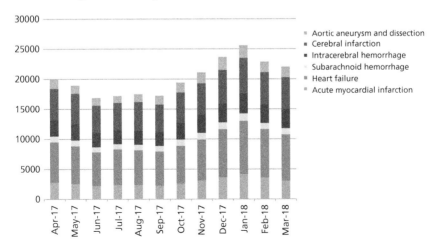

Figure 2.29 Cardiovascular disease mortality by month of the year (Ministry of Health, Labor and Welfare: Vital Statistics Monthly Report (Apr 2017–Mar 2018).

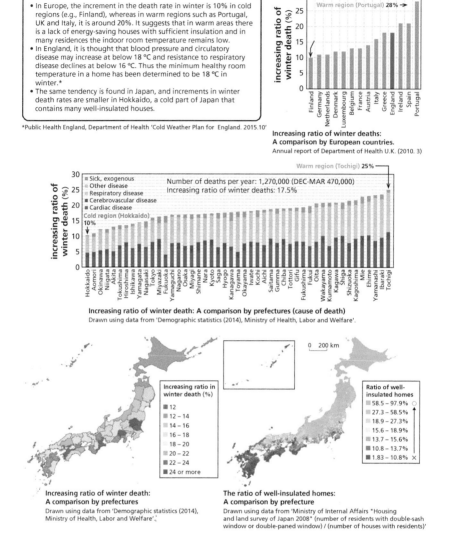

- In Europe, the increment in the death rate in winter is 10% in cold regions (e.g., Finland), whereas in warm regions such as Portugal, UK and Italy, it is around 20%. It suggests that in warm areas there is a lack of energy-saving houses with sufficient insulation and in many residences the indoor room temperature remains low.
- In England, it is thought that blood pressure and circulatory disease may increase at below 18 °C and resistance to respiratory disease declines at below 16 °C. Thus the minimum healthy room temperature in a home has been determined to be 18 °C in winter.*
- The same tendency is found in Japan, and increments in winter death rates are smaller in Hokkaido, a cold part of Japan that contains many well-insulated houses.

*Public Health England, Department of Health 'Cold Weather Plan for England. 2015.10'

Increasing ratio of winter deaths:
A comparison by European countries.
Annual report of Department of Health U.K. (2010. 3)

Increasing ratio of winter death: A comparison by prefectures (cause of death)
Drawn using data from 'Demographic statistics (2014), Ministry of Health, Labor and Welfare'.

Increasing ratio of winter death:
A comparison by prefectures
Drawn using data from 'Demographic statistics (2014),
Ministry of Health, Labor and Welfare'.

The ratio of well-insulated homes:
A comparison by prefecture
Drawn using data from 'Ministry of Internal Affairs "Housing
and land survey of Japan 2008" (number of residents with double-sash
window or double-paned window) / (number of houses with residents)'

Figure 2.30 Winter mortality rates tend to be lower in areas where residents are more likely to have sufficient thermal insulation (data from Italy and Japan). *Source*: Ikaga 2017.

events (Figure 2.30). The World Health Organization (WHO) recommends that room temperature is maintained at above 18°C to maintain healthy conditions.

In the J-HOP study, there was significant seasonal variation in home BP control status. Morning home BP and the prevalence of the masked uncontrolled morning hypertension were highest in the cold winter (Figure 2.31), while nighttime home BP level and the prevalence of masked uncontrolled nocturnal hypertension were highest in the hot summer (Figure 2.32) [214].

Using data obtained using the HEM-7252G-HP HBPM device, which includes a thermosensor, we defined "thermosensitive hypertension" as hypertension

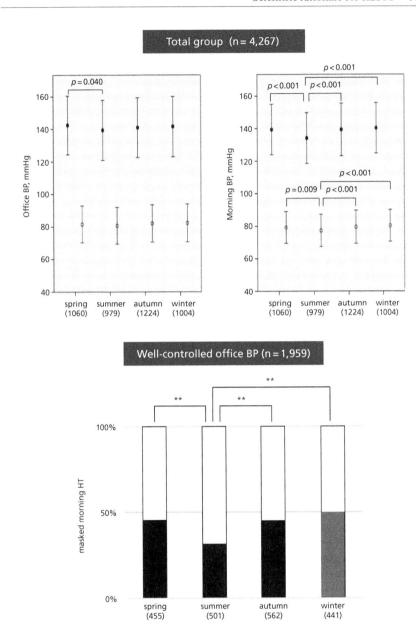

Figure 2.31 Seasonal variation in home blood pressure (BP) and the prevalence of masked hypertension in a post hoc analysis of data from the Japan Morning Surge-Home Blood Pressure (J-HOP) study of patients with cardiovascular disease risk factors. **$p < 0.001$. *Source*: Narita et al. Am J Hypertens. 2020; 33: 620–628 [214]. Reprinted by permission of Oxford University Press.

where home BP is closely related to seasonal changes in temperature (e.g. $R^2 > 0.3$, change of morning SBP >10 mmHg per 10°C temperature change) [37]. Morning BP appears to be more closely associated with cold temperature than evening BP (Figure 2.33) [215]. The Nationwide Smart Wellness Housing Survey in Japan,

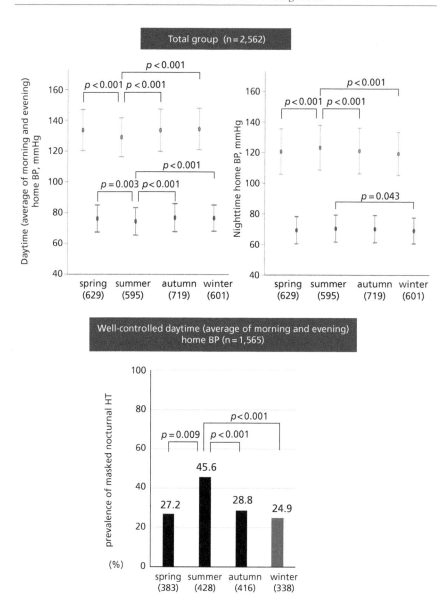

Figure 2.32 Seasonal variation in masked nocturnal hypertension in a post hoc analysis of the Japan Morning Surge-Home Blood Pressure (J-HOP) Nocturnal Blood Pressure study of patients with cardiovascular disease risk factors. BP, blood pressure. *Source*: Narita et al. Am J Hypertens. 2020; 33: 620–628 [214]. Reprinted by permission of Oxford University Press.

the first largest nationwide survey on home BP and indoor temperature, showed that SBP in the morning was more sensitive to changes in indoor temperature than evening SBP (increase of 8.2 vs. 6.5 mmHg per 10°C temperature decrease), and the slope of this association was steeper in the elderly (Figure 2.34) [216]. In addition, we confirmed the morning BP-lowering effect of retrofitted house insulation, showing a reduction in home BP, especially morning home BP, in patients

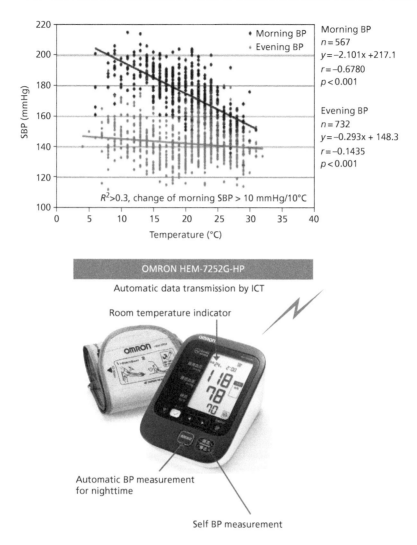

Figure 2.33 A case of thermosensitive hypertension (measured between 7 Mar and 18 Dec, 2015). BP, blood pressure; ICT, information and communication technology; SBP, systolic BP. *Source*: Kario. Essential Manual on Perfect 24-Hour Blood Pressure Management from Morning to Nocturnal Hypertension: Up-to-date for Anticipation Medicine. Wiley, 2018: 1–309 [24].

with hypertension. Indoor morning temperature rose by 1.4°C after retrofitting of insulation, and morning home SBP was significantly reduced by 3.1 mmHg. Furthermore, there was heterogeneity in the effect of insulation retrofitting on morning home SBP in patients with hypertension compared with normotensive subjects (−7.7 vs. −2.2 mmHg, *p*-value for interaction, 0.043) [217].

Alcohol

Regular alcohol consumption is a risk for masked morning hypertension (Figure 2.35) [95].

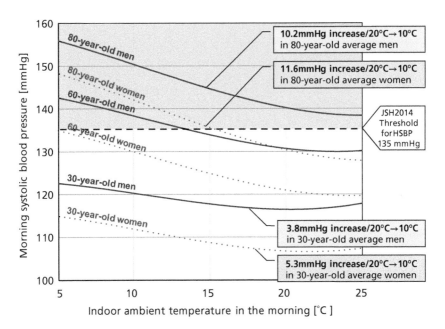

Figure 2.34 Sensitivity of morning systolic blood pressure (SBP) to indoor temperature (*n* = 3,775; mean age 57 years). JSH, The Japanese Society of Hypertension. *Source*: Umishio et al. Hypertension. 2019; 74: 756–766 [216].

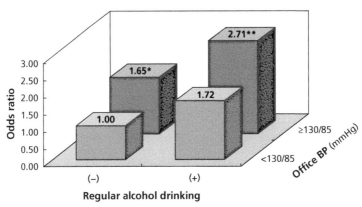

Logistic regression analysis: adjusted by age, sex, BMI, smoking, number of antihypertensive drug classes, and calcium channel blocker use. Odds ratio: vs regular alcohol drinking (–) and office BP <130/85 mmHg group, *$p<0.05$, **$p<0.01$

Figure 2.35 Risk of having masked morning hypertension based on alcohol consumption and office blood pressure (BP); logistic regression analysis adjusted for age, sex, body mass index, number of antihypertensive drug classes, and use of a calcium channel blocker. Reference group was those without regular alcohol consumption and a BP of <130/85 mmHg. *$p < 0.05$, **$p <0.01$. *Source*: Ishikawa et al. Hypertens Res. 2006; 29: 679–86 [95].

Daytime hypertension (stress hypertension)

During the daytime, everyday stressors can contribute to elevated BP, including work and psychological stress, along with temperature and physical activity. The response to the different stressors varies between individuals and may also vary within the same individual on different days.

The workplace is one potentially stressful environment. A study from Japan showed that average worksite SBP was significantly higher than the morning home SBP (by nearly 5 mmHg; p = 0.026); this was largely due to a significantly higher worksite BP vs. morning home BP in participants with office BP < 140/90 mmHg (by >6 mmHg for SBP [p < 0.001], and by >3.5 mmHg for DBP [p = 0.013]), whereas these differences were not observed in those with office BP ≥140/90 mmHg or those using antihypertensive medication(Figure 2.36) [218]. Significant correlations were observed between worksite, office and morning SBP, and the left ventricular mass index (all p < 0.0001), and a weaker correlation was observed between nighttime SBP and LVMI (p = 0.010) (Figure 2.37) [218]. Another study investigated the stress-induced BP variability measured by a recently developed wrist-type HBPM. The watch-type wearable BP device used in this study has been validated against both recognized standards and ABPM (Figures 2.38 and 2.39) [219, 220].

Using a wearable BP monitoring device, BP was found to be significantly higher during periods with negative emotions (e.g. anxiety or tension) compared with positive emotions (happy or calm), and these differences were greater than BP changes during mild or moderate exercise (Figure 2.40) [222]. Differences in BP during negative and positive emotion periods remained statistically significant after adjustment for age, sex, body mass index, location, measurement time, body position, and intensity of physical activity. Both negative emotions and worksite stress were significant predictors of SBP on wearable BP monitoring [222]. Overall, there are a variety of factors that contribute to the 24-hour BP profile and BP surges for each individual, and these can synergistically combine to elevate BP to a significant extent (Figure 2.41) [221].

Nighttime HBPM

In the past, nighttime BP was measured using ABPM. However, more recently, nocturnal HBPM devices are available for use in clinical practice to facilitate the diagnosis of nocturnal hypertension.

Cutting-edge of HBPM

ABPM has historically been the gold standard for measuring nighttime BP. However, newer HBPM devices can also be used to evaluate nighttime BP, with results that are comparable to those of ABPM. The Jichi Medical University and Omron Healthcare Co., Ltd. (Kyoto, Japan) have been conducting cutting-edge collaboration program projects in the SURGE (SUper ciRculation monitorinG with high tEchnology) research and development center to develop new home BP variability monitoring systems and define a new clinically relevant index of BP

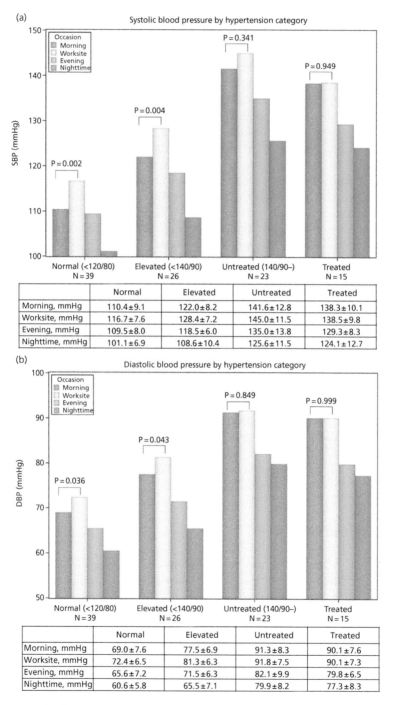

(a)	Normal	Elevated	Untreated	Treated
Morning, mmHg	110.4±9.1	122.0±8.2	141.6±12.8	138.3±10.1
Worksite, mmHg	116.7±7.6	128.4±7.2	145.0±11.5	138.5±9.8
Evening, mmHg	109.5±8.0	118.5±6.0	135.0±13.8	129.3±8.3
Nighttime, mmHg	101.1±6.9	108.6±10.4	125.6±11.5	124.1±12.7

(b)	Normal	Elevated	Untreated	Treated
Morning, mmHg	69.0±7.6	77.5±6.9	91.3±8.3	90.1±7.6
Worksite, mmHg	72.4±6.5	81.3±6.3	91.8±7.5	90.1±7.3
Evening, mmHg	65.6±7.2	71.5±6.3	82.1±9.9	79.8±6.5
Nighttime, mmHg	60.6±5.8	65.5±7.1	79.9±8.2	77.3±8.3

Figure 2.36 Blood pressure across hypertension categories based on office blood pressure levels. Data are mean ± standard deviation. *Source*: Tomitani et al. J Clin Hypertens (Greenwich). 2021; 23: 53–60 [218].

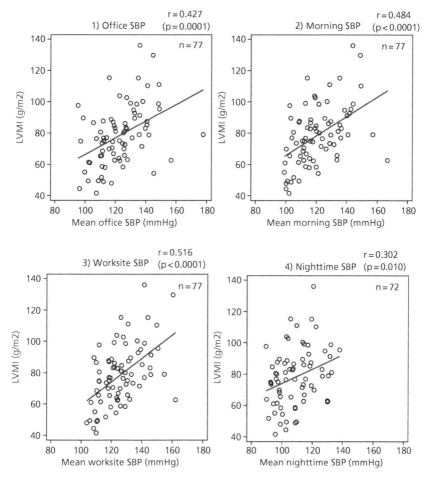

Figure 2.37 Relationships between the left ventricular mass index (LVMI) and office, morning, worksite, and nighttime systolic blood pressure (SBP). Source: Tomitani N, et al. J Clin Hypertens (Greenwich). 2021; 23: 53-60 [218].

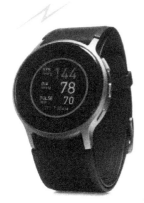

- 115g, diameter 48 mm, thickness 14 mm
- "Silent" oscillometric measurement
- Additional functions
  - Position sensing
  - Step counting
  - Sleep quantity and quality
  - Event button
  - Bluetooth function
- Mean difference ±SD; ≤5 ±≤8 mmHg
- Fulfilled the validation criteria 1 and 2 of ANSI/AAI/ISO 81060-2: 2013

Figure 2.38 Newly developed "wearable" wrist-watch blood pressure monitoring device (FDA approved in 2018). SD, standard deviation. Source: Kuwubara et al. J Clin Hypertens. 2019; 21: 853–858 [219]; Kario et al. J Clin Hypertens. 2020;22:135–141 [220].

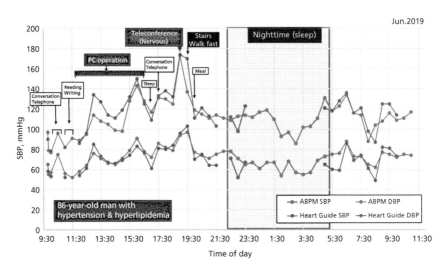

Figure 2.39 Comparison showing simultaneous monitoring with a wearable device (HeartGuide; Omron Healthcare Co., Ltd.) and ambulatory blood pressure monitoring (ABPM). DBP, diastolic blood pressure; PC, personal computer; SBP, systolic blood pressure. *Source*: Kario. Hypertension. 2020; 76: 640–650 [221].

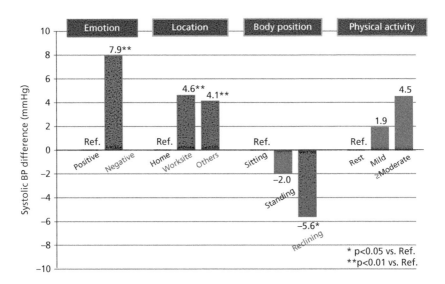

Figure 2.40 Stress-induced blood pressure (BP) elevation self-measured using a wearable watch-type device (50 outpatients with ≥1 cardiovascular risk factor, 642 BP readings). Self-reported emotions are positive ("happy" or "calm") or negative ("anxious" or "tense"). Mixed-effect model adjusted for age, sex, body mass index, emotional location, body position, and intensity of physical activity. *Source*: Created based on data from Tomitani et al. Am J Hypertens. 2021; 34: 377–382 [222].

variability (Table 2.4) (Table 2.5) [156, 157, 223–243]. Nocturnal HBPM is now available in clinical practice [244].

Recent advance was a wrist-type nocturnal HBPM device that provides less discomfort and low measurement noise. In addition, the latest device (HEM-

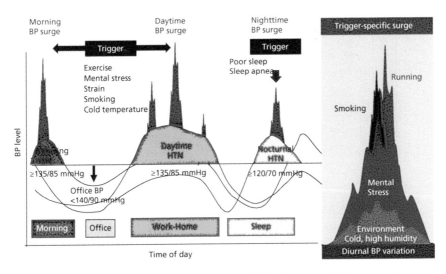

Figure 2.41 Synergistically accumulated trigger-specific blood pressure (BP) surges and diurnal variation. HTN, hypertension. *Source*: Kario. Hypertension. 2020; 76: 640–650 [221].

Table 2.4 Cutting-edge nighttime blood pressure (BP) monitoring at home (Jichi Medical University – Omron Healthcare Co., Ltd).

Nighttime home BP monitoring (brachial/wrist)
Trigger nighttime BP monitoring (TNP)
Wearable beat-by-beat surge BP monitoring (WSP)

Source: Kario. Essential Manual on Perfect 24-Hour Blood Pressure Management from Morning to Nocturnal Hypertension: Up-to-date for Anticipation Medicine. Wiley, 2018: 1–309 [24].

9601T) equipped with different algorithms for the sitting and supine positions improved the accuracy of nighttime BP readings.

Basic nighttime home BP monitoring (Medinote)

Medinote, a semiautomatic HBPM device was developed, with the function of allowing automatic fixed-interval BP measurement during sleep (Figure 2.42) [224]. BP data are stored in the device memory. Development of the Medinote device was the first step in detecting basic nighttime BP information using at-home, self-measured BP monitoring rather than ABPM. The Medinote device has now undergoing further development to an information technology (IT)-based new nighttime HBPM device, HEM-9700T (Omron Healthcare).

Clinical evidence using nocturnal HBPM: J-HOP nocturnal BP study

The J-HOP study (Table 2.1) was the first and largest nationwide nocturnal home BP cohort, and used the Medinote monitoring device with data memory to successfully measure nighttime home BP once each at three time points during sleep (2:00 AM, 3:00 AM, 4:00 AM), and three times each in the morning and evening for 14 days [190, 226]. Data from 2562 participants indicated that self-measurement of nighttime BP at home was feasible [226]. There was no difference between

Table 2.5 Research and development of nighttime home blood pressure monitoring devices and evidence (Jichi Medical University School of Medicine).

Year	Source	Device	Major device function	ICT-based	Validation	Competing device
2010 2012 2014 2015	Kario et al.[223] Ishikawa et al.[224] Ishikawa et al.[225] Kario et al.[226]	Medinote® (HEM-5041) (Omron Healthcare)	Automatic BP monitoring during sleep with fixed intervals function	Not available	Coleman et al.[240]	Watch BP Home N (microlife)
2017 2018	Kario et al.[227] Fujiwara et al.[228]	HEM-7252G-HP (Omron Healthcare)	Automatic BP monitoring during sleep with fixed intervals function, timer function after going to bed and built-in 3rd generation mobile communication facility	Available	Takahashi et al.[241]	Watch BP Home N (microlife)
2006 2011 2014 2017 2018	Shirasaki et al.[229] Shirasaki et al.[230] Kario et al.[231] Kuwabara et al.[232] Kuwabara et al.[243]	Triggered nighttime blood pressure monitoring (TNP)	Automatic BP monitoring during sleep with fixed intervals function and triggered BP function which initiates BP monitoring when oxygen saturation falls threshold or low heart rate period during the sleep	Not available	Viera AJ et al.[242]	None
2014 2015 2016	Kario et al.[231] Kario et al.[233] Yoshida et al.[234]	Information and communication technology (ICT)-based TNP (ITNP)	TNP with built-in 3rd generation mobile communication facility (nigh-by-night evaluation)	Available	None	None
2016 2018	Kario [156] Kario [235]	Wearable beat-by-beat surge BP monitoring (WSP)	Wrist-type continuous BP monitoring based on the tonometry method	Not available	None	None
2019 2020 2021 2021	Kuwabara et al [236] Kuwabara et al [237] Kario et al [238] Tomitani et al [239]	HEM-9600/01T (Omron Healthcare)	Automatic oscillometric device for measuring BP at the wrist (9601T; supine algorithm-equipped wrist nocturnal home blood pressure monitoring device with an upper arm device)	Available	None	None

Source: Kario Hypertension. 2018; 71(6): 997–1009 [1].

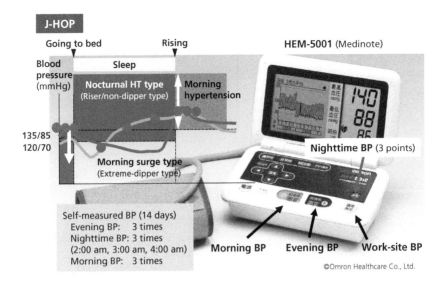

Figure 2.42 Semiautomatic home blood pressure (BP) monitoring device (Medinote). HT, hypertension. *Source*: Kario. Essential Manual on Perfect 24-Hour Blood Pressure Management from Morning to Nocturnal Hypertension: Up-to-date for Anticipation Medicine. Wiley 2018, 1–309 [24].

nighttime home SBP at 2:00 AM and 3:00 AM, but SBP at 4:00 AM was slightly higher (by an average of 1.5 mmHg; $p < 0.0001$) (Figure 2.43) [226]. We defined nighttime home BP as the average of three nighttime BP readings measured at 2:00 AM, 3:00 AM, and 4:00 AM.

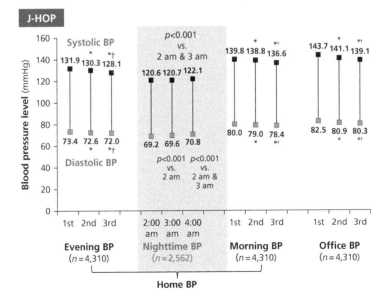

Figure 2.43 Home blood pressure (BP) levels in the Japan Morning Surge-Home Blood Pressure (J-HOP) study. *p < 0.001 vs first measurement; † vs. second measurement by paired t-test. *Source*: Kario. J Clin Hypertens. 2015;17:340–348 [226].

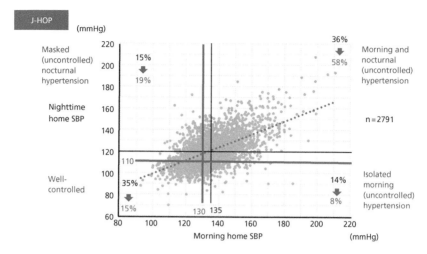

Figure 2.44 Shift in the prevalence of nocturnal hypertension classified by the new American Heart Association/American College of Cardiology 2017 guidelines (shown in red) vs. those classified based on the previous Seventh Report of the Joint National Committee on Prevention, Detection, Evaluation and Treatment of High Blood Pressure guidelines (shown in black) in subjects from the Japan Morning Surge-Home Blood Pressure Study (2,791 medicated patients with hypertension). SBP, systolic blood pressure. *Source*: Kario. Hypertension. 2018; 71: 979–984 [148].

In the J-HOP Nocturnal BP study, the prevalence of uncontrolled nocturnal hypertension (nighttime SBP $\geq$120 mmHg) was 51%, and that of masked nocturnal was 15% (Figure 2.44). Of those with well-controlled morning home SBP (<130 mmHg), 30% remained uncontrolled at a threshold of SBP $\geq$120 mmHg [147].

Organ damage and biomarkers

In the J-HOP study, nighttime home SBP was significantly correlated with the UACR, LVMI, baPWV, maximum carotid IMT, and plasma levels of NT-proBNP and hs-cTnT (Figure 2.45) [226]. In addition, nighttime home BP was significantly correlated with organ damage independently of office, morning, and evening BP readings. Even in those with well-controlled morning home SBP/DBP (<135/85 mmHg), 27% had "masked home nocturnal hypertension" with nighttime home SBP $\geq$120 mmHg (Figure 2.46) [226]. These patients had higher UACR and NT-proBNP, indicating that masked home nocturnal hypertension is associated with advanced organ damage but remains unrecognized by conventional HBPM. A subanalysis of J-HOP data showed that nighttime home BP was almost comparable to that measured using ABPM (Figure 2.47) [224], and the association with organ damage (LVH and microalbuminuria) was greater for nighttime home SBP than nighttime SBP detected by ABPM (Figure 2.48) [224].

Cardiovascular prognosis

In the J-HOP Nocturnal BP Study, a 10 mmHg increase in nighttime home SBP was associated with an increased risk of cardiovascular events (hazard ratio 1.201)

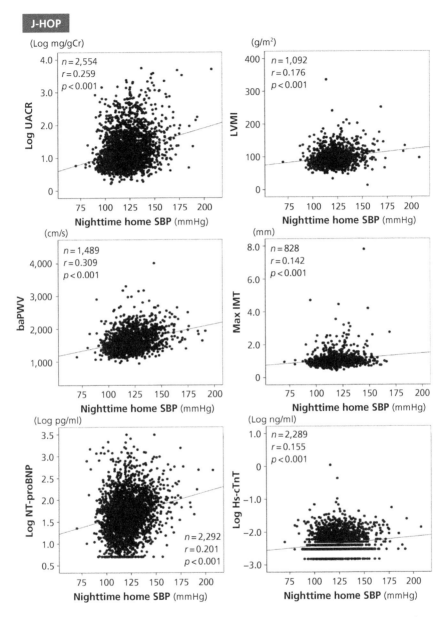

Figure 2.45 Association between nighttime home blood systolic blood pressure (SBP) and target organ damage in the Japan Morning Surge-Home Blood Pressure (J-HOP) study. baPWV, brachial-artery pulse wave velocity; hs-cTNT, high-sensitivity cardiac troponin T; IMT, intima-media thickness; LVMI, left ventricular mass index; NT-proBNP, N-terminal pro-brain natriuretic peptide; UACR, urinary albumin-creatinine ratio. *Source*: Kario. J Clin Hypertens. 2015;17:340–348 [226].

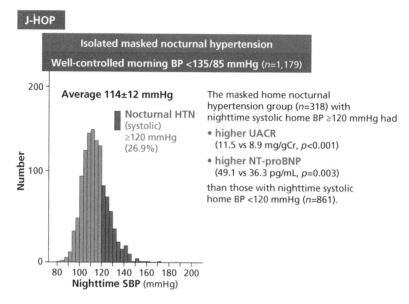

Figure 2.46 Distribution of nighttime home systolic blood pressure (SBP) levels in the Japan Morning Surge-Home Blood Pressure (J-HOP) study. BP, blood pressure; HTN, hypertension; NT-proBNP, amino terminal pro B-type natriuretic peptide; UACR, urinary albumin-creatinine ratio. *Source*: Kario. J Clin Hypertens. 2015;17:340–348 [226].

after adjustments for covariates including office and morning home SBP values. Patients with the nocturnal home SBP in the highest quintiles were at increased risk of experiencing both stroke and CAD events (Figure 2.49) [190].

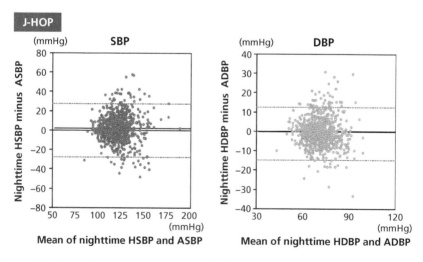

Figure 2.47 Bland-Altman plots of nighttime blood pressure (BP) measured using home BP monitoring and ambulatory BP monitoring in the Japan Morning Surge-Home Blood Pressure (J-HOP) study. ADBP, ambulatory diastolic BP; ASBP, ambulatory systolic BP; DBP, diastolic BP; HDBP, home diastolic BP; HSBP, home systolic BP; SBP, systolic BP. *Source*: Ishikawa et al. Hypertension. 2012; 60: 921–928 [224].

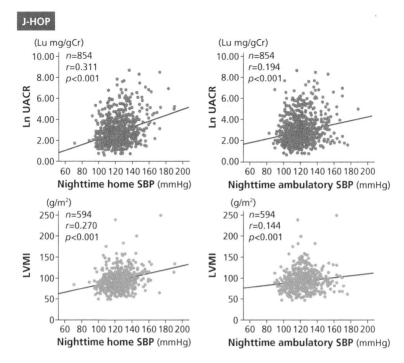

Figure 2.48 Nighttime systolic blood pressure (SBP) and target organ damage. LVMI, left ventricular mass index; UACR, urinary albumin-creatinine ratio. *Source*: Ishikawa et al. Hypertension. 2012; 60: 921–928 [224].

Masked nocturnal hypertension and prognosis

Patients with masked uncontrolled nocturnal hypertension had a significantly increased risk of cardiovascular events, approaching that in patients with sustained hypertension, while the presence of isolated daytime hypertension without nocturnal hypertension did not significantly increase cardiovascular risk (Figure 2.50) [245].

HBPM- vs. ABPM-defined nocturnal hypertension

The J-HOP Nocturnal BP study was the first to directly compare the prognostic power of nocturnal hypertension detected by HBPM vs. ABPM for predicting future cardiovascular events [246]. Nocturnal hypertension was defined as nighttime home or ambulatory SBP of ≥120 mmHg. The number of participants with nocturnal hypertension defined by HBPM and ABPM was 564 (56.1%) and 469 (46.7%), respectively (Figure 2.51). Nocturnal hypertension defined by HBPM was associated with increased risk of future cardiovascular events: total cardiovascular events (CAD and stroke events; 1.78 [1.00–3.15]) and stroke (2.65 [1.14–6.20]), independent of office SBP (Figure 2.52). No such associations were seen for nocturnal hypertension defined by ABPM.

Nighttime home BP was also a better indicator of the impact of BP control on organ damage during antihypertensive treatment than ABPM. In the Japan

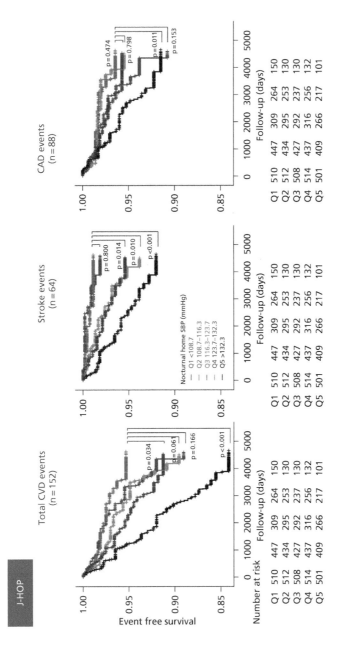

Figure 2.49 Kaplan-Meier curves showing the risk of cardiovascular events by quintile (Q) of nighttime home systolic blood pressure (SBP) in the Japan Morning Surge-Home Blood Pressure (J-HOP) Nocturnal Blood pressure study (*n* = 2,545, mean age 63 years). CAD, coronary artery disease; CVD, cardiovascular disease. *Source*: Kario et al. Hypertension. 2019; 73: 1240–1248 [190].

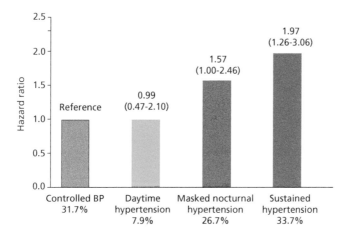

Figure 2.50 Cardiovascular event risks associated with masked nocturnal hypertension defined by home blood pressure (HBP) monitoring in the Japan Morning Surge-Home Blood Pressure (J-HOP) Nocturnal Blood pressure study (n = 2,745 high-risk patients, mean age 64 years, 82.7% receiving antihypertensive therapy; mean follow-up 7.6 years). Values are hazard (95% confidence interval). *Source*: Fujiwara et al. Hypertension. 2020; 76: 259–266 [245].

Morning Surge-Target Organ Protection (J-TOP) study, the reduction of nighttime home BP was more closely associated with the regression of LVH evaluated by cardiac echography and electrocardiography; these associations were absent with nocturnal hypertension defined by ABPM (Figure 2.53) [225].

Trigger nighttime BP monitoring

Another advance was the development of trigger nighttime BP monitoring (TNP). This was based on the automated fixed interval-measurement technique of the Medinote device, with an added trigger function that initiates BP measurement when oxygen desaturation falls below a variable threshold continuously monitored by pulse oximetry (Figure 2.54) [157].

Obstructive sleep apnea syndrome (OSAS) is characterized by uncontrolled nocturnal hypertension with increased BP variability (both morning and night-time BP surges) (Figure 2.55) [233, 247]. TNP can detect the specific nighttime BP surges triggered by hypoxic episodes in patients with OSAS (Figure 2.56) [230, 248, 249]. However, neither earlier HBPM devices nor ABPM with fixed time-interval measurement was able to detect the nighttime BP surge specific to each sleep apnea episode. Furthermore, a pulse rate-trigger function was added to TNP to detect the "basal nighttime BP," which is determined by the circulating volume and structural cardiovascular system without any increase in sympathetic tonus. This double TNP is a brand-new concept for evaluating the pathogenic pressor mechanism of nighttime BP.

Figure 2.57 shows nighttime BP parameters obtained from TNP [231]. The distribution and reproducibility of hypoxia-triggered nighttime BP parameters were evaluated and compared with those of fixed-interval nighttime BP parameters for two consecutive nights in 147 patients with OSA. The mean and distribution

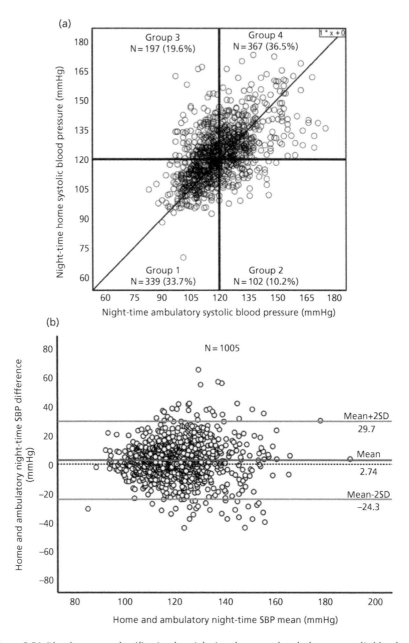

Figure 2.51 Blood pressure classification by nighttime home and ambulatory systolic blood pressure (SBP); and Bland Altman plot for the difference between nighttime SBP measured by home and ambulatory blood pressure monitoring devices in the Japan Morning Surge-Home Blood Pressure (J-HOP) Nocturnal Blood pressure study. SD, standard deviation. *Source*: Mokwatsi et al. Hypertension. 2020; 76: 554–561 [246].

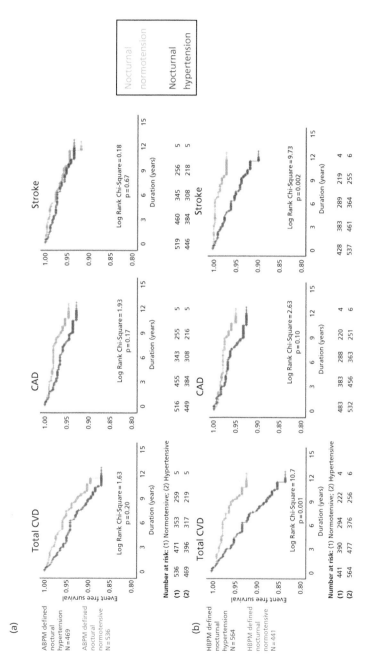

Figure 2.52 Kaplan-Meier curve of cardiovascular disease (CVD) events in participants with and without nocturnal hypertension defined using ambulatory blood pressure monitoring (ABPM: a) or home blood pressure monitoring (HBPM: b) in the Japan Morning Surge-Home Blood Pressure (J-HOP) Nocturnal Blood pressure study (1005 high CVD risk patients; mean 7.6 years' follow-up). CAD, coronary artery disease. *Source:* Mokwatsi et al. Hypertension. 2020; 76: 554–561 [246].

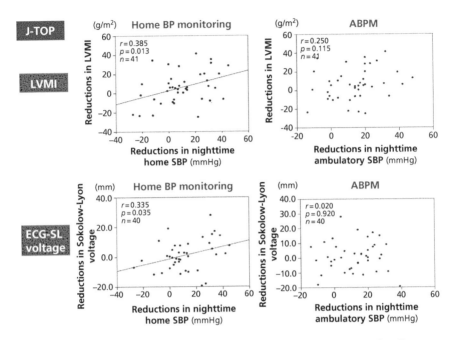

Figure 2.53 Association between the reduction in nighttime blood pressure (BP) and cardiac hypertrophy during antihypertensive treatment. ABPM, ambulatory BP monitoring; LVMI, left ventricular mass index; SBP, systolic BP. *Source*: Ishikawa et al. J Hypertens. 2014; 32: 82–89 [225].

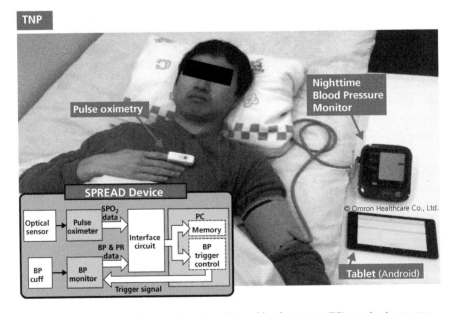

Figure 2.54 Information technology-based nighttime blood pressure (BP) monitoring system with oxygen and pulse rate (PR) triggers and a cloud-based system (Jichi Medical University, Omron Healthcare Co., Ltd., Kyoto, Japan). PC, personal computer; SpO_2, oxygen saturation. *Source*: Kario et al. J Clin Hypertens. 2015;17: 682–685 [233].

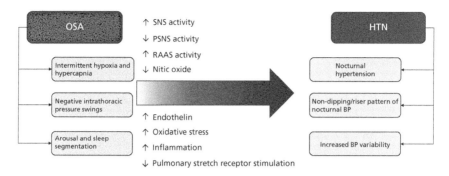

Figure 2.55 Mechanistic links between obstructive sleep apnea (OSA) and hypertension (HTN). BP, blood pressure; PSNS, parasympathetic nervous system; RAAS, renin-angiotensin aldosterone system; SNS, sympathetic nervous system. *Source*: Kario et al. Hypertension. 2021;77:1047–1060 [247].

(standard deviation [SD]) of the hypoxia-peak SBP were significantly greater than that of the mean nighttime SBP (148.8 ± 20.5 vs. 123.4 ± 14.2 mmHg, $p < 0.001$) (Figure 2.58) [232]. The repeatability coefficient (expressed as % MV) of hypoxia-peak SBP between night one and night two was comparable to that of mean nighttime SBP (43% vs. 32%). In conclusion, hypoxia-peak nighttime BP was much higher than mean nighttime BP, and it was as reproducible as mean nighttime BP. In the patients with nocturnal hypertension (mean nighttime SBP ≥ 120 mmHg), approximately 50% had increased hypoxia-induced nighttime BP surge ≥ 160 mmHg (Figure 2.59) [232].

Figure 2.60 shows nighttime BP readings detected by TNP in two cases with drug-resistant hypertension and OSAS [157]. Although patients had comparable

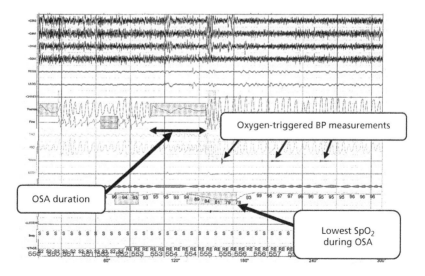

Figure 2.56 Polysomnography and the timing of blood pressure (BP) measurement during trigger nocturnal home BP monitoring. OSA, obstructive sleep apnea; SpO_2, oxygen saturation. *Source*: Sasaki et al. Hypertension. 2018; 72: 1133–1140 [249].

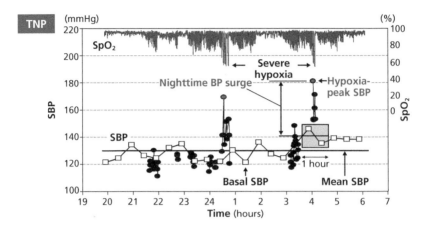

Figure 2.57 Definition of nighttime blood pressure (BP) parameters by trigger nighttime BP monitoring (TNP). SBP, systolic BP; SpO$_2$, oxygen saturation. *Source*: Kario et al. J Clin Hypertens. 2014; 16: 459–466 [231].

OSAS severity (based on the apnea-hypopnea index [AHI]), the trigger function of TNP revealed quite different nighttime BP surges between these patients. It is well known that cardiovascular events occur more frequently during sleep periods in patients with OSAS. The hypoxia-induced nighttime BP surge could trigger sleep-onset cardiovascular events in these patients. Using this TNP device, it is possible to specifically identify OSAS patients at high risk for sleep-onset cardiovascular events.

There may be a different mechanism for nocturnal hypertension in different patients, even average nighttime BP readings are the same: peak nighttime BP

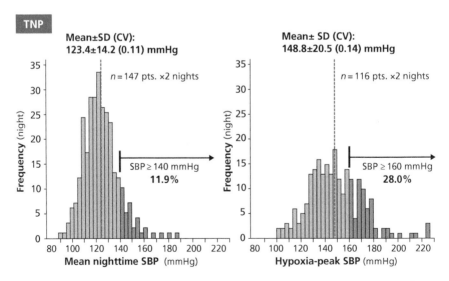

Figure 2.58 Distribution of higher mean level and hypoxia-induced peak nighttime systolic blood pressure (SBP) in patients with suspected sleep apnea. CV, coefficient of variation. *Source*: Kuwubara et al. J Clin Hypertens. 2017; 19: 30–37 [232].

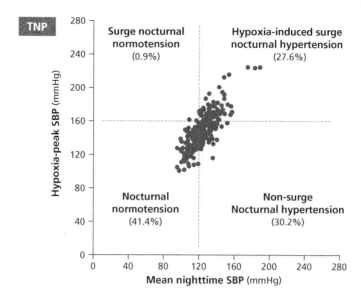

Figure 2.59 Prevalence of hypoxia-induced surge nocturnal hypertension in patients with suspected sleep apnea. SBP, systolic blood pressure. *Source*: Kuwabara et al. J Clin Hypertens. 2017; 19: 30–37 [232].

levels measured by hypoxia trigger may be attributed to sympathetic overdrive, while basal nighttime BP levels measured by lowest heart rate trigger may be determined by circulating volume and vascular structure (Figure 2.61) [37]. The former BP component of nocturnal hypertension may be suppressed by nighttime dosing of sympatholytic drugs, while the latter component would be better managed using diuretics, calcium channel blocker, and/or renin-angiotensin system (RAS) inhibitors.

IT-based trigger nighttime BP monitoring system and the SPREAD study

Finally, an IT-based nighttime BP monitoring system (ITNP) with oxygen saturation and heart rate triggers, and a 3G web system, has been developed with our colleagues at Omron Healthcare Co., Ltd. (Toshikazu Shiga, Takahide Tanaka, Mitsuo Kuwabara, Osamu Shirasaki, Yutaka Kobayashi). The ITNP system is a cloud computing-based composite management and analysis system for data sent from the BP device in the patient's home. The most important benefit of this system is to detect day-by-day variation in nighttime and morning BP, and nighttime BP surges associated with sleep apnea episodes, the extent of which can be influenced by daily environmental changes. Using this ITNP, the prospective study of sleep pressure and disordered breathing in resistant hypertension and cardiovascular disease (SPREAD) has been started. It is a registry to evaluate the clinical implications of nighttime BP and nighttime BP surges in high-risk patients with resistant hypertension and/or cardiovascular disease.

In the SPREAD study, ITNP detected the exaggerated nighttime BP surges triggered by sleep apnea-related hypoxia in a 36-year-old man. The patient developed

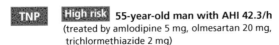

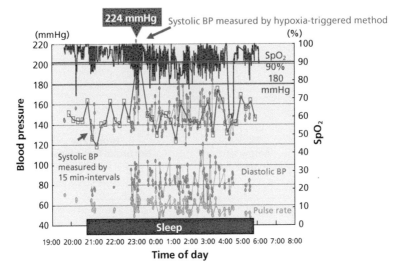

Evening systolic BP (before going to bed): 146 mmHg
Nighttime systolic BP (measured by hypoxia-triggered BP monitoring):
 Average 150 mmHg; SD 17.0 mmHg; Peak 224 mmHg

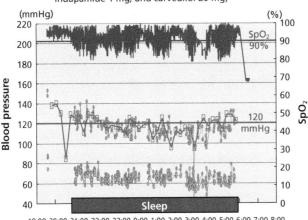

Evening systolic BP (before going to bed) 151 mmHg
Nighttime systolic BP (measured by hypoxia-triggered BP monitoring):
 Average 114 mmHg; SD 8.3 mmHg; Peak 136 mmHg

Figure 2.60 Different nighttime blood pressure (BP) surges in two patients with resistant hypertension and obstructive sleep apnea syndrome. AHI, apnea-hypopnea index; SD, standard deviation; SpO$_2$, oxygen saturation. *Source*: Kario. Hypertens Res. 2013; 36: 478–484 [157].

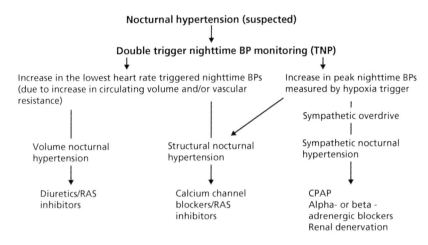

Figure 2.61 Three types of nocturnal hypertension and targeted antihypertensive treatment options based on data obtained using double-trigger nighttime blood pressure (BP) monitoring. CPAP, continuous positive airway pressure; RAS, renin-angiotensin system. *Source*: Kario. Essential Manual of 24-Hour Blood Pressure Management from Morning to Nocturnal Hypertension. UK: Wiley Blackwell; 2015:1–138 [37].

sleep-onset ischemic and hemorrhagic stroke on three occasions (Figure 2.62) [234]. In a 74-year-old woman with OSAS, even when the average of nighttime BP levels measured by ABPM at fixed 30-minute intervals was <120/70 mmHg (Figure 2.63), ITNP detected repetitive exaggerated nighttime BP surges (Figure 2.64) [233].

The assessment of SAS was repeated using ITNP in a real-life setting and was found to increase the sensitivity of the diagnosis of SAS and related nighttime BP surge. Using polysomnography in alcohol-prohibited conditions in hospitals may underestimate the severity of OSAS and may misdiagnose patients with moderate OSAS. SPREAD study participants with mild-to-moderate OSAS showed significant night-by-night variability in the number of apnea/hypopnea episodes. Apnea-hypopnea episodes, nighttime BP, and BP surge all increased on the day of alcohol intake (Figure 2.65). ITNP will help to detect high-risk OSAS patients with nocturnal hypertension and/or nighttime BP surge and assess the quality of BP control during continuous positive airway pressure (CPAP) and/or antihypertensive treatment (Figure 2.66) [37]. Strict BP control throughout a 24-hour period, including nighttime BP and hypoxia-induced peak, could attenuate the development of organ damage and help to prevent cardiovascular events in patients with OSA, and the ITNP system would contribute to achieving this goal.

CPAP adherence and nighttime BP surge

CPAP treatment almost eliminates nighttime BP surge in patients with OSAS (Figure 2.67) [248, 250]. However, cardiovascular protection and the BP-lowering effect of CPAP are not perfect, and OSAS patients may still develop cardiovascular events [251, 252]. The 2017 AHA/ACC guidelines state that the effectiveness of CPAP to reduce BP in adults with hypertension and OSAS is not well established, with a Class IIb level of evidence [178]. It is possible that good adherence to CPAP therapy may be the key for this treatment approach to be effective.

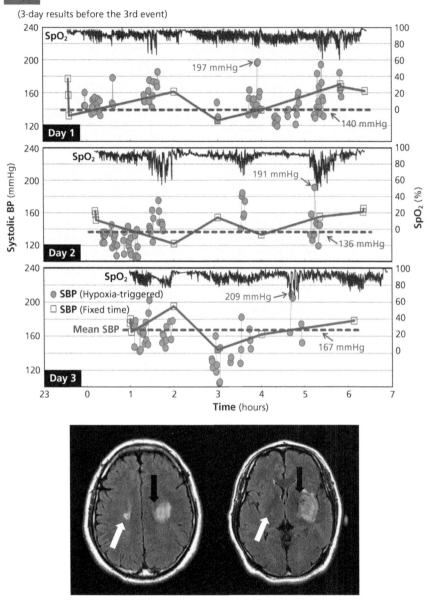

Figure 2.62 A 36-year-old patient with hypertension developed three hemorrhagic strokes. Upper figure: close circles represent systolic blood pressure (SBP) measured by an oxygen-triggered function. Open boxes represent SBP values measured by the fixed-point function. The hypoxia-related nighttime SBP surges were observed on all three days. Lower figure: brain magnetic resonance imaging at the time of the third event. All three events occurred during sleep. Red arrows represent the sites of acute left putaminal hemorrhage. Black arrows represent the sites of an earlier left putaminal hemorrhage. White arrows represent an old lacunar infarction. SpO_2, oxygen saturation monitored by pulse oximetry. Source: Yoshida et al. J Am Soc Hypertens. 2016;10:201–204 [234], with permission from Elsevier.

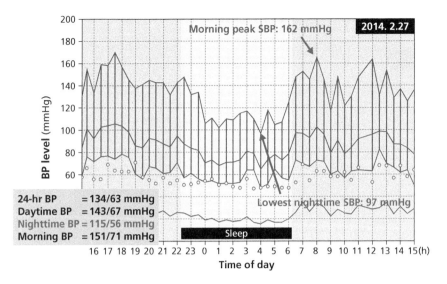

Figure 2.63 Exaggerated morning blood pressure (BP) surge detected by ambulatory blood pressure monitoring in a 76-year-old women with obstructive sleep apnea syndrome. Nighttime BP was <120/70 mmHg. SBP, systolic BP. *Source*: Kario et al. J Clin Hypertens. 2015;17:682–685 [233].

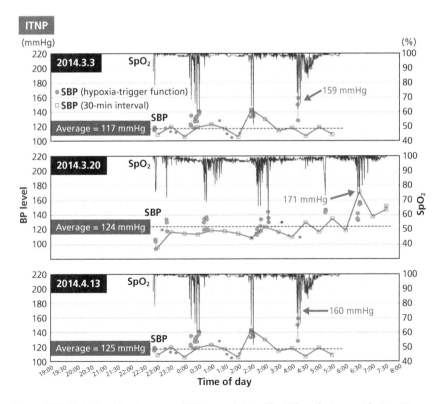

Figure 2.64 Nighttime blood pressure (BP) surge detected by IT based trigger nighttime BP monitoring (ITNP). SBP, systolic BP; SpO$_2$, oxygen saturation. *Source*: Kario et al. J Clin Hypertens. 2015;17: 682–685 [233].

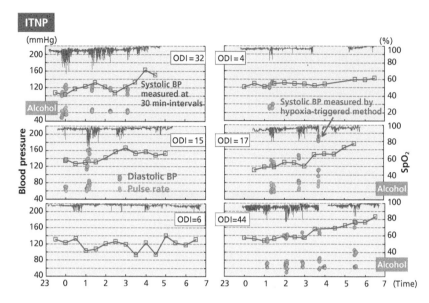

Figure 2.65 Nighttime blood pressure measured by IT based trigger nighttime blood pressure monitoring (ITNP) on different days in a patient from the sleep pressure and disordered breathing in resistant hypertension and cardiovascular disease (SPREAD) registry. ODI, oxygen desaturation index; SpO₂, oxygen saturation. Source: Kario. Essential Manual of 24-Hour Blood Pressure Management from Morning to Nocturnal Hypertension. UK: Wiley Blackwell; 2015:1–138 [37].

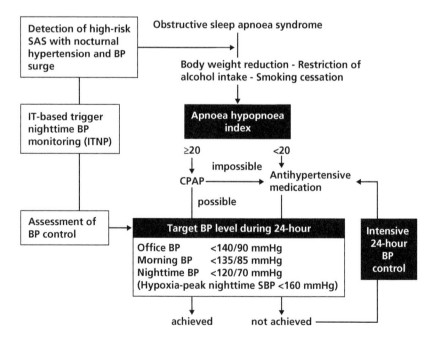

Figure 2.66 Management of blood pressure (BP) variability using information technology-based trigger nighttime BP monitoring (ITNP) in sleep apnea. CPAP, continuous positive airway pressure; SAS, sleep apnea syndrome. *Source*: Kario. Essential Manual of 24-Hour Blood Pressure Management from Morning to Nocturnal Hypertension. UK: Wiley Blackwell; 2015:1–138 [37].

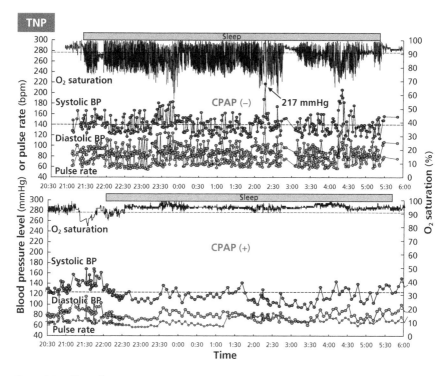

Figure 2.67 Effect of continuous positive airway pressure (CPAP) on nighttime blood pressure (BP) measured using trigger nighttime BP monitoring (TNP) in a patient with hypertension and sleep apnea syndrome. O_2, oxygen. *Source*: Kario. Hypertens Res. 2009; 32: 428–432 [248].

ITNP could be used to evaluate adherence to, and efficacy of, CPAP on a day-by-day basis. Even in OSAS using CPAP every night, the mask may be off the face (Figure 2.68) and the pressure of CPAP may be insufficient in the presence of other conditions such as upper tract infection and allergic rhinitis (Figures 2.68 and 2.69). Effective CPAP can reduce mean nighttime SBP by 8 mmHg (Figure 2.70), and by up to 42 mmHg when evaluated based on hypoxia peak nighttime SBP (Figure 2.71). These results suggest that ITNP could be a useful tool for assessing the therapeutic efficacy of CPAP therapy.

Antihypertensive medication on nighttime BP surge

Only a small dose of doxazosin reduced nighttime BP surge and basal nighttime BP in patients with OSAS, while the cluster of hypoxic episodes was similar at baseline and during treatment (Figure 2.72) [248], indicating that OSAS-induced nocturnal hypertension and nighttime BP surge are at least partly attributable to sympathetic overdrive caused by nocturnal hypoxia. In a recent study using TNP, bedtime dosing of nifedipine and carvedilol significantly reduced all nighttime BP measures (Figure 2.73) [231], while nighttime BP-lowering properties differed between the two drugs. Carvedilol reduced peak nighttime BP to a similar extent as nifedipine, but had less effect in reducing

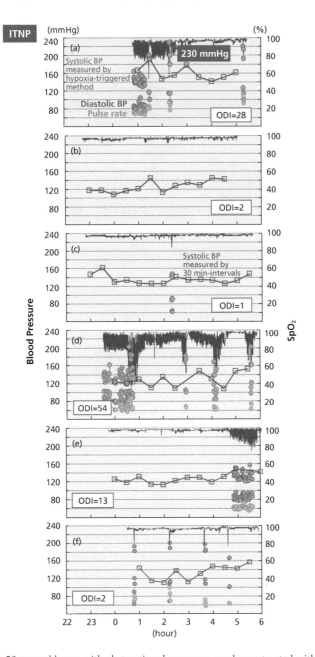

Figure 2.68 A 58-year-old man with obstructive sleep apnea syndrome treated with continuous positive airway pressure (CPAP) who developed cardiopulmonary arrest during a sleep period at home. Figures (a) to (f) are blood pressure (BP) data from six different days during IT-based trigger nighttime BP monitoring (ITNP). (a) Short sleep-triggered marked nighttime BP surge that reached 230 mmHg. After rising with this episode, CPAP was initiated. (b), (c) well treated with CPAP. (d) The CPAP mask was not worn for the total duration of the sleep period. Marked nighttime BP surges were detected with severe hypoxic clusters. (e) CPAP mask was no longer in place 1.5 hours before rising in the morning. (f) Spike hypoxic episodes triggered marked nighttime BP surges even when well treated with CPAP. This is the day the patient developed severe rhinorrhea. ODI, oxygen desaturation index; SpO_2, oxygen saturation. Source: Kario. Essential Manual of 24-Hour Blood Pressure Management from Morning to Nocturnal Hypertension. UK: Wiley Blackwell; 2015:1–138 [37].

Table 2.6 Morning and nighttime systolic blood pressure (SBP) values at baseline, and after administration of carvedilol or nifedipine in the effects of vasodilating vs. sympathloytic antihypertensives on sleep blood pressure in hypertensive patients with sleep apnea syndrome (VASSPS) study.

	Baseline	Carvedilol	Nifedipine
Morning SBP	150.8	137.4[b]	118.2[c,f]
Morning heart rate	61.8	57.0[b]	64.7[f]
Nighttime SBP	137.3	121.8[c]	112.8[c,d]
Nighttime heart rate	59.8	57.2[a]	62.4[f]
Maximum SBP	164.7	143.0[b]	138.0[b]
Minimum nighttime SBP	113.6	99.6[c]	88.6[c,e]
Nighttime SBP surge (mmHg)	30.8	18.6[a]	22.1

Data are mean values in mmHg.
[a] $p < 0.05$, [b] $p < 0.01$, [c] $p < 0.001$ vs. baseline, by paired t-test.
[d] $p < 0.05$, [e] $p < 0.01$, [f] $p < 0.001$ vs. carvedilol-added phase, by paired t-test.
Source: Kario et al. J Clin Hypertens. 2014; 16: 459–466 [231].

basal BP, resulting in significant suppression of the hypoxia-induced nighttime BP surge (Table 2.6) [231]. Even in a patient with OSAS who had well-controlled mean nighttime SBP, 55% of hypoxia-triggered peak nighttime SBP values were >140 mmHg (Figure 2.74) [231]; bedtime dosing of nifedipine reduced both mean and hypoxia-peak SBP.

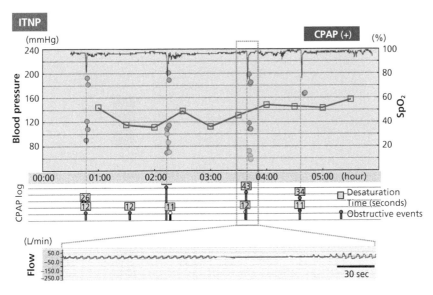

Figure 2.69 A 58-year-old man who developed cardiopulmonary arrest during sleep at home. On a day when spike hypoxic episodes triggered marked nighttime BP surges even when well treated with continuous positive airway pressure (CPAP), CPAP log data were measured concurrently with triggered blood pressure (BP) monitoring. In harmony with nighttime blood pressure surges during desaturation episodes, the flags of obstructive sleep apnea events and decreased nasal air flow are clearly observed in CPAP log data. SpO_2, oxygen saturation. *Source*: Kario. Essential Manual of 24-Hour Blood Pressure Management from Morning to Nocturnal Hypertension. UK: Wiley Blackwell; 2015:1–138 [37].

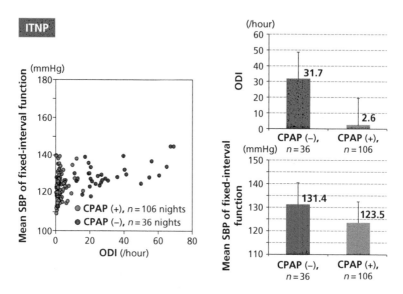

Figure 2.70 Mean nighttime systolic blood pressure (SBP) measured by IT based trigger nighttime blood pressure monitoring (ITNP) in a patient registered in the sleep pressure and disordered breathing in resistant hypertension and cardiovascular disease (SPREAD) registry. CPAP, continuous positive airway pressure; ODI, oxygen desaturation index. *Source*: Kario. Essential Manual of 24-Hour Blood Pressure Management from Morning to Nocturnal Hypertension. UK: Wiley Blackwell; 2015:1–138 [37].

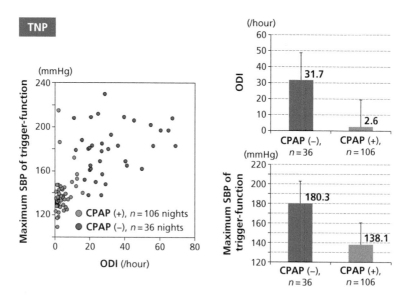

Figure 2.71 Hypoxia-peak nighttime systolic blood pressure (SBP) measured by trigger nighttime blood pressure monitoring (TNP) in a patient from the sleep pressure and disordered breathing in resistant hypertension and cardiovascular disease (SPREAD) registry. CPAP, continuous positive airway pressure; ODI, oxygen desaturation index. *Source*: Kario. Essential Manual of 24-Hour Blood Pressure Management from Morning to Nocturnal Hypertension. UK: Wiley Blackwell; 2015:1–138 [37].

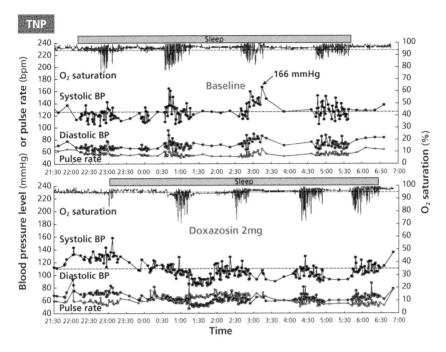

Figure 2.72 Effect of an evening dose of doxazosin on nighttime blood pressure (BP) measured by trigger nighttime BP monitoring (TNP) in a patient with hypertension. O₂, oxygen. *Source*: Kario. Hypertens Res. 2009; 32: 428–432 [248].

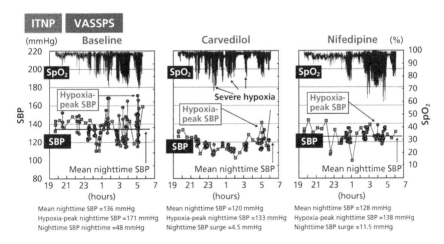

Figure 2.73 Typical case of nighttime blood pressure (BP) parameters measured by trigger nighttime BP monitoring (TNP) at baseline and on nights after administration of carvedilol or nifedipine. Red circles indicate systolic BP (SBP) values measured by an oxygen-triggered function, and green boxes indicate SBP values measure by the fixed-interval (every 30 minutes) function in the Effects of Vasodilating vs. sympathloytic antihypertensives on sleep blood pressure in hypertensive patients with sleep apnea syndrome (VASSPS) study. SpO₂, oxygen saturation. *Source*: Kario et al. J Clin Hypertens. 2014; 16: 459–466 [231].

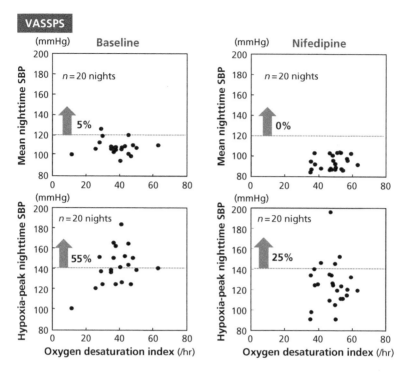

Figure 2.74 Change in nighttime systolic blood pressure (SBP) parameters at baseline and on nifedipine-administered nights in a patient with hypertension and sleep apnea in the effects of vasodilating vs. sympatholytic antihypertensives on sleep blood pressure in hypertensive patients with sleep apnea syndrome (VASSPS) study. *Source*: Kario et al. J Clin Hypertens. 2014; 16: 459–466 [231].

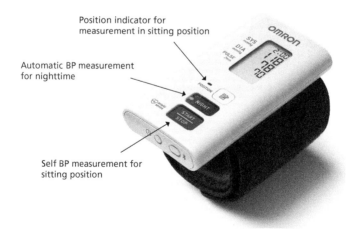

Figure 2.75 The Omron HEM-9601T wrist-type nocturnal home blood pressure (BP) monitoring device (NightView). *Source*: Kario et al. J Clin Hypertens (Greenwich). 2021; 23: 793–801 [238].

Wrist home HBPM and WISDOM Night study

A nocturnal HBPM device that accurately measures nighttime BP with less sleep disturbance is needed for the 24-hour management of hypertension. We conducted the first comparison study of simultaneous self-monitoring by both a supine position algorithm-equipped wrist nocturnal HBPM device (HEM-9601T, NightView; Omron Healthcare) (Figure 2.75) with a similar upper-arm device (HEM-9700T; Omron Healthcare) in 50 patients with hypertension (mean age 68.9 years) [238]. Both devices were worn on the same nondominant arm during sleep over two nights. The patients self-measured their nighttime BP by starting nocturnal measurement mode just before going to bed. In total, 694 paired measurements were obtained over two nights (7.2 ± 1.5 measurements per night), and the mean differences ($\pm$SD) in SBP between the devices was 0.2 ± 10.2 mmHg ($p = 0.563$), with good agreement (Figure 2.76). In addition, in the comparison of nighttime BP indices, the difference in average SBP at 2:00 AM, 3:00 AM, and 4:00 AM and the average SBP of 1-hour interval measurements was -0.5 ± 5.5 mmHg ($p = 0.337$), with good agreement (Figure 2.77). Evidence from the J-HOP Nocturnal BP study, which measured BP at 2:00 AM, 3:00 AM, and 4:00 AM using brachial nocturnal HBPM could be applicable to the wrist device. In addition, the wrist-based device is completely silent even at the time of the BP measurements and substantially reduces sleep disturbance compared with the upper-arm-type device. Thus, the newly developed HEM-9601T (NightView) can accurately measure BP during sleep without reducing sleep quality and could be useful in clinical practice. We are now conducting the WISDOM Night study, the first observational study to establish the clinical implications of wrist-measured nocturnal BP.

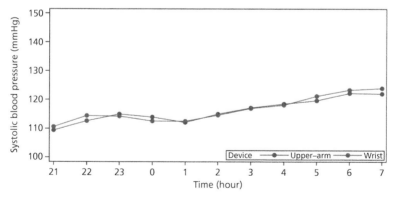

Time (hour)	21:00	22:00	23:00	0:00	1:00	2:00	3:00	4:00	5:00	6:00	7:00
Number of measurements	10	30	60	75	85	89	86	84	82	57	21
Wrist SBP, mmHg	110.6	114.5	114.3	112.6	112.5	114.7	117.0	118.1	121.2	123.3	123.9
Upper-arm SBP, mmHg	109.4	112.7	115.0	114.0	112.1	115.0	117.2	118.5	119.7	122.2	122.0
Difference at each time, mmHg	1.2	1.8	−0.7	−1.4	0.4	−0.4	−0.2	−0.4	1.5	1.1	1.9
P for difference	0.806	0.524	0.720	0.442	0.806	0.826	0.991	0.816	0.369	0.584	0.573

Figure 2.76 Mixed-effects analysis of time trend in systolic blood pressure (SBP) measured using a wrist-type and upper-arm-type device ($n = 679$). *Source*: Kario et al. J Clin Hypertens (Greenwich). 2021; 23: 793–801 [238].

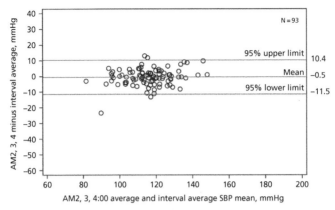

	Average of 2:00, 3:00 and 4:00	Average of interval measures	Difference	P for difference
Average per one night (N = 93 average values from 50 patients)				
Number of measurements	2.8 ± 0.5	7.4 ± 1.3		
SBP, mmHg	115.8 ± 13.4	116.3 ± 12.3	−0.5 ± 5.5	0.337
DBP, mmHg	66.8 ± 8.0	67.1 ± 8.0	−0.2 ± 3.7	0.530
Heart rate, bpm	59.9 ± 6.7	60.7 ± 6.6	−0.8 ± 2.7	0.007

Figure 2.77 Comparison of individual average of wrist device blood pressure measurements at 2:00 AM, 3:00 AM, and 4:00 AM with those measured at one-hour intervals throughout one night. DBP, diastolic blood pressure; SBP, systolic blood pressure. *Source*: Kario et al. J Clin Hypertens (Greenwich). 2021; 23: 793–801 [238].

CHAPTER 3

Practical use of ABPM and HBPM

Concept and positioning of ABPM and HBPM in guidelines

Recent guidelines

All recent hypertension guidelines, including those from the Japanese Society of Hypertension (JSH 2019) [253], European Society of Hypertension/European Society of Cardiology (ESH/ESC 2018) [254], and the 2017 American Heart Association/American College of Cardiology (AHA/ACC) [178], recommend the practical use of out-of-office BP measurement for the diagnosis and management of hypertension. In particular, the JSH 2019 guidelines strongly recommend a home blood pressure measurement (HBPM)-guided approach as the first step for the management of hypertension [253].

There are four different options for measuring blood pressure (BP) available in clinical practice (office BP, automated office BP [AOBP], HBPM, and ambulatory BP monitoring [ABPM]) (Figure 3.1) [180]. Each approach reflects different pressor effects (Figure 3.1) [156, 180]. However, all out-of-office BP measurements are superior to routine office BP measurements for predicting cardiovascular events. After achieving a universal BP goal of 130/80 mmHg, the ideal goal of white-coat effect-excluding BP may be <125 mmHg.

Diagnosis of masked and white-coat hypertension

Masked hypertension is defined as normotension based on office BP readings and hypertension based on out-of-office BP measurement, while white-coat hypertension is defined as normotension based on out-of-office BP and hypertension based on office BP (Figure 3.2) [37]. Detection of masked and white-coat hypertension by using the out-of-office BP monitoring devices is important to improve the quality of BP control and reduce the cardiovascular event risk (Figure 3.3) [41]. Table 3.1 [37] highlights different office, home, and ambulatory BP value thresholds for the definition of hypertension. The 2017 AHA/ACC guidelines recommend a universal threshold of 130/80 mmHg for office, home, and daytime ABPM (Table 3.2).

Essential Manual of 24-Hour Blood Pressure Management: From Morning to Nocturnal Hypertension, Second Edition. Kazuomi Kario.
© 2022 John Wiley & Sons Ltd. Published 2022 by John Wiley & Sons Ltd.

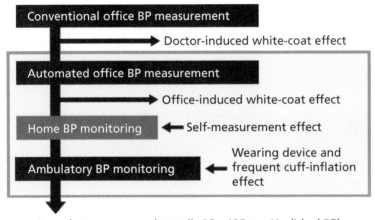

Non-doctor measured systolic BP <125 mmHg (Ideal BP)

Figure 3.1 Different approaches to blood pressure (BP) measurement and influencing factors. *Source:* Kario. Curr Hypertens Rev. 2016;12:2–10 [180]. Copyright (2017) Bentham Science Publishers Ltd. Republished with permission of Bentham Science Publishers Ltd.

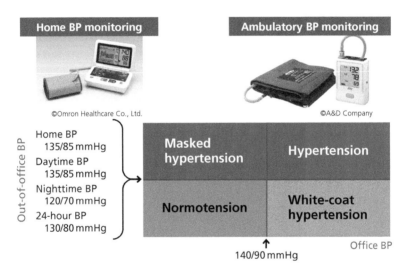

Figure 3.2 Out-of-office blood pressure (BP) monitoring. *Source:* Modified from Kario. Essential Manual of 24-Hour Blood Pressure Management from Morning to Nocturnal Hypertension. UK: Wiley Blackwell; 205: 1–138 [37].

Definition of morning hypertension

The broad definition of "morning hypertension" is having an average morning systolic BP (SBP) ≥135 mmHg and/or average morning diastolic BP (DBP) ≥85 mmHg, regardless of office BP (Table 3.3) [24, 38]. In addition, the strict definition of "morning hypertension" includes those with a morning–evening home BP difference (ME-dif; morning SBP—evening SBP) of ≥20 mmHg [38, 51]. Morning hypertension (ambulatory morning hypertension) can also be diagnosed

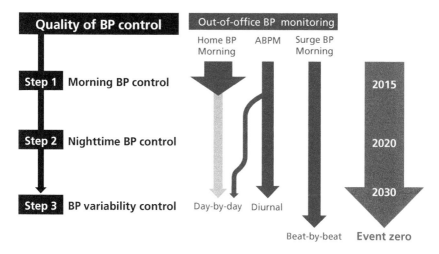

Figure 3.3 ICT-based strategy for "Zero Cardiovascular Events." ABPM, ambulatory blood pressure monitoring. *Source:* Kario. J Hum Hypertens. 2017; 31: 231–243 [41].

Table 3.1 Different blood pressure thresholds for the diagnosis of hypertension.

Blood pressure (mmHg)	Systolic	Diastolic
Office (automated office)	140 (140)	90 (90)
Home		
Morning	135	85
Daytime (awake)	135	85
Evening	135	85
Nighttime (sleep)	120	70
Ambulatory		
24 hour	130	80
Daytime (awake)	135	85
Nighttime (sleep)	120	70
Morning	135	85

Source: Kario. Essential Manual of 24-Hour Blood Pressure Management from Morning to Nocturnal Hypertension. London: Wiley–Blackwell; 2015: 1–138 [37].

Table 3.2 Corresponding values of systolic/diastolic blood pressure for office, home, and daytime, nighttime, and 24-hour ambulatory blood pressure measurements.

Office	HBPM	Daytime ABPM	Nighttime ABPM	24-hour ABPM
120/80	120/80	120/80	100/65	115/75
130/80	130/80	130/80	110/65	125/75
140/90	135/85	135/85	120/70	130/80
160/100	145/90	145/90	140/85	145/90

ABPM, ambulatory blood pressure monitoring; HBPM, home blood pressure monitoring.
Source: Whelton et al. Hypertension. 2018; 71: 1269–1324 [178]. Copyright (2017), with permission from Elsevier.

Table 3.3 Definition of morning hypertension.

Morning hypertension (home BP monitoring)	
Wide definition	Average of self-measured morning home BPs ≥135 mmHg systolic and/or ≥85 mmHg diastolic
Specific definition	Above definition plus ME difference (morning BP minus evening BP) ≥20 mmHg
Ambulatory morning hypertension (ABPM)	Average of ambulatory BPs during 2-hours after rising ≥135 mmHg systolic and/or ≥85 mmHg diastolic
Masked morning hypertension	Morning hypertension with office BP <140/90 mmHg

BP, blood pressure.
Source: Kario. Essential Manual on Perfect 24-Hour Blood Pressure Management from Morning to Nocturnal Hypertension: Up-to-date for Anticipation Medicine. Wiley, 2018: 1–309 [24].

using ABPM [51]. Masked morning hypertension is defined as morning hypertension when office BP is <140/90 mmHg.

Definition of nocturnal hypertension

Nocturnal hypertension is defined as average nighttime SBP ≥120 mmHg and/or DBP ≥70 mmHg (Table 3.4). Nighttime BP is that measured from bedtime to rising or over the period 1:00 AM to 6:00 AM by ABPM or HBPM (at least three readings per night for at least two days). Office-masked nocturnal hypertension is defined as nocturnal hypertension with office BP <140/90 mmHg, while morning-masked nocturnal hypertension is defined as nocturnal hypertension with morning home BP <135/85 mmHg. Isolated nocturnal hypertension is defined as nocturnal hypertension with office BP 140/90 mmHg and morning home BP values <135/85 mmHg.

When to use HBPM and ABPM

Clinical use of HBPM and ABPM increases the quality of hypertension management. HBPM is easily implemented in clinical practice. However, HBPM only measures BP at a specific time (morning and/or evening) and in a specific

Table 3.4 Definition of nocturnal hypertension.

Nocturnal hypertension
Average of nighttime BP readings[a] ≥120 mmHg systolic and/or ≥70 mmHg diastolic
Office-masked noctural hypertension
Nocturnal hypertension with office BP <140/90 mmHg
Morning-masked nocturnal hypertension
Nocturnal hypertension with morning home BP <135/85 mmHg
Isolated nocturnal hyptertension
Nocturnal hypertension with both office BP <140/90 mmHg and morning home BP <135/85 mmHg

ABPM, ambulatory blood pressure monitoring; BP, blood pressure; HBPM, home BP monitoring.
[a] Nighttime BP is the average of BP readings measured from bedtime to rising or from 1 am to 6 am by ABPM or by HBPM (at least 3 readings per night, and over at least 2 days)
Source: Kario. Essential Manual on Perfect 24-Hour Blood Pressure Management from Morning to Nocturnal Hypertension: Up-to-date for Anticipation Medicine. Wiley, 2018: 1–309 [24].

condition (resting while sitting), while ABPM measures dynamic ambulatory BP changes during the day and nighttime BP during sleep periods. This allows detection of both dynamic nighttime BP changes and masked nocturnal hypertension. Thus, the best clinical practice would include usage of both HBPM and ABPM [181]. Morning BP can be measured using both HBPM and ABPM. HBPM is self-measured at home while the patient is seated, and ABPM measures BP regularly at 15–30-minute intervals throughout each 24-hour period. ABPM used to be the only option for measuring BP overnight, but recent HBPM device design advances mean that nighttime home BP can be measured during sleep. The advantages of HBPM over ABPM include convenience and less discomfort.

HBPM is recommended for all medicated hypertensive patients, those with elevated BP (office SBP 120–129 mmHg and DBP <80 mmHg), or individuals with prehypertension who have an estimated two-year risk of new-onset hypertension of ≥40% (calculated by the Genki–Jichi hypertension prediction model [255]) (Figure 3.4 and Table 3.5).

ABPM is recommended for high-risk patients with hypertension who have any of the following: (1) home BP ≥120/80 mmHg; (2) history of cardiovascular events; (3) organ damage (e.g. left ventricular hypertrophy [LVH], albuminuria, N-terminal pro-brain natriuretic peptide [NT-proBNP] level >125 pg/mL);

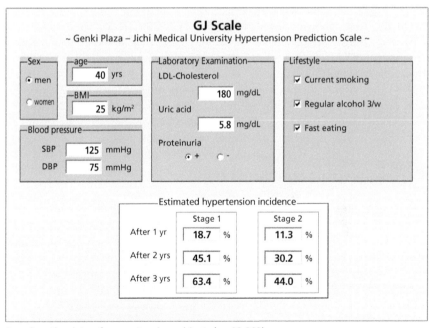

Based on the data of normotensive subjects (n = 93,303)
examined at Genki Plaza health check examination in 2005

Figure 3.4 Genki-Jichi Hypertension prediction simulation (based on data from normotensive subjects [n = 93,303] examined at Genki Plaza health check examination in 2005.
Source: Kario. Essential Manual on Perfect 24-Hour Blood Pressure Management from Morning to Nocturnal Hypertension: Up-to-date for Anticipation Medicine. Wiley, 2018: 1–309 [24].

Table 3.5 Individuals for whom out-of-office blood pressure (BP) is recommended.

Home BP monitoring	• All medicated patients with hypertension • Individuals with office BP ≥120/80 mmHg • Individuals with prehypertension and an estimated 2-year risk of new-onset hypertension of ≥40%[a]
Ambulatory BP monitoring/ nocturnal home BP monitoring	**High-risk patients with hypertension with:** • Home BP ≥120/80 mmHg • History of cardiovascular events • Target organ damage (LVH, albuminuria, NT-proBNP level >125 pg/mL, etc) • Suspected nocturnal hypertension comorbidities (sleep apnea syndrome, CKD, diabetes, etc) • Suspected SHATS

CKD, chronic kidney disease; LVH, left ventricular hypertrophy; NT-proBNP, N-terminal pro-brain natriuretic peptide; SHATS, systemic hemodynamic atherothrombotic syndrome.
[a]Based on the Genki-Jichi hypertension prediction simulator [255].
Source: Modified from: Kario. Essential Manual on Perfect 24-Hour Blood Pressure Management from Morning to Nocturnal Hypertension: Up-to-date for Anticipation Medicine. Wiley, 2018: 1–309 [24].

(4) nocturnal hypertension-suspected comorbidities (sleep apnea syndrome, diabetes, chronic kidney disease [CKD]); or (5) suspected systematic hemodynamic atherothrombotic syndrome (SHATS).

In the Trial of Preventing Hypertension (TROPHY) [256], the incidence of new-onset Stage 2 hypertension in patients with Stage 1 hypertension (office BP 130–140/85–90 mmHg) was 40.4% at the two-year follow-up, and 63.0% at the four-year follow-up. However, the average home BP at baseline was already 134/83 mmHg, indicating that at least half of the subjects already had hypertension diagnosed based on home BP readings. In a recent analysis, subjects with elevated office BP (120–129/<80 mmHg) had >3 times the risk of hypertension than those with normal (optimal) BP (Figure 3.5) [257, 258].

Clinically suspected SHATS

The novel contribution of SHATS is the synergistic combination of various types of BP variability and hemodynamic stress in relation to vascular disease [57, 58, 157]. That is, SHATS is defined by both vascular (one or more clinical/subclinical vascular diseases) and BP components (one or more phenotypes of BP variability), although the precise definition and criteria of SHATS are not yet clearly established [57, 58, 157–159]. Nonetheless, the concept highlights the fact that, in clinical practice, clinicians should recognize the synergistic risk posed by exaggerated BP variability and vascular damage (Figure 3.6).

The clinical relevance of SHATS is different for younger and older subjects. SHATS is clinically important for predicting future-sustained hypertension in younger subjects, and early detection of SHATS in this setting may allow early intervention to prevent target organ damage. In older subjects, SHATS is important as a direct trigger for cardiovascular events, and therefore suppression of SHATS could directly reduce the cardiovascular event burden.

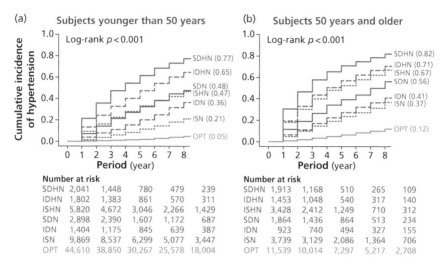

Figure 3.5 Incidence of new onset of hypertension in normotensive subjects in the Genki Plaza Medical Center for Health Care. (a) Subjects younger than 50 years. (b) Subjects 50 years and older. Blood pressure (BP) was divided into seven categories: (1) Optimal BP (OPT), SBP/DBP <120/80 mmHg; (2) Isolated systolic normal BP (ISN), 120–129/<80 mmHg; (3) Isolated diastolic normal BP (IDN), <120/80–84 mmHg; (4) Systolic diastolic normal BP (SDN), 120–129/80–84 mmHg; (5) Isolated systolic high-normal BP (ISHN), 130–139/<85 mmHg; (6) Isolated diastolic high-normal BP (IDHN), <130/85–89 mmHg; and (7) Systolic diastolic high-normal BP (SDHN), 130–139/85–89 mmHg. The label of each line is the BP category and (in parentheses) the cumulative incidence of hypertension. The log-rank test was used to calculate p-values. *Source:* Reproduced with permission, from Kanegae et al. J Clin Hypertens (Greenwich). 2017; 19: 603–610 [258].

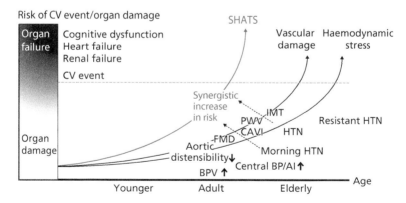

Figure 3.6 Effect of the systematic atherothrombotic syndrome (SHATS) on cardiovascular (CV) event and organ damage worsened by the vicious cycle of hemodynamic stress and vascular damage. AI, augmentation index; BPV, blood pressure variability; CAVI, cardio-ankle vascular index; FMD, flow-mediated dilatation of brachial artery; HTN, hypertension; IMT, intima-media thickness of carotid artery; PWV, pulse wave velocity. *Source:* Kario. J Clin Hypertens (Greenwich). 2015; 17: 328–331 [155].

Cardio-ankle vascular index (CAVI)

As a measure of SHATS, we use the cardio-ankle vascular index (CAVI), which is an index of arterial stiffness that is less dependent on BP than pulse wave velocity (PWV). The cardiac and vascular screening system, VaSera device (Fukuda Denshi Co., Ltd., Tokyo, Japan), measures the following four parameters to evaluate cardiovascular damage: ECG, cardiac sound, and brachial and ankle pulse waves (Figure 3.7). These measures are useful to evaluate hypertensive heart disease, aortic valvular disease, central pressure, cardiac function, and the ankle-brachial index (ABI) to calculate BP-independent value for CAVI at one examination. This system stores the intracuff pressure wave form of four different extremities. There reference values for CAVI are as follows: <8.0, normal; >8.0 and <9.0, borderline; and >9.0, abnormal (Figure 3.8) [259]. CAVI predicts the development of hypertension (Figure 3.9) [260], and is associated with small artery retinopathy [260] (Figure 3.10).

Coupling study

We are now conducting a nationwide cohort study (the Cardiovascular Prognostic COUPLING study – the COUPLING Registry) to determine the effect of vascular disease and BP variability on cardiovascular prognosis [261] (Figure 3.11). Cross-sectional data from this study show that CAVI increases with age [261] (Figure 3.12) and is higher in patients with diabetes and in current smokers [262] (Figure 3.13).

ABPM and/or nocturnal HBPM is recommended to detect SHATS and high-risk hypertension when CAVI is >9 and office or home SBP variability increased.

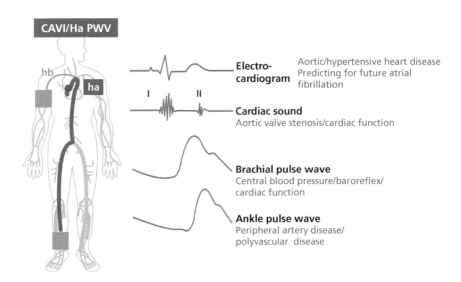

Figure 3.7 Development of a device for predicting future heart failure by analyzing wave forms obtained from three modalities. CAVI, cardio-ankle vascular index. *Source:* Kario. Essential Manual on Perfect 24-Hour Blood Pressure Management from Morning to Nocturnal Hypertension: Up-to-date for Anticipation Medicine. Wiley, 2018: 1–309 [24].

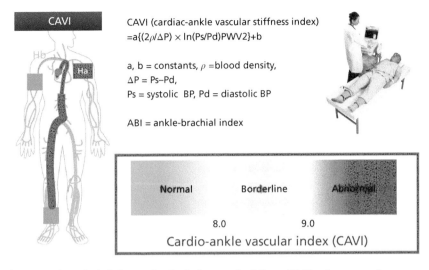

CAVI (cardiac-ankle vascular stiffness index)
=a{(2ρ/ΔP) × ln(Ps/Pd)PWV2}+b

a, b = constants, ρ =blood density,
ΔP = Ps–Pd,
Ps = systolic BP, Pd = diastolic BP

ABI = ankle-brachial index

Figure 3.8 Physiological diagnostic criteria for vascular failure. BP, blood pressure. *Source:* Tanaka et al. Hypertension. 2018; 72: 1060–1071 [259].

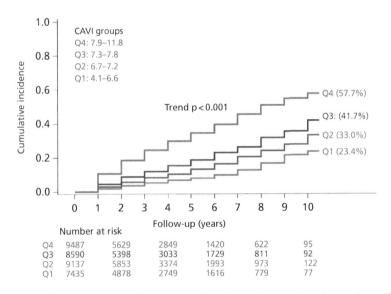

Figure 3.9 Incidence of new-onset hypertension in patient subgroups based on cardio-ankle vascular index (CAVI) quartiles (Q) at baseline. *Source:* Kario et al. Hypertension. 2019; 73: 75–83 [260].

How to measure home BP

Table 3.6 demonstrates the difference in home BP measurements between international and Japanese guidelines. The timing of morning BP measurement is the same, but timing of the evening measurement is different [263]. Figure 2.1 shows

p for trend < 0.001
Prevalence (%)
5
4
3
2
1
0
0.1
0.3
0.7
2.9
Q1
4.1–6.6
Q2
6.7–7.2
Q3
7.3–7.8
Q4
7.9–11.8
CAVI
Fundus(+) 6 24 62 266
Fundus(–) 7,400 9,045 8,437 8,868

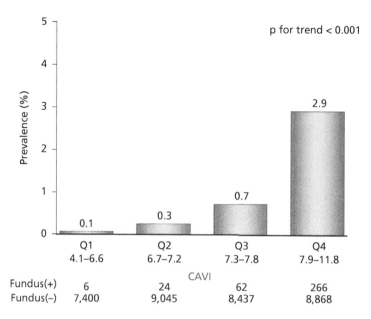

Figure 3.10 Prevalence of small artery retinopathy in patient subgroups based on cardio-ankle vascular index (CAVI) quartiles (Q) at baseline ($n = 34{,}108$). *Source:* Kario et al. Hypertension. 2019; 73: 75–83 [260].

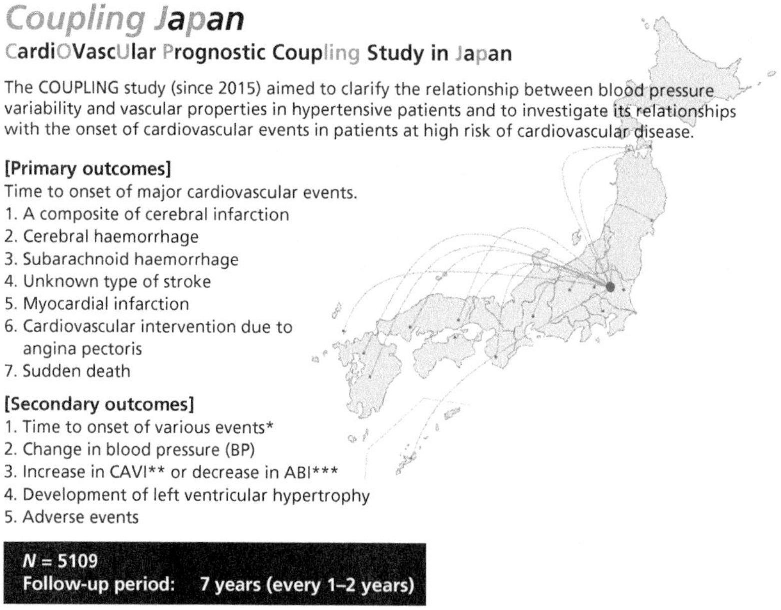

Coupling Japan
CardiOVascUlar Prognostic Coupling Study in Japan
The COUPLING study (since 2015) aimed to clarify the relationship between blood pressure variability and vascular properties in hypertensive patients and to investigate its relationships with the onset of cardiovascular events in patients at high risk of cardiovascular disease.
[Primary outcomes]
Time to onset of major cardiovascular events.
1. A composite of cerebral infarction
2. Cerebral haemorrhage
3. Subarachnoid haemorrhage
4. Unknown type of stroke
5. Myocardial infarction
6. Cardiovascular intervention due to angina pectoris
7. Sudden death
[Secondary outcomes]
1. Time to onset of various events*
2. Change in blood pressure (BP)
3. Increase in CAVI** or decrease in ABI***
4. Development of left ventricular hypertrophy
5. Adverse events
N = 5109
Follow-up period: 7 years (every 1–2 years)

Figure 3.11 The COUPLING study. *Each fatal and nonfatal cardiovascular event, hospitalization for angina pectoris or heart failure, aortic dissection, peripheral arterial disease, end-stage renal disease; doubling of serum creatinine level; new onset of atrial fibrillation, dementia, need of nursing care; total death. **CAVI (cardiac-ankle vascular stiffness index) = $a\{(2\rho/\Delta P)\times\ln(Ps/Pd)PWV2\}+b$. a and b, constants; ρ, blood density; ΔP, Ps–Pd; Ps, systolic BP; Pd, diastolic BP. ***ABI, ankle-brachial index. *Source:* Kario. Prog Cardiovasc Dis. 2016; 59: 262–281 [156].

Coupling Japan

CardiOVascUlar Prognostic Coupling Study in Japan

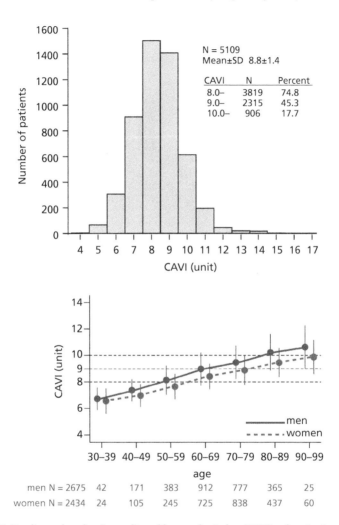

Figure 3.12 Baseline values for the cardio-ankle vascular index (CAVI) values in Coupling Japan study. Left: distribution of baseline CAVI values in the population at baseline; Right: mean baseline CAVI values in 10-year age categories by patient sex (values are mean ± standard deviation). *Source:* Kario et al. J Clin Hypertens (Greenwich). 2020; 22: 465–474 [261].

the standard method of self-measured home BP monitoring (HBPM) based on Asian recommendations [183–185]. European Society of Hypertension (ESH) guidelines [111] recommend measuring evening BP before dinner, while JSH 2019 guidelines and the AHA/ASH/PCNA Statement on Home BP Monitoring recommend measuring evening BP before going to bed [253, 264]. There is no

Coupling Japan

CardiOVascUlar Prognostic Coupling Study in Japan

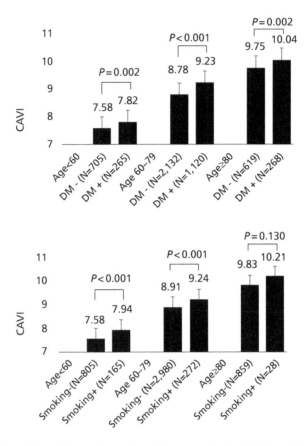

Figure 3.13 Associations between the cardio-ankle vascular index (CAVI) and diabetes/glucose tolerance disorder (left) or smoking status (right) by age group. DM, diabetes mellitus. *Source:* Kabutoya et al. J Clin Hypertens (Greenwich). 2020; 22: 1208–1215 [262].

significant difference in the morning BP and evening BP measured before dinner. However, bathing and alcohol consumption significantly decrease evening BP measured at bedtime (Figure 3.14) [263]. In addition, reproducibility of home BP is better for morning BP than for evening BP. There is no significant correlation between morning home BP and office BP self-measured in the waiting room before examination (waiting-room BP), and office BP measured by the doctor (examining-room BP) (Figure 3.15) [265]. Thus, to simplify home BP measurement in clinical practice, we recommend measurement of morning BP.

Table 3.6 Comparison of Eastern and Asian hypertension guidelines for home blood pressure monitoring (HBPM).

	Timing	Frequency/ occasion	Duration
AHA/ACC 2017	• Morning (before taking medications) • Evening (before supper)	≥Twice (1 min apart)	• Ideally 7 days
ESH/ESC 2018	• Morning • Evening	Twice (1–2 min apart)	• ≥3 days • Preferably for 6–7 consecutive days before each clinic visit
NICE/BHS 2011	• Twice daily • Ideally morning and evening	Twice (≥1 min apart)	• ≥4 days • Ideally 7 days
AHA/ASH/ PCNA statement on HBPM (Pickering TG et al. [264])	• Morning before drug intake • Evening (at bedtime)	Twice to three times (1 min apart)	• 7 days
JSH 2019	• Morning (within 1 h after waking up, after urination, before dosing in the morning, before breakfast • Evening (at the bedtime) According to instructions: before dinner, before dosing in the evening, before bathing, or before alcohol consumption. Others (if necessary): in the presence of symptoms, during the daytime on holidays, during sleep at night (Home sphygmomanometers that facilitate automatic blood pressure measurement during sleep at night are available.)	Twice	• 7 days (at least 5 days)
HOPE Asia Network*	• Morning (before taking medications) • Evening (at bedtime)	Twice(≥2 min apart)	• ≥3 days

ACC, American College of Cardiology; AHA, American Heart Association; ASH, American Society of Hypertension; BHS, British Hypertension Society; ESC, European Society of Cardiology; ESH, European Society of Hypertension; HOPE, Hypertension Cardiovascular Outcome Prevention and Evidence; JSH, Japanese Society of Hypertension; NICE, National Institute for Health and Care Excellence; PCNA, Preventive Cardiovascular Nursing Association.
Source: Kario. Essential Manual on Perfect 24-Hour Blood Pressure Management from Morning to Nocturnal Hypertension: Up-to-date for Anticipation Medicine. Wiley, 2018: 1–309 [24].

Nighttime home BP measurement schedule

There is no consensus about the standard measurement of nighttime home BP. Table 3.7 provides suggested protocol for measuring nighttime home BP. A validated home BP monitor should be used, and patients should be shown how to put

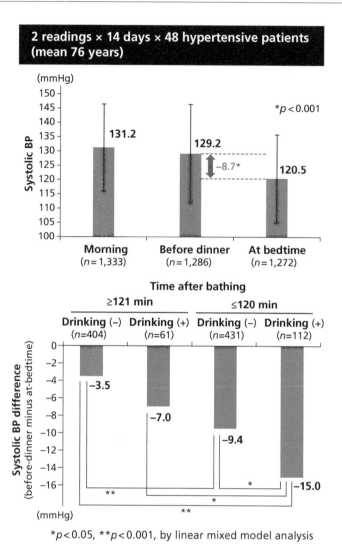

Figure 3.14 Different evening home systolic blood pressure (BP) readings before dinner and at bedtime. *Source:* Fujiwara et al. J Clin Hypertens (Greenwich). 2017; 19: 731–739 [263].

the cuff of the BP monitor on the upper arm or wrist. Automatic BP measurements should be set for 2–3 times (at least twice) during sleep at either of the following time intervals: (1) fixed time (2:00 AM, 3:00 AM, 4:00 AM), (2) individual behavior (bedtime-based) time (2–4 hours after going to bed) for two or more nights. The average of at least six measures is required to provide a reliable measure of home BP. Nocturnal hypertension is diagnosed when nighttime home BP is ≥120/70 mmHg.

Data from a crossover showed two nights (six readings) in one week with a measurement achievement rate of over 90%, and that there were no significant differences between the fixed-time measurement and the phase bedtime-based measurement (Figures 3.16 and 3.17) [266]. On the other hand, another study

- Hypertensive patients (*n* = 113, 78.8 years)
- **Home BP**: mean morning BP values for ≥7 days
- **Waiting-room BP**: measured by patients themselves
- **Examining-room BP**: measured by a physician

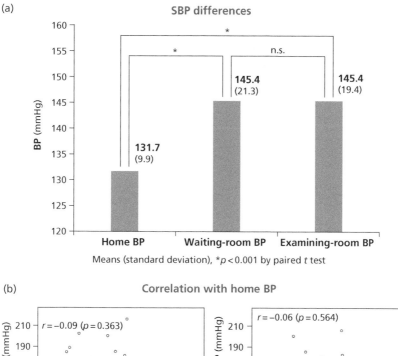

(a)

SBP differences

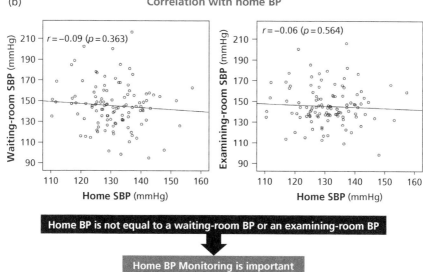

(b) Correlation with home BP

Figure 3.15 Home blood pressure (BP) vs. waiting-room and examining-room BP. SBP, systolic BP. *Source:* Fujiwara et al. J Clin Hypertens (Greenwich). 2017; 19: 1051–1053 [265].

using a newly developed wrist BP monitoring (HEM-9601T; Omron Healthcare) showed that the average of three fixed-time measurements (2:00 AM, 3:00 AM, and 4:00 AM) was comparable to the average of all the 60-min interval measurements throughout a night, while the average of the three bed-time measurements at 2,

Table 3.7 Nighttime home blood pressure (BP) measurement.

Nighttime home BP measurement is performed as follows Set the cuff of BP monitoring on the upper arm or wrist Set automatic BP measurements 2–3 times during sleep
Timing of measurements (at least twice) 1) 2:00 AM, 3:00 AM, 4:00 AM 2) 2-4 hours after going to bed
Days 2 or more nights
Calculation Average of ≥6 measures

Source: Kario. Essential Manual on Perfect 24-Hour Blood Pressure Management from Morning to Nocturnal Hypertension: Up-to-date for Anticipation Medicine. Wiley, 2018: 1–309 [24].

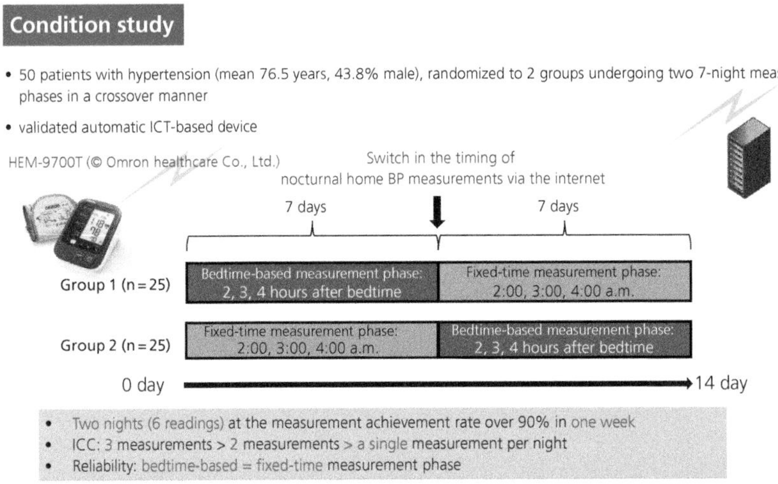

Condition study

- 50 patients with hypertension (mean 76.5 years, 43.8% male), randomized to 2 groups undergoing two 7-night measurement phases in a crossover manner

- validated automatic ICT-based device

- Two nights (6 readings) at the measurement achievement rate over 90% in one week
- ICC: 3 measurements > 2 measurements > a single measurement per night
- Reliability: bedtime-based = fixed-time measurement phase

Figure 3.16 Study protocol of the Condition study (Comparison of different schedules of nocturnal home BP measurement: bedtime-based measurement vs. fixed-time measurement). ICC, intraclass correlation coefficient; ICT, information and communication technology. *Source:* Fujiwara et al. J Clin Hypertens (Greenwich). 2018; 20: 1633–1641 [266].

3, and 4 hours after going to bed was significantly lower than all the 60-min interval average [239].

ABPM parameters

ABPM allows more extensive assessment of the 24-hour ambulatory BP profile of individual patients, including BP variability. Figure 3.18 and Tables 3.8–3.11 show ambulatory BP and BP variability parameters calculated from ambulatory BP measurements obtained from one ABPM recording [2, 37].

Condition study

- Two nights (6 readings) at the measurement achievement rate over 90% in one week

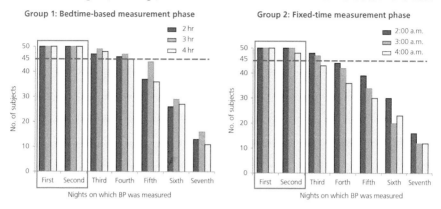

Figure 3.17 Numbers of participants who measured their nocturnal home blood pressure (BP). In the bedtime-based measurement phase, the number of participants who measured their nocturnal home BP fell significantly on the fourth night. In the fixed-time measurement phase, the number of participants who measured their nocturnal home BP dropped significantly on the third night. *Source:* Fujiwara et al. J Clin Hypertens (Greenwich). 2018; 20: 1633–1641 [266].

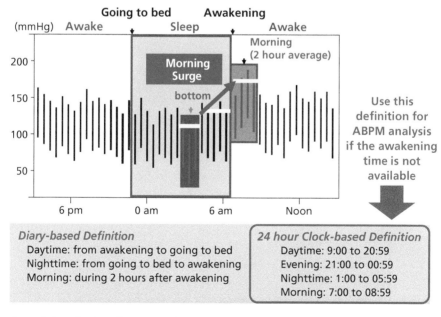

Figure 3.18 Definition of time period for calculating ambulatory blood pressure monitoring (ABPM) parameters. *Source:* Kario et al. Circulation. 2003; 107: 1401–1406 [2].

Table 3.8 Diary-based definition of morning and nighttime blood pressure (BP) parameters.

Morning BP parameters	
Average morning SBP	– 2-hour average of morning SBPs during 2 hours after rising
Moving peak morning SBP	– Highest 1-hour moving average of consecutive SBPs during 2 hours after rising
Maximum morning SBP	– Maximum morning SBP (one SBP) during 2 hours after rising
Nighttime BP parameters	
Average nighttime SBP	– Average of nighttime SBPs from going to bed to rising
Average peak nighttime SBP	– Average of highest three different nighttime SBPs from going to bed to rising
Maximum nighttime SBP	– Maximum nighttime SBP (1 SBP) from going to bed to rising
Minimum nighttime SBP	– Minimum nighttime SBP (1 SBP) from going to bed to rising
Moving lowest nighttime SBP	– Lowest 1-hour moving average of consecutive SBPs from going to bed to rising
Pre-wakening nighttime SBP	– 2-hour average of nighttime SBPs during 2 hours before rising
Daytime BP parameters	
Average daytime SBP	– Average of daytime SBPs from rising to going to bed

SBP, systolic BP.
Source: Kario. Essential Manual on Perfect 24-Hour Blood Pressure Management from Morning to Nocturnal Hypertension: Up-to-date for Anticipation Medicine. Wiley, 2018: 1–309 [24].

Table 3.9 Diary-based definition of morning and nighttime blood pressure (BP) surge parameters.

Morning BP surge parameters	
Sleep-trough morning surge	– Average morning SBP minus moving lowest nighttime SBP
Dynamic morning surge	– Moving peak morning SBP minus moving lowest nighttime SBP
Maximum dynamic morning surge	– Maximum morning SBP minus minimum nighttime SBP
Pre-wakening morning surge	– Average morning SBP minus pre-wakening nighttime SBP
Nighttime BP surge parameters	
Average nighttime surge	– Average peak nighttime SBP minus average nighttime SBP
Dynamic nighttime surge	– Average peak nighttime SBP minus moving lowest nighttime SBP
Maximum dynamic nighttime surge	– Maximum nighttime SBP minus minimum nighttime SBP
Nighttime BP dipping parameters	
Nighttime dipping (%)	– (1 minus average nighttime SBP/average daytime SBP) × 100
Subgroup classification based on nighttime SBP dipping (%)	– Extreme-dipper: ≥20%; Dipper: <20%, ≥10%; Non-dipper: <10%, ≥0%; Riser: <0%

SBP, systolic BP.
Source: Kario. Essential Manual on Perfect 24-Hour Blood Pressure Management from Morning to Nocturnal Hypertension: Up-to-date for Anticipation Medicine. Wiley, 2018: 1–309 [24].

Table 3.10 Twenty-four-hour clock-based definition of morning and nighttime blood pressure (BP) parameters.

Morning BP parameters

Average morning SBP	– 2-hour average of morning SBPs between 7 am and 9 am
Moving peak morning SBP	– Highest 1-hour moving average of consecutive SBPs between 6 am and 10 am
Maximum morning SBP	– Maximum morning SBP (one SBP) between 6 am and 10 am
Minimum morning SBP	– Minimum morning SBP (one SBP) between 5 am and 9 am before maximum morning SBP
Moving lowest pre-wakening morning SBP	– Lowest 1-hour moving average of consecutive SBPs between 5 am and 9 am before moving peak morning SBP

Nighttime BP parameters

Average nighttime SBP	– Average of nighttime SBPs between 1 am and 6 am
Average peak nighttime SBP	– Average of highest 3 different nighttime SBPs between 1 am and 6 am
Maximum nighttime SBP	– Maximum nighttime SBP (1 SBP reading) between 1 am and 6 am
Minimum nighttime SBP	– Minimum nighttime SBP (1 SBP reading) between 1 am and 6 am
Moving lowest nighttime SBP	– Lowest 1-hour moving average of consecutive SBP reading between 1 am and 6 am

SBP, systolic BP.
Source: Kario. Essential Manual on Perfect 24-Hour Blood Pressure Management from Morning to Nocturnal Hypertension: Up-to-date for Anticipation Medicine. Wiley, 2018: 1–309 [24].

Table 3.11 Twenty-four-hour-clock-based definition of morning and nighttime blood pressure (BP) surge parameters.

Morning BP surge parameters

Average morning surge	– Average morning SBP minus average nighttime SBP
Dynamic morning surge	– Moving peak morning SBP minus moving lowest nighttime SBP
Dynamic pre-wakening morning surge	– Moving peak morning SBP minus moving lowest pre-wakening morning SBP
Maximum dynamic morning surge	– Maximum morning SBP minus minimum nighttime SBP
Maximum pre-wakening morning surge	– Maximum morning SBP minus minimum morning SBP

Nighttime BP surge parameters

Average nighttime surge	– Average peak nighttime SBP minus average nighttime SBP
Dynamic nighttime surge	– Average peak nighttime SBP minus moving lowest nighttime SBP
Maximum dynamic nighttime surge	– Maximum nighttime SBP minus minimum nighttime SBP

Daytime BP parameters

Average daytime SBP	– Average of daytime SBPs between 9 am and 9 pm

SBP, systolic BP.
Source: Kario. Essential Manual on Perfect 24-Hour Blood Pressure Management from Morning to Nocturnal Hypertension: Up-to-date for Anticipation Medicine. Wiley, 2018: 1–309 [24].

24-hour BP

Twenty-four-hour BP is the average of BP readings during a 24-hour period and is the most important BP parameter in terms of cardiovascular risk [88].

Daytime BP and nighttime BP

Daytime BP and nighttime BP are calculated from the average of BP readings measured during daytime and nighttime, respectively. The time periods used to define daytime, nighttime, and morning ambulatory BP values are based on a diary of an individual's behavior or based on 24-hour clock time (Figure 3.18 and Tables 3.8–3.11) [2, 37]. The diary-based definition of daytime and nighttime BP is superior to the 24-hour clock time definition because the majority of ambulatory BP values are determined by the patient's timing of getting up in the morning and going to bed.

Morning BP parameters

Morning BP parameters are defined as follows: average morning SBP—2-hour average of morning SBP values during the two hours after rising or between 7 AM and 9 AM; moving peak morning SBP –highest 1-hour moving average of consecutive SBPs during the two hours after rising, or between 6:00 AM and 10:00 AM; and maximum morning SBP—maximum morning SBP (one reading) during the two hours after rising or between 6:00 AM and 10:00 AM.

Nighttime BP parameters

Nighttime BP parameters are defined as follows: average nighttime SBP—average of nighttime SBP values; average peak nighttime SBP—average of three highest different nighttime SBP values; maximum nighttime SBP—one SBP reading; minimum nighttime SBP—one SBP reading; moving lowest nighttime SBP—lowest one-hour moving average of consecutive nighttime SBP values; and pre-wakening nighttime SBP—two-hour average of nighttime SBP values during the two hours before rising.

MBPS parameters

Sleep-trough morning surge is calculated as the average morning SBP minus the moving lowest nighttime SBP; prewakening morning surge is calculated as the average morning SBP minus prewakening morning SBP. Dynamic morning surge is calculated as the moving peak morning SBP minus moving lowest nighttime SBP, and maximum dynamic morning surge is calculated as the maximum morning SBP minus minimum nighttime SBP. The prewakening morning SBP (diary) or minimal (or moving prewakening) morning SBP (clock-based) between 5:00 AM and 9:00 AM is used to calculate the prewakening morning SBP surge.

Nighttime BP surge parameters

Average nighttime surge is calculated as the average peak nighttime SBP minus the average nighttime SBP, dynamic nighttime surge as the average peak nighttime SBP minus moving lowest nighttime SBP, and maximum dynamic nighttime surge as the maximum nighttime SBP minus minimum nighttime SBP. In addition to an increase in nighttime BP, increased BP variability during sleep (standard deviation of nighttime SBP) is an independent and synergistic risk factor for cardiovascular events.

Nighttime BP dipping parameters

Nighttime SBP dipping (%) is calculated as (1 minus average nighttime SBP/average daytime SBP) ×100. Subgroups are classified as follows: extreme dipper: ≥20%; dipper: <20%, ≥10%; non-dipper: <10%, ≥0%; riser: <0% [7, 8].

ABPM-defined hypertension subtypes

Figure 3.19 shows a normotensive dipping pattern of BP in patients with white-coat hypertension. Individuals with either this pattern or a normal pattern show normal diurnal BP rhythm with a nighttime BP fall of 10–19% compared with daytime BP. Figure 3.20 shows a hypertensive extreme-dipper pattern, with excessive nighttime fall in BP of at least 20%, and a hypertensive dipper pattern with adequate nighttime BP fall (of 10–19%). Figure 3.21 shows patients with nocturnal hypertension, including those with a non-dipper pattern with reduced nighttime BP fall (0–9%), and a riser pattern with higher nighttime BP than daytime BP (>0% increase).

Home and ambulatory BP-guided management of hypertension

Home BP control <135/85 mmHg is the standard first step. Figure 3.22 shows a recommended strategy for those already receiving antihypertensive therapy based on office BP, HBPM, and ABPM [192]. For individuals with office BP ≥130/80 mmHg, HBPM should be conducted to exclude white coat uncontrolled hypertension; uncontrolled hypertension is diagnosed if home BP is ≥135/85 mmHg. If white-coat uncontrolled hypertension is suspected, or there is evidence of target organ damage in individuals with home BP <135/85 mmHg, ABPM should be performed. BP control is defined as 24-hour BP on ABPM of <130/80 mmHg. For the detection of masked uncontrolled hypertension, HBPM may also performed in individuals with treated hypertension who have office BP <130/80 mmHg and a high baseline level of cardiovascular risk.

STEpwise-Personalized 24-hour BP control approach (STEP24 approach)

This approach is summarized in (Figure 3.23) [1].

Targeting morning hypertension (Step 1)

Controlling morning home SBP to <145 mmHg is the first step in reducing relatively short-term risk, with the goal being morning home BP <135 mmHg (and ideally <125 mmHg) (Figure 3.24) [37]. In the JSH 2019 guidelines, recommended

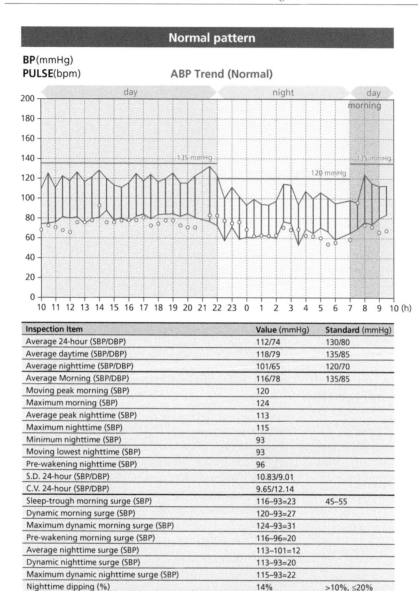

Inspection Item	Value (mmHg)	Standard (mmHg)
Average 24-hour (SBP/DBP)	112/74	130/80
Average daytime (SBP/DBP)	118/79	135/85
Average nighttime (SBP/DBP)	101/65	120/70
Average Morning (SBP/DBP)	116/78	135/85
Moving peak morning (SBP)	120	
Maximum morning (SBP)	124	
Average peak nighttime (SBP)	113	
Maximum nighttime (SBP)	115	
Minimum nighttime (SBP)	93	
Moving lowest nighttime (SBP)	93	
Pre-wakening nighttime (SBP)	96	
S.D. 24-hour (SBP/DBP)	10.83/9.01	
C.V. 24-hour (SBP/DBP)	9.65/12.14	
Sleep-trough morning surge (SBP)	116–93=23	45–55
Dynamic morning surge (SBP)	120–93=27	
Maximum dynamic morning surge (SBP)	124–93=31	
Pre-wakening morning surge (SBP)	116–96=20	
Average nighttime surge (SBP)	113–101=12	
Dynamic nighttime surge (SBP)	113–93=20	
Maximum dynamic nighttime surge (SBP)	115–93=22	
Nighttime dipping (%)	14%	>10%, ≤20%
Subgroup classification based on nighttime SBP dipping (%)	Dipper	

Figure 3.19 Typical blood pressure (BP) pattern (normal pattern; See next page for white-coat hypertension pattern) evaluated by ambulatory BP monitoring (ABPM). bpm, beats/minute; C.V., coefficient of variation; DBP, diastolic BP; SBP, systolic BP; S.D., standard deviation. *Source:* Kario. Essential Manual on Perfect 24-Hour Blood Pressure Management from Morning to Nocturnal Hypertension: Up-to-date for Anticipation Medicine. Wiley, 2018: 1–309 [24].

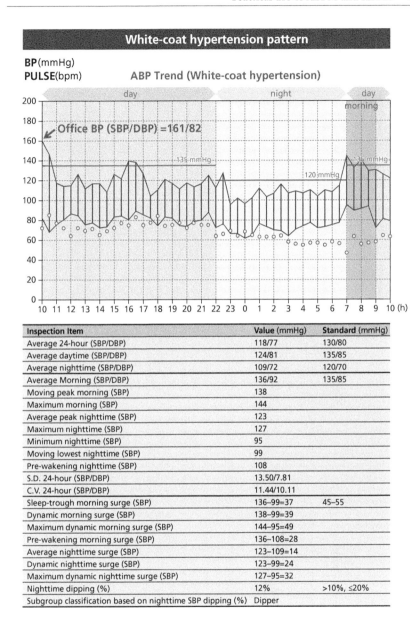

White-coat hypertension pattern

BP(mmHg)
PULSE(bpm)   ABP Trend (White-coat hypertension)

Inspection Item	Value (mmHg)	Standard (mmHg)
Average 24-hour (SBP/DBP)	118/77	130/80
Average daytime (SBP/DBP)	124/81	135/85
Average nighttime (SBP/DBP)	109/72	120/70
Average Morning (SBP/DBP)	136/92	135/85
Moving peak morning (SBP)	138	
Maximum morning (SBP)	144	
Average peak nighttime (SBP)	123	
Maximum nighttime (SBP)	127	
Minimum nighttime (SBP)	95	
Moving lowest nighttime (SBP)	99	
Pre-wakening nighttime (SBP)	108	
S.D. 24-hour (SBP/DBP)	13.50/7.81	
C.V. 24-hour (SBP/DBP)	11.44/10.11	
Sleep-trough morning surge (SBP)	136−99=37	45−55
Dynamic morning surge (SBP)	138−99=39	
Maximum dynamic morning surge (SBP)	144−95=49	
Pre-wakening morning surge (SBP)	136−108=28	
Average nighttime surge (SBP)	123−109=14	
Dynamic nighttime surge (SBP)	123−99=24	
Maximum dynamic nighttime surge (SBP)	127−95=32	
Nighttime dipping (%)	12%	>10%, ≤20%
Subgroup classification based on nighttime SBP dipping (%)	Dipper	

Figure 3.19 *(Continued)*

target BP levels are <130/80 mmHg for office BP, and <125/75 mmHg for home BP for all patients with hypertension apart from elderly patients aged >75 years without any complication, those with bilateral carotid or major cerebral artery stenosis, or CKD patients without albuminuria (Table 3.12) [253]. The HOPE Asia Network recommends targeting home SBP to <125 mmHg in high-risk Asian patients, especially those with diabetes, CKD, and/or cardiovascular disease (Table 3.13) [183].

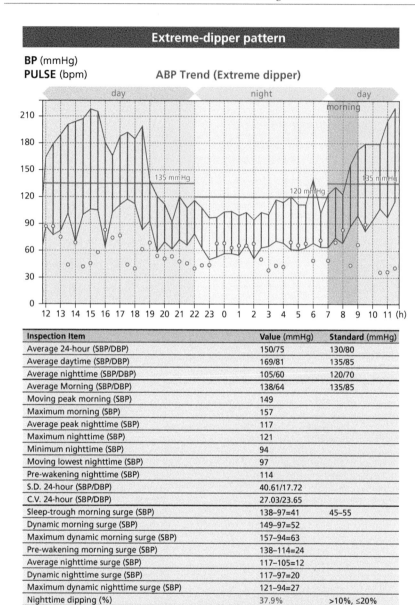

Inspection Item	Value (mmHg)	Standard (mmHg)
Average 24-hour (SBP/DBP)	150/75	130/80
Average daytime (SBP/DBP)	169/81	135/85
Average nighttime (SBP/DBP)	105/60	120/70
Average Morning (SBP/DBP)	138/64	135/85
Moving peak morning (SBP)	149	
Maximum morning (SBP)	157	
Average peak nighttime (SBP)	117	
Maximum nighttime (SBP)	121	
Minimum nighttime (SBP)	94	
Moving lowest nighttime (SBP)	97	
Pre-wakening nighttime (SBP)	114	
S.D. 24-hour (SBP/DBP)	40.61/17.72	
C.V. 24-hour (SBP/DBP)	27.03/23.65	
Sleep-trough morning surge (SBP)	138–97=41	45–55
Dynamic morning surge (SBP)	149–97=52	
Maximum dynamic morning surge (SBP)	157–94=63	
Pre-wakening morning surge (SBP)	138–114=24	
Average nighttime surge (SBP)	117–105=12	
Dynamic nighttime surge (SBP)	117–97=20	
Maximum dynamic nighttime surge (SBP)	121–94=27	
Nighttime dipping (%)	37.9%	>10%, ≤20%
Subgroup classification based on nighttime SBP dipping (%)	Extreme dipper	

Figure 3.20 Typical blood pressure (BP) pattern (extreme-dipper pattern; See next page for dipper pattern[normal]) evaluated by ambulatory BP monitoring (ABPM). bpm, beats/minute; C.V., coefficient of variation; DBP, diastolic BP; S.D., standard deviation; SBP, systolic BP. *Source:* Kario. Essential Manual on Perfect 24-Hour Blood Pressure Management from Morning to Nocturnal Hypertension: Up-to-date for Anticipation Medicine. Wiley, 2018: 1–309 [24].

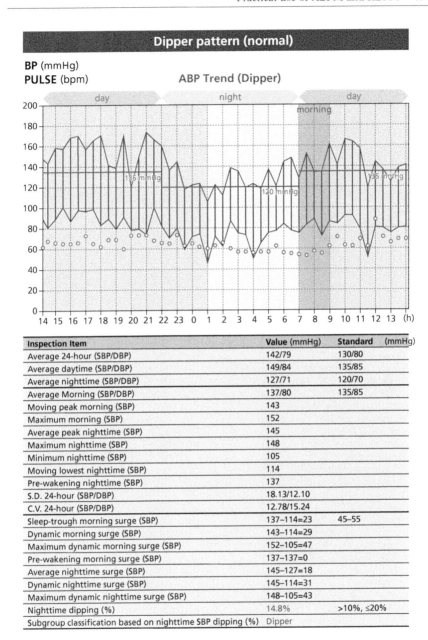

Dipper pattern (normal)

Inspection Item	Value (mmHg)	Standard (mmHg)
Average 24-hour (SBP/DBP)	142/79	130/80
Average daytime (SBP/DBP)	149/84	135/85
Average nighttime (SBP/DBP)	127/71	120/70
Average Morning (SBP/DBP)	137/80	135/85
Moving peak morning (SBP)	143	
Maximum morning (SBP)	152	
Average peak nighttime (SBP)	145	
Maximum nighttime (SBP)	148	
Minimum nighttime (SBP)	105	
Moving lowest nighttime (SBP)	114	
Pre-wakening nighttime (SBP)	137	
S.D. 24-hour (SBP/DBP)	18.13/12.10	
C.V. 24-hour (SBP/DBP)	12.78/15.24	
Sleep-trough morning surge (SBP)	137−114=23	45–55
Dynamic morning surge (SBP)	143−114=29	
Maximum dynamic morning surge (SBP)	152−105=47	
Pre-wakening morning surge (SBP)	137−137=0	
Average nighttime surge (SBP)	145−127=18	
Dynamic nighttime surge (SBP)	145−114=31	
Maximum dynamic nighttime surge (SBP)	148−105=43	
Nighttime dipping (%)	14.8%	>10%, ≤20%
Subgroup classification based on nighttime SBP dipping (%)	Dipper	

Figure 3.20 (*Continued*)

Targeting nocturnal hypertension (Step 2)

After morning home BP is well controlled (<135/85 mmHg on antihypertensive treatment), nighttime BP should be measured by ABPM or nocturnal HBPM. When nighttime SBP is ≥120 mmHg or nighttime DBP is ≥70 mmHg, this residual, uncontrolled nocturnal hypertension is the next target of antihypertensive treatment (Step 2) Figure 3.23 [1].

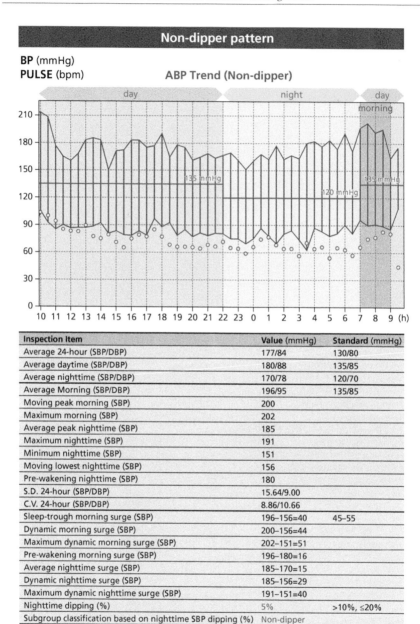

Inspection Item	Value (mmHg)	Standard (mmHg)
Average 24-hour (SBP/DBP)	177/84	130/80
Average daytime (SBP/DBP)	180/88	135/85
Average nighttime (SBP/DBP)	170/78	120/70
Average Morning (SBP/DBP)	196/95	135/85
Moving peak morning (SBP)	200	
Maximum morning (SBP)	202	
Average peak nighttime (SBP)	185	
Maximum nighttime (SBP)	191	
Minimum nighttime (SBP)	151	
Moving lowest nighttime (SBP)	156	
Pre-wakening nighttime (SBP)	180	
S.D. 24-hour (SBP/DBP)	15.64/9.00	
C.V. 24-hour (SBP/DBP)	8.86/10.66	
Sleep-trough morning surge (SBP)	196–156=40	45–55
Dynamic morning surge (SBP)	200–156=44	
Maximum dynamic morning surge (SBP)	202–151=51	
Pre-wakening morning surge (SBP)	196–180=16	
Average nighttime surge (SBP)	185–170=15	
Dynamic nighttime surge (SBP)	185–156=29	
Maximum dynamic nighttime surge (SBP)	191–151=40	
Nighttime dipping (%)	5%	>10%, ≤20%
Subgroup classification based on nighttime SBP dipping (%)	Non-dipper	

Figure 3.21 Typical blood pressure (BP) pattern (left: non-dipper pattern; right: riser pattern) evaluated by ambulatory BP monitoring (ABPM). bpm, beats/minute; DBP, diastolic BP; SBP, systolic BP. *Source:* Kario. Essential Manual on Perfect 24-Hour Blood Pressure Management from Morning to Nocturnal Hypertension: Up-to-date for Anticipation Medicine. Wiley, 2018: 1–309 [24].

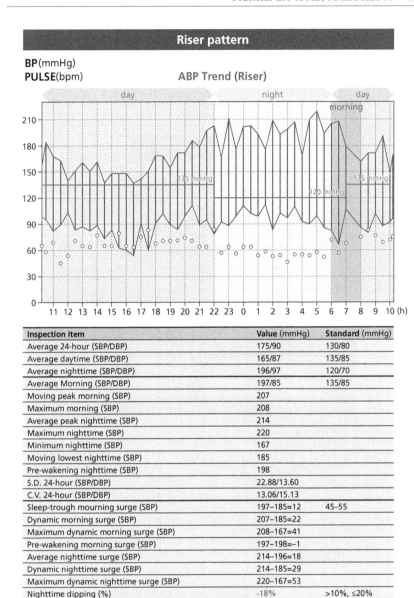

Inspection Item	Value (mmHg)	Standard (mmHg)
Average 24-hour (SBP/DBP)	175/90	130/80
Average daytime (SBP/DBP)	165/87	135/85
Average nighttime (SBP/DBP)	196/97	120/70
Average Morning (SBP/DBP)	197/85	135/85
Moving peak morning (SBP)	207	
Maximum morning (SBP)	208	
Average peak nighttime (SBP)	214	
Maximum nighttime (SBP)	220	
Minimum nighttime (SBP)	167	
Moving lowest nighttime (SBP)	185	
Pre-wakening nighttime (SBP)	198	
S.D. 24-hour (SBP/DBP)	22.88/13.60	
C.V. 24-hour (SBP/DBP)	13.06/15.13	
Sleep-trough mourning surge (SBP)	197–185=12	45–55
Dynamic morning surge (SBP)	207–185=22	
Maximum dynamic morning surge (SBP)	208–167=41	
Pre-wakening morning surge (SBP)	197–198=–1	
Average nighttime surge (SBP)	214–196=18	
Dynamic nighttime surge (SBP)	214–185=29	
Maximum dynamic nighttime surge (SBP)	220–167=53	
Nighttime dipping (%)	-18%	>10%, ≤20%
Subgroup classification based on nighttime SBP dipping (%)	Riser	

Figure 3.21 (*Continued*)

Pressor mechanism-based nighttime BP management strategy

To achieve perfect 24-hour BP control, the pressor mechanism for individual patients needs to be considered (Figure 3.23).

An increase in basal BP is dependent on increased circulating volume or advanced vascular disease (increased vascular stiffness and increased vascular resistance because of small artery remodeling (Figure 3.23). The treatments of

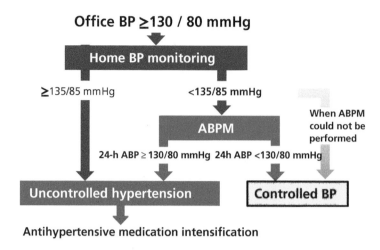

Figure 3.22 Follow-up strategy for treated individuals with uncontrolled office hypertension. ABP, ambulatory blood pressure; ABPM, ambulatory blood pressure monitoring; BP, blood pressure. *Source:* Kario et al. Hypertension. 2019; 74: 229–236 [192].

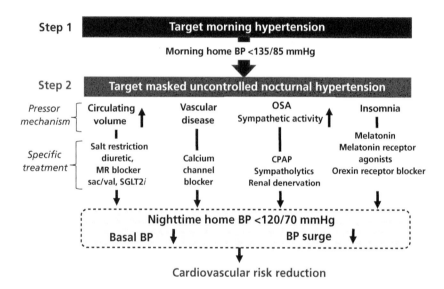

Figure 3.23 STEpwise-Personalized 24-hr blood pressure control approach (STEP24 approach). BP, blood pressure; CPAP, continuous positive airway pressure; MR, mineralocorticoid receptor; OSA, obstructive sleep apnea; sac/val, sacubitril/valsartan; SGLT2i, sodium glucose cotransporter 2 inhibitor. *Source:* Modified from Kario. Hypertension. 2018;71:997–1009 [1].

choice for patients with increased circulating volume should be salt restriction, diuretics, mineralocorticoid receptor antagonists (aldosterone blockers), sacubitril/valsartan, and sodium-glucose cotransporter 2 inhibitors (SGLT2i), while those with advanced vascular disease are theoretically more likely to benefit from

Morning systolic blood pressure (mmHg)

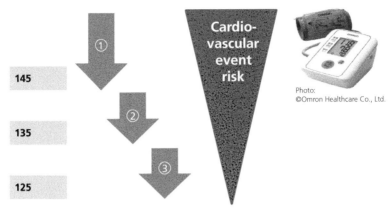

Figure 3.24 Home blood pressure-based antihypertensive strategy for morning hypertension. *Source:* Modified from Kario Essential Manual of 24-Hour Blood Pressure Management from Morning to Nocturnal Hypertension, Wiley -Blackwell, 2015: 1–138 [37].

Table 3.12 Target blood pressure (BP) levels for BP control (Japanese Society of Hypertension 2019 guidelines).

	Office BP	Home BP
Young, middle-aged, and early elderly patients	<130/80 (age <75 years)	<125/75 (age <75 years)
Late-elderly patients	<140/90 (age ≥75 years)	<135/85 (age ≥75 years)
Patients with diabetes	<130/80	<125/75
Patients with CAD	<130/80	<125/75
Patients with cerebrovascular disease	<130/80 (no bilateral carotid artery stenosis or occlusion of major cerebral artery)	<125/75 (no bilateral carotid artery stenosis or occlusion of major cerebral artery)
	<140/90 (present or undiagnosed bilateral carotid artery stenosis or occlusion of major cerebral artery)	<135/85 (present or undiagnosed bilateral carotid artery stenosis or occlusion of major cerebral artery)
Patients with CKD	<130/80 (proteinuria positive)	<125/75 (proteinuria positive)
	<140/90 (proteinuria negative)	<135/85 (proteinuria negative)
Patients currently taking antithrombotic drugs	<130/80	<125/75

CAD, coronary artery disease; CKD, chronic kidney disease.
Source: Modified from Umemura et al. Hypertens Res. 2019; 42: 1235–1481 [253].

Table 3.13 Home blood pressure targets for Asian patients with hypertension from the Hypertension Cardiovascular Outcome Prevention and Evidence (HOPE) Asia Network.

HOPE Asia network		
	Class of recommendation	Level of evidence
Antihypertensive strategies should target a home SBP of <135/85 mmHg	I	B
Strict antihypertensive treatment targeting a home SBP of <125 mmHg may have benefit in high-risk Asian patients with hypertension, especially those with diabetes or CKD, and/or cardiovascular disease	IIa	B

SBP, systolic blood pressure.
Source: Park et al. J Hum Hypertens. 2018; 32: 249–258 [183].

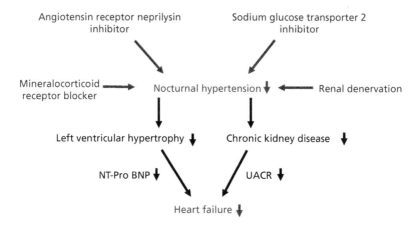

Figure 3.25 New drug classes and renal denervation lower nighttime blood pressure, resulting in regression of left ventricular hypertrophy, renal protection and a reduction in heart failure risk. ARNi, angiotensin receptor neprilysin inhibitors; CKD, chronic kidney disease; LVH, left ventricular hypertrophy; MR, mineralocorticoid receptor; NT-proBNP, N-terminal pro-brain natriuretic peptide; RDN, renal denervation; SGLT2i, sodium-glucose cotransport inhibitors; UACR, urinary albumin-creatinine ratio. *Source:* Kario K, Williams B. Nocturnal Hypertension and Heart Failure: Mechanisms, Evidence, and New Treatments. Hypertension. 2021; 78:564–577.

calcium channel blocker monotherapy or calcium channel blocker therapy combined with a renin–angiotensin system inhibitor [37, 227, 267–275]. Recent clinical outcome trials have clearly demonstrated that sacubitril/valsartan improved cardiovascular prognosis [276, 277] and that SGLT2i reduced the rate of cardiovascular events (especially in patients with heart failure) and prevented decline in renal function [278–280] (Figure 3.25). Sympatholytic treatment using β-/α-blockers [157, 231, 248] and renal denervation are effective for reducing the average and the peak of night-time BPs, especially in patients with OSA [281, 282]. Hypnotics, such as melatonin, melatonin receptor agonists, and orexin receptor antagonists [283], might be preferable for patients with sleep disorders [24, 284].

CHAPTER 4

BP targets, when to initiate antihypertensive therapy, and nonpharmacological treatment

Clinical implications of antihypertensive treatment

Recent guidelines have lowered the target threshold for defining blood pressure (BP) control during antihypertensive therapy (Table 4.1) [178, 185, 253, 254].

SPRINT and automated office BP

The most striking evidence directly influencing the 2017 AHA/ACC guidelines [178] was the results of the Systolic Blood Pressure Intervention Trial (SPRINT) study [179]. This trial clearly demonstrated the benefit of strict BP lowering to a systolic blood pressure (SBP) target of <120 mmHg in patients with hypertension. Rates of cardiovascular events and all-cause mortality were lower in the strict BP control group than in the standard BP control group (SBP <140 mmHg). After this intervention study, the direction of BP management has been clearly set. However, the evidence from SPRINT was obtained using automated office blood pressure (AOBP) measurement, which is different from routine office BP measurement. AOBP measurement uses an automated device and readings are taken after the patient has been in a sitting position for five minutes since the physician left the office. AOBP values for SBP are about 10–15 mmHg lower than those measured using standard office BP techniques. The AOBP approach may exclude the physician-associated white-coat effect but cannot eliminate the pressor effect of the office setting [180].

Meta-analysis of antihypertensive trials

A recent meta-analysis of data from 123 studies ($n = 613\,815$) showed that, regardless of baseline BP, a 10-mmHg reduction in SBP significantly reduced the rate of major cardiovascular events by 20%, coronary heart disease by 17%, stroke by 27%, heart failure by 28%, and all-cause of death by 13%. No effect of BP reduction on chronic kidney disease was identified (Figure 4.1) [285]

Essential Manual of 24-Hour Blood Pressure Management: From Morning to Nocturnal Hypertension,
Second Edition. Kazuomi Kario.
© 2022 John Wiley & Sons Ltd. Published 2022 by John Wiley & Sons Ltd.

Table 4.1 Guideline-defined office blood pressure targets (mmHg) during antihypertensive therapy.

	JSH 2019 [253]	ACC/AHA 2017 [178]	ESC/ESH 2018 [254]	HOPE Asia Network [185]
Young, middle-aged, and early elderly patients	<130/80 (age <75 years)	<130/80 (age <65 years)	SBP <130, ≥120 (age <65 years)	<130/80
Late-elderly patients	<140/90 (age ≥75 years)	<130/80 (age ≥65 years)	SBP <140, ≥130 (age ≥65 years)	<140/90 (elderly)
Patients with diabetes	<130/80	<130/80	SBP <130, ≥120	<130/80
Patients with CAD	<130/80	<130/80	SBP <130, ≥120	—
Patients with cerebrovascular disease	<130/80	<130/80	SBP <130, ≥120	—
Patients with CKD	<130/80 (proteinuria positive) <140/90 (proteinuria negative)	130/80 (with/ without proteinuria)	SBP <140, ≥130	—

ACC, American College of Cardiology; AHA, American Heart Association; CAD, coronary artery disease; CKD, chronic kidney disease; ESC, European Society of Cardiology; ESH, European Society of Hypertension; HOPE, Hypertension Cardiovascular Outcome Prevention and Evidence.
Source: Kario K. Essential Manual of 24 Hour Blood Pressure Management: From Morning to Nocturnal Hypertension, Second Edition. Wiley, 2022.

When to initiate antihypertensive therapy

Hypertension develops with advancing age. The predominant pressor effect in younger patients is neurohumoral activation, which is related to obesity and metabolic factors. Structural changes in both small and large arteries and increased salt sensitivity due to reduced renal function are important causes of hypertension as age increases (Figure 4.2) [286].

Lifestyle modification is the first intervention to target BP and should be stated when office BP is 130/80 mmHg or morning home BP is 125/75 mmHg. Strict BP control at the early stage of hypertension is important to prevent cardiovascular remodeling, organ damage, and cardiovascular events. For example, in patients with atrial fibrillation (AF), history of hypertension, and poor BP control before the onset of AF are significant risk factors for the occurrence of cardiovascular events after AF onset (Figure 4.3) [287].

Patient preference

The benefits of BP-lowering interventions are due to the reductions in BP per se, regardless of the methods used to achieve these decreases (including lifestyle modifications, drug therapy, and device usage) (Figure 4.4). This means that real-world management of hypertension can include options based on patient preference to maximize the BP reductions achieved during therapy.

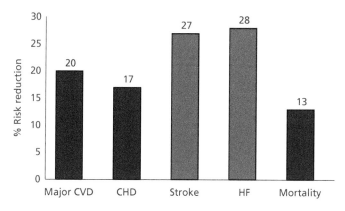

Figure 4.1 Percentage risk reduction associated with a 10-mmHg decrease in SBP during antihypertensive therapy (meta-analysis data; $n = 613815$). CHD, coronary heart disease; CVD, cardiovascular disease; HF, heart failure. *Source:* Created based on data from Ettehad et al. Lancet. 2016; 387(10022): 957–967 [285].

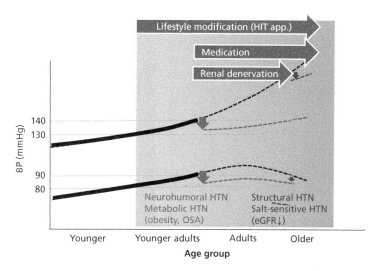

Figure 4.2 Age-related timing of antihypertensive therapy initiation (renin-angiotensin system inhibitors for younger patients with metabolic hypertension, and calcium channel blockers for older patients with structural and salt-sensitive hypertension. eGFR, estimated glomerular filtration rate; HIT, health information technology; HTN, hypertension; OSA, obstructive sleep apnea. *Source:* Republished with permission of Bentham Science Publishers, from Kario. Curr Hypertens Review. 2018; 14: 2–5 [286]; permission conveyed through Copyright Clearance Center, Inc.

Sodium intake

Salt restriction is the most effective nonpharmacological treatment approach in patients with hypertension, regardless of antihypertensive medication. A recent intervention study demonstrated that strict salt restriction prescribed by a nutritionist lowered salt intake (estimated by 24-hour urine sodium excretion) by an

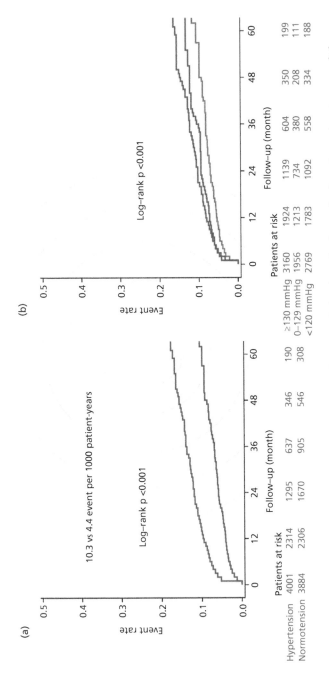

Figure 4.3 Kaplan-Meier curves showing the rate of cardiovascular events (ischemic stroke, hemorrhagic stroke, and acute myocardial infarction) in nonvalvular atrial fibrillation (NVAF) patients with vs. without preexisting hypertension before the onset of NVAF, overall (a), and in subgroups based on systolic blood pressure before NVAF onset (b). Data from 7885 patients from a Japanese database. *Source:* Kario et al. J Clin Hypertens. 2020; 22: 431–437 [287].

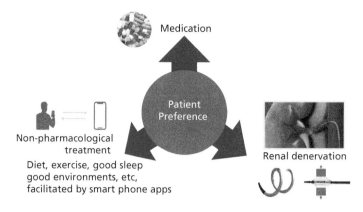

Figure 4.4 Patient preference-based approach for the management of hypertension. *Source:* Republished with permission of Bentham Science Publishers, from Kario. Curr Hypertens Rev. 2016; 12: 2–10 [180]. Permission conveyed through Copyright Clearance Center, Inc.

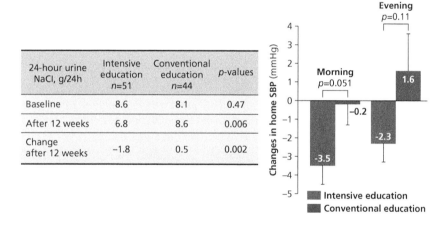

24-hour urine NaCl, g/24h	Intensive education n=51	Conventional education n=44	p-values
Baseline	8.6	8.1	0.47
After 12 weeks	6.8	8.6	0.006
Change after 12 weeks	−1.8	0.5	0.002

Figure 4.5 Effect of strict salt restriction prescribed by a nutritionist on urinary sodium (NaCl) excretion and home systolic blood pressure (SBP) in medicated patients with hypertension. *Source:* Nakano et al. J Clin Hypertens. 2016;18:385–392 [288].

additional 1.8 g/day in medicated patients with hypertension compared with conventional education by physicians. As a result, morning home SBP was marginally reduced (Figure 4.5), and ambulatory BP was significantly reduced throughout the 24-hour period, including daytime, nighttime, and morning (Figure 4.6) [288]. The between-group difference in the reduction of 24-hour SBP was at least 7 mmHg.

Other dietary requirements

A balanced, healthy diet plays an important role in helping to control BP. Key minerals include potassium, magnesium, and calcium.

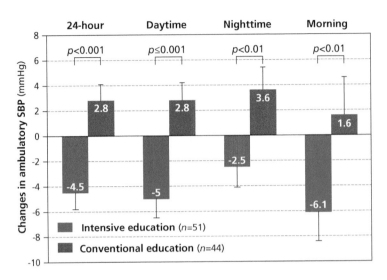

Figure 4.6 Effect of strict salt restriction prescribed by a nutritionist on ambulatory systolic blood pressure (SBP) in medicated patients with hypertension. *Source:* Nakano et al. J Clin Hypertens. 2016;18:385–392 [288].

Potassium has a strong relationship with sodium, the main regulator of extracellular fluid volume, including plasma volume. Low potassium intake increases the risk of hypertension, especially when combined with high sodium intake [289–292]. Conversely, higher potassium intake may help to decrease BP, secondary to increased vasodilation and urinary sodium excretion which reduces plasma volume, and these effects might be more pronounced in salt-sensitive individuals [293–295]. Specifically, meta-analysis data from 25 randomized controlled trials showed that potassium supplementation for 4–15 weeks was associated with reductions in SBP (–4.48 mmHg) and DBP (–2.96 mmHg) [296]. However, a Cochrane review that included the six highest-quality trials reported that reductions in SBP and DBP with potassium supplementation were nonsignificant [297]. However, caution needs to be exercised with potassium supplementation due to the increased risk of arrhythmias and other adverse events associated with hyperkalemia [298]. Fruits and vegetables have a higher concentrations of potassium than cereals and meats, therefore, a healthy diet high in fruit and vegetables is recommended to reduce the risk of hypertension.

Both magnesium and calcium play a role in vascular relaxation, meaning that deficiencies in these minerals could contribute to arterial stiffness, leading to hypertension. A comprehensive meta-analysis of randomized, double-blind, placebo-controlled trials found a significant reduction in both SBP and DBP during magnesium supplementation (weighted mean difference vs. placebo of –2.00 mmHg for SBP and –1.78 mmHg for DBP) (Figure 4.7) [299]. Similarly, systematic reviews of randomized trials investigating the effects of calcium supplementation [300, 301] on have shown a consistent decrease in BP (–2.5 mmHg for SBP in patients with hypertension, and –1.4 mmHg in normotensive individuals)

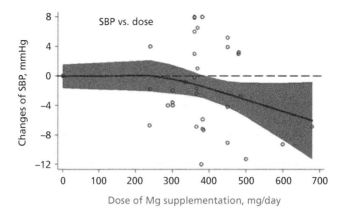

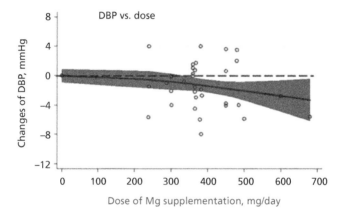

Figure 4.7 Overall effect of magnesium supplementation on systolic blood pressure (SBP; upper) and diastolic blood pressure (DBP; lower) in participants with or without hypertension. *Source:* Zhang et al. Hypertens. 2016;68:324–333 [299].

[300, 301]. Thus, ensuring adequate dietary intake of these key minerals as part of a healthy balanced diet is an important part of nonpharmacological strategies to prevent and manage hypertension.

Exercise

Regular physical activity can help to prevent hypertension and is part of strategies to reduce BP in patients with hypertension. Exercise prescription is a key component of lifestyle modification recommendations and can also be combined with antihypertensive drug therapy to help achieve target BP. Although there is a transient increase in BP during exercise, BP drops after exercise (in proportion to exercise intensity (Figure 4.8), contributing to lower overall BP [302].

Hypertension guidelines recommend regular, moderate-intensity dynamic aerobic exercise on 5–7 days per week, with advice to add resistance exercises

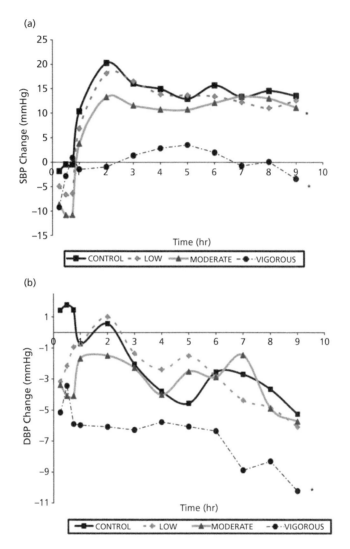

Figure 4.8 Awake systolic blood pressure (SBP; a) and diastolic blood pressure (DBP; b) change from baseline (mean ± standard deviation) at hourly intervals over 9 hours after control and different intensity exercise (control refers to seated rest). *p,0.001 for exercise vs. control. *Source:* Reprinted from Eicher et al. Am Heart J. 2010; 160: 513–520 [302], Copyright (2010), with permission from Elsevier.

on 2–3 days/week [254]. Regular medium-to-high intensity aerobic activity may reduce BP in patients with hypertension by a mean of 11/5 mmHg [303]. For healthy adults, the recommendation is for up to 300 minutes per week of aerobic physical activity or 150 minutes per week of vigorous-intensity aerobic physical activity, or equivalent combinations of the two forms of exercise [254]. Appropriate exercise therapy can also be recommended for elderly patients with hypertension [253].

Sleep hygiene

Sleep disturbance is closely associated with hypertension, metabolic disease, and various types of cardiovascular disease (Figure 4.9) [37,156,181,235,304,305]. Sleep disturbance includes sleep deprivation, shift-working, insomnia, obstructive sleep apnea syndrome (OSAS), restless leg syndrome, and narcolepsy. Nighttime BP and its variability could be the new hemodynamic cardiovascular risk indicator of these sleep-related disorders. Both not enough and too much sleep have been associated with attenuated nighttime BP dipping [306]. Sleep duration of 6–8 hours with good sleep quality is associated with lower cardiovascular risk [307–311]; therefore, good sleep hygiene should be encouraged in patients with hypertension.

Housing condition

Cold temperatures in the winter increase BP, especially in the morning, triggering cardiovascular events. Improving housing conditions by retrofitting insulation increased room temperature, and was associated with a significant BP reduction in the winter (Table 4.2) [217].

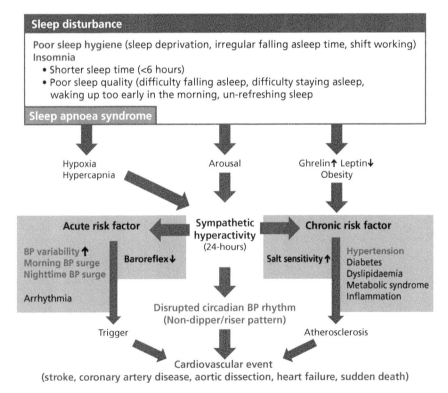

Figure 4.9 Sleep disturbance and related mechanisms of cardiovascular disease. BP, blood pressure. *Source:* Kario. Sleep and circadian cardiovascular Medicine. In: Encyclopedia of Cardiovascular Research and Medicine (Vasan R., Sawyer D., eds). Amsterdam, Netherlands. Elsevier 2018, pp. 424–437 [235], with permission from Elsevier.

Table 4.2 Effect of intervention and change in indoor temperature on home blood pressure in the morning and evening.

Predictor	Unadjusted			Model-1[a]			Model-2[b]		
	β	95% CI	P	β	95% CI	P	β	95% CI	P
Change in morning HSBP from the baseline survey (mmHg)									
Intervention vs. control	−2.6	−4.3 to −1.0	0.001	−3.1	−4.6 to −1.5	<0.001	−2.7	−4.2 to −1.1	0.001
Change in Temp$_{in}$ (°C)	—	—	—	—	—	—	−0.64	−0.78 to −0.49	<0.001
Change in morning HDBP from the baseline survey (mmHg)									
Intervention versus control	−1.8	−2.9 to −0.7	0.001	−2.1	−3.2 to −1.1	<0.001	−1.9	−3.0 to −0.9	<0.001
Change in Temp$_{in}$ (°C)	—	—	—	—	—	—	−0.29	−0.39 to −0.19	<0.001
Change in evening HSBP from the baseline survey (mmHg)									
Intervention versus control	−1.5	−3.2 to 0.1	0.069	−1.8	−3.4 to −0.2	0.029	−1.6	−3.1 to −0.0	0.046
Change in Temp$_{in}$ (°C)	—	—	—	—	—	—	−0.73	−0.88 to −0.57	<0.001
Change in evening HDBP from the baseline survey (mmHg)									
Intervention vs. control	−1.3	−2.4 to −0.1	0.028	−1.5	−2.6 to −0.4	0.006	−1.4	−2.5 to −0.3	0.010
Change in Temp$_{in}$ (°C)	—	—	—	—	—	—	−0.34	−0.44 to −0.23	<0.001

CI, confidence interval; HDBP, home diastolic blood pressure; HSBP, home systolic blood pressure; Temp$_{in}$, indoor ambient temperature.

[a] Model-1 included the treatment condition (intervention versus control) as a predictor, and was adjusted for HSBP/HDBP at the baseline survey, change in age, change in body mass index and change in outdoor temperature from baseline.

[b] Model-2 included the treatment condition (intervention versus control) and change in indoor temperature as predictors, and was adjusted for HSBP/HDBP at the baseline survey, change in age, change in body mass index, and change in outdoor temperature from baseline.

Source: Umishio et al. J Hypertens. 2020; 38: 2510–2518 [217].

Applications and algorithms to facilitate lifestyle modification: CureAPP

Digital therapeutics is a new approach to treat hypertension via using software programs such as smartphone apps and/or device algorithms. We have developed a new interactive smartphone app (HERB Mobile) associated with a web-based patient management console (HERB Console). This is designed to help achieve reductions in BP based on an algorithm that promotes lifestyle modifications in conjunction with medically validated nonpharmacological interventions [312].

The app can assess the personality, behavior characteristics, and hypertension determinants for each individual patient and provide appropriate, targeted. This app-supported lifestyle modification includes three steps—Step 1: input and education; Step 2: app-based recommendations for salt intake, body weight control, smoking cessation, alcohol restriction, exercise, sleep hygiene, and stress management; and Step 3—planning and evaluation (Figure 4.10) [312].

A feasibility study using this system and found that it had potential to facilitate a reduction in 24-hour BP. Therefore, a randomized, controlled, multicenter, open-label trial "HERB-DH1 (HERB digital hypertension 1)" was conducted to assess the efficacy of the HERB system in patients with essential hypertension. In this pivotal study, patients are allocated to the intervention group (HERB system + standard lifestyle modification) or control group (standard lifestyle modification alone). The mean change from baseline to 12 weeks in 24-h SBP on ABPM (primary outcome) was significantly greater in the digital therapeutics vs. control group [–4.9 vs. –2.5mmHg; between-group difference –2.4, 95% confidence interval (CI) –4.5 to –0.3, p = 0.024] (Figure 4.11) [313].

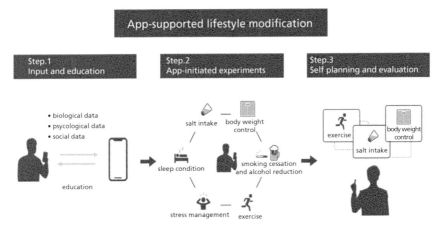

Figure 4.10 App-supported lifestyle modification in "HERB Mobile". The "HERB Mobile" uses a 3-step approach to ensure lifestyle modification: input and education, app-initiated experiments, and self-planning and evaluation. Through this process, app users can change their behavior to reduce their blood pressure. *Source:* Kario K et al. J Clin Hypertens. 2020; 22: 1713–1722 [312].

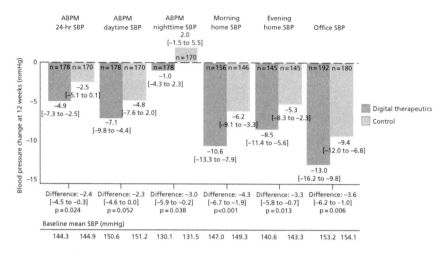

Figure 4.11 Changes from baseline to 12weeks in 24-h, daytime, and nighttime systolic blood pressure based on ambulatory blood pressure monitoring, morning and evening home systolic blood pressure, and office systolic blood pressure. Values are reported as mean [95% confidence interval]. ABPM, ambulatory blood pressure monitoring; SBP, systolic blood pressure. *Source*: Kario K et al. 2021 [313].

CHAPTER 5
Antihypertensive medication

Concept of 24-hour BP lowering including nighttime and morning BPs

To achieve perfect 24-hour blood pressure (BP) control, selection of long-acting antihypertensive agents is essential. The BP-lowering effect of short-acting drugs is attenuated from midnight through the early morning hours, while that of long-acting agents persist until the next morning drug dosage (Figure 5.1) [314]. In masked uncontrolled hypertension, reduction of morning home BP decreased important markers of target organ damage, including the urinary albumin-creatinine ratio (UACR), pulse wave velocity (PWV), and left ventricular hypertrophy (LVH) even though office BP did not change (Figure 5.2) [315].

Chronotherapy

Use of long-acting antihypertensive agents is required for perfect 24-hour BP control of morning and nocturnal hypertension (Table 5.1) [37]. Longer-acting antihypertensives are better at controlling nighttime and morning BP levels. These drugs are usually administered once daily in the morning, and provide continuous BP reduction over a 24-hour period to attenuate the exaggerated morning BP surge (MBPS).

Specific chronological treatment is based on the timing of antihypertensive dosing and selection of antihypertensive agent drug class(es). Specific treatment of the MBPS can be achieved using antihypertensive medication that reduces the pressor effect of neurohumoral factors potentiated in the morning (Figure 1.58) [106], such as agents that inhibit sympathetic activity or the renin-angiotensin-aldosterone system (RAAS) (Table 5.1) [37].

Bedtime dosing of antihypertensive drugs, especially calcium channel blockers (CCBs), alpha-blockers, and RAAS inhibitors, suppresses the exaggerated MBPS without excessive nocturnal hypotension during sleep. These treatments are also effective for nocturnal hypertension. On the other hand, specific drugs for reducing nighttime BP are those that reduce circulating volume, such as diuretics

Essential Manual of 24-Hour Blood Pressure Management: From Morning to Nocturnal Hypertension,
Second Edition. Kazuomi Kario.
© 2022 John Wiley & Sons Ltd. Published 2022 by John Wiley & Sons Ltd.

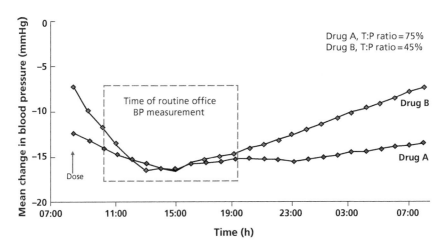

Figure 5.1 Twenty-four-hour blood pressure (BP)-lowering profiles of different antihypertensive agents. Although both may appear to have similar antihypertensive effects based on office BP, the two have very different profiles over 24 hours, as measured by ambulatory BP monitoring, with Drug A showing a more consist effect throughout the 24-hour dosing interval. *Source*: Based on Elliott et al. J Hypertens Suppl. 1996; 14: S15–S19 [314].

(including thiazide-type diuretics), indapamide, mineralocorticoid receptor blockers, sacubitril/valsartan, and sodium-glucose cotransporter (SGLT2) inhibitors.

Antihypertensive drug choice

In addition to BP-lower efficacy, selection of the appropriate antihypertensive drug(s) needs to take into account any concomitant conditions (Table 5.2) [253]. With respect to the effects of antihypertensive drug classes on cardiovascular event rates, beta-blockers provide less-effective prophylaxis of major cardiovascular events and stroke compared with other antihypertensive agents, while CCBs and angiotensin receptor blockers (ARBs) are the most effective agents for reducing the risk of stroke (Figure 5.3) [285]. However, diuretics appear to be superior to CCBs for preventing the development of heart failure (Figure 5.3) [285]. However, it is important to note that beta-blocker studies included in the meta-analysis used conventional agents that were available from the 1980s through to the early 2000s, such as propranolol and atenolol. Therefore, the effects of newer beta-blockers such as carvedilol and bisoprolol also need to be investigated.

Calcium channel blockers

CCBs have potent BP-lowering effects on morning BP when their antihypertensive effect persists for 24 hours. The most important characteristic of the BP-lowering effects of CCBs is that the extent of BP reduction almost always depends on pretreatment baseline BP. The higher the baseline BP, the greater the BP

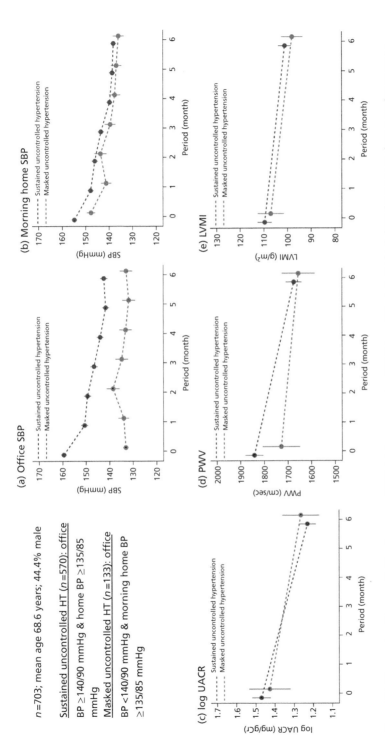

Figure 5.2 Changes in office systolic blood pressure (SBP) (a), home morning SBP (b), and the extent of subclinical CVD (c–e) during antihypertensive therapy in patients with sustained uncontrolled hypertension (HT) or masked uncontrolled HT. BP, blood pressure; CVD, cardiovascular disease; LVMI, left ventricular mass index; PWV, pulse wave velocity; SBP, systolic blood pressure; UACR, urinary albumin-creatinine ratio. Office SBP decreased only in the sustained uncontrolled HT group ($p < 0.001$ vs. baseline). Morning home SBP decreased significantly from baseline in both groups ($p < 0.001$). All indices of subclinical CVD were reduced during the study period in both groups (all $p < 0.001$). *Source:* Reprinted from Hoshide et al. J Am Coll Cardiol. 2018; 71: 2858–2859 [315]. Copyright (2015), with permission from Elsevier.

Table 5.1 Antihypertensive treatment to target morning and nocturnal hypertension.

	Non-specific	Specific
Morning hypertension (exaggerated morning BP surge)	Long-acting drug	Bedtime dosing of calcium channel blocker, RAS inhibitors, alpha-blocker
Nocturnal hypertension (Riser/non-dipper)	Long-acting drug	Diuretics (thiazides, mineral corticoid blocker) Bedtime dosing of RAS inhibitors, calcium channel blocker, alpha-blocker, Sacubitril/ valsartan (LCZ696) SGLT2 inhibitor

BP, blood pressure; RAS, renin-angiotensin system; SGLT2, sodium glucose cotransporter 2.
Source: Modified from Kario. Essential Manual of 24-Hour Blood Pressure Management from Morning to Nocturnal Hypertension. UK: Wiley Blackwell; 2015:1–138 [37].

Table 5.2 Indications for specific antihypertensive therapies based on the presence of comorbidities (based on 2019 recommendations from the Japanese Society of Hypertension).

	CCBs	ARB/ACEi	Thiazide diuretics	β-blockers
Left ventricular hypertrophy	●	●		
Heart failure with reduced ejection fraction		●[a]	●	●[a]
Tachycardia	● (non-dihydropyridines)			●
Angina	●			●[b]
Post-myocardial infarction		●		●
CKD patients with microalbuminuria and proteinuria		●		

[a]Start with low doses, increase gradually with due care and attention.
[b]Watch for coronary vasospastic angina.
ACEi, angiotensin converting-enzyme inhibitor; ARB, angiotensin receptor blocker; CCBs, calcium channel blockers; CKD, chronic kidney disease.
Source: Umemura et al. Hypertens Res. 2019;42:1235–1481 [253].

reduction achieved. The fact that CCBs do not lower BP extensively when baseline levels are lower means that these agents are ideally suited to reducing BP variability. In patients with a morning surge-type of morning hypertension, higher morning BP is reduced to a greater extent while lower nighttime BP is not reduced, resulting in an improved circadian BP pattern. In patients with nocturnal hypertension (non-dipper/riser type of nighttime BP), both higher nighttime BP and daytime BP could be similarly reduced by CCBs.

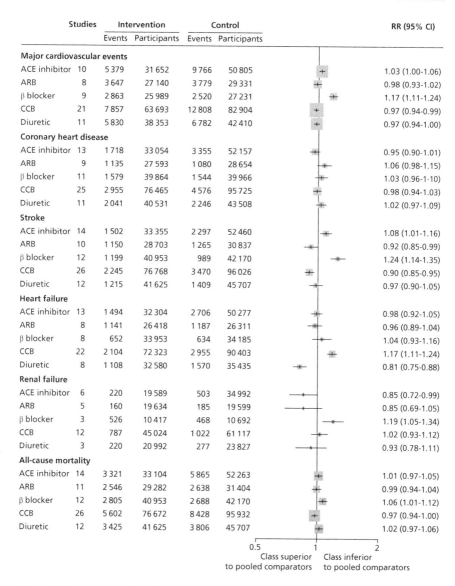

Studies	Intervention		Control		RR (95% CI)
	Events	Participants	Events	Participants	
Major cardiovascular events					
ACE inhibitor 10	5 379	31 652	9 766	50 805	1.03 (1.00-1.06)
ARB 8	3 647	27 140	3 779	29 331	0.98 (0.93-1.02)
β blocker 9	2 863	25 989	2 520	27 231	1.17 (1.11-1.24)
CCB 21	7 857	63 693	12 808	82 904	0.97 (0.94-0.99)
Diuretic 11	5 830	38 353	6 782	42 410	0.97 (0.94-1.00)
Coronary heart disease					
ACE inhibitor 13	1 718	33 054	3 355	52 157	0.95 (0.90-1.01)
ARB 9	1 135	27 593	1 080	28 654	1.06 (0.98-1.15)
β blocker 11	1 579	39 864	1 544	39 966	1.03 (0.96-1·10)
CCB 25	2 955	76 465	4 576	95 725	0.98 (0.94-1.03)
Diuretic 11	2 041	40 531	2 246	43 508	1.02 (0.97-1.09)
Stroke					
ACE inhibitor 14	1 502	33 355	2 297	52 460	1.08 (1.01-1.16)
ARB 10	1 150	28 703	1 265	30 837	0.92 (0.85-0.99)
β blocker 12	1 199	40 953	989	42 170	1.24 (1.14-1.35)
CCB 26	2 245	76 768	3 470	96 026	0.90 (0.85-0.95)
Diuretic 12	1 215	41 625	1 409	45 707	0.97 (0.90-1.05)
Heart failure					
ACE inhibitor 13	1 494	32 304	2 706	50 277	0.98 (0.92-1.05)
ARB 8	1 141	26 418	1 187	26 311	0.96 (0.89-1.04)
β blocker 8	652	33 953	634	34 185	1.04 (0.93-1.16)
CCB 22	2 104	72 323	2 955	90 403	1.17 (1.11-1.24)
Diuretic 8	1 108	32 580	1 570	35 435	0.81 (0.75-0.88)
Renal failure					
ACE inhibitor 6	220	19 589	503	34 992	0.85 (0.72-0.99)
ARB 5	160	19 634	185	19 599	0.85 (0.69-1.05)
β blocker 3	526	10 417	468	10 692	1.19 (1.05-1.34)
CCB 12	787	45 024	1 022	61 117	1.02 (0.93-1.12)
Diuretic 3	220	20 992	277	23 827	0.93 (0.78-1.11)
All-cause mortality					
ACE inhibitor 14	3 321	33 104	5 865	52 263	1.01 (0.97-1.05)
ARB 11	2 546	29 282	2 638	31 404	0.99 (0.94-1.04)
β blocker 12	2 805	40 953	2 688	42 170	1.06 (1.01-1.12)
CCB 26	5 602	76 672	8 428	95 932	0.97 (0.94-1.00)
Diuretic 12	3 425	41 625	3 806	45 707	1.02 (0.97-1.06)

0.5   1   2
Class superior   Class inferior
to pooled comparators   to pooled comparators

Figure 5.3 Event-controlling effect by antihypertensive drug class. ACE, angiotensin converting enzyme; ARB, angiotensin receptor blocker; CCB, calcium channel blocker; CI, confidence interval; RR, relative risk. *Source*: Reprinted from Ettehad et al. Lancet. 2016; 387: 957–967 [285], with permission from Elsevier.

There are several types of calcium channel in the body (Table 5.3) [316], and CCBs predominantly block L-type channels to antagonize vascular smooth muscle contraction, resulting in BP reduction. Cilnidipine and azelnidipine also have activity at N-type and L-type channels, respectively, resulting in a unique profile of 24-hour BP-lowering effect.

Table 5.3 Properties of calcium channels.

Type	Location	Location/Function
L-type	Vascular smooth muscle	Contraction of smooth muscle of blood vessels Contraction of myocardium Causes vasoconstriction
N-type	Neurons Brain	Regulates the release of norepinephrine from neuronal endings
T-type	Heart Kidney Adrenal glands	In heart, regulates pacemaker activity Dilates the afferent & efferent arterioles in the kidneys Stimulates the release of aldosterone
P-/Q-/R-type	Neurons	Neurotransmitter release

Source: Created based on data from Triggle. Biochemical Pharmacology. 2007 30;74:1–9 [316].

Amlodipine

Amlodipine, the CCB with the longest half-life, is the best drug for facilitating morning BP control when it is administered once daily in the morning. Amlodipine monotherapy was more effective than valsartan, a short-acting renin-angiotensin system (RAS) inhibitor, in controlling 24-hour ambulatory BP and morning BP in patients with hypertension (Figure 5.4) [317]. In addition, the prevalence of non-reactor patients (showing no reduction in morning BP) was reduced to a greater extent in the amlodipine group than in the valsartan group. The higher the baseline morning BP, the greater the difference between the two agents in morning BP-lowering effect.

In a titration study of amlodipine, 10 mg/day in a patient with uncontrolled hypertension treated with amlodipine 5 mg/day, similar characteristics of

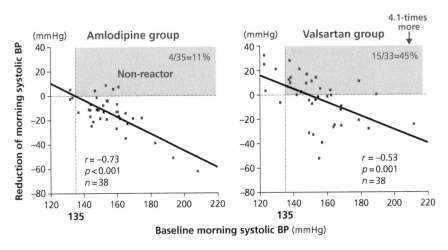

Figure 5.4 Ambulatory morning blood pressure (BP)-lowering effects of amlodipine vs. valsartan. *Source*: Created based on data from Eguchi et al. Am J Hypertens. 2004;17:112–117 [317].

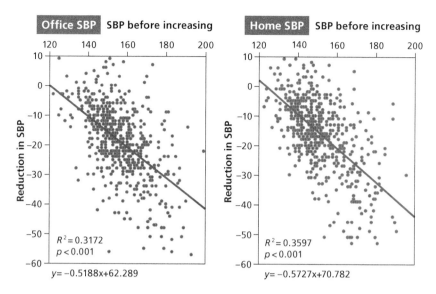

Figure 5.5 Systolic blood pressure (SBP)-lowering effect of increasing the dose of amlodipine from 5 to 10 mg once daily in 583 patients with uncontrolled hypertension in the Amlodipine Cohort study by Internet-based research for Evaluation of Efficacy (ACHIEVE) study. *Source*: Kario et al. Curr Hypertens Rev. 2011;7:102–110 [318]. Republished with permission of Bentham Science Publishers Ltd.

amlodipine were found even when the dosage was increased [318]. The BP-lowering effect of amlodipine titration from 5 to 10 mg/day is highly dependent on baseline BP both for office BP and home BP (Figure 5.5) [318]. This office- and home BP-lowering effect of amlodipine titration has been shown to be comparable in patients previously treated with amlodipine 5 mg monotherapy, amlodipine 5 mg in combination with an ARB, and amlodipine 5 mg combined with both an ARB and diuretics (Figure 5.6) [318].

Amlodipine has been shown to significantly reduce higher daytime BP, but not lower nighttime BP in extreme dippers, while in non-dippers, amlodipine reduced higher nighttime BP as well as higher daytime BP (Figure 5.7) [319]. In a meta-analysis of Asian studies (two crossover and nine parallel controlled studies), where ten studies used amlodipine and one used nifedipine gastrointestinal therapeutic system (GITS), the ambulatory BP-lowering effect of CCBs was greater than that of RAS inhibitors, and the slope of the regression lines was comparable for both nighttime and daytime BP measurements (Figure 5.8) [320].

Nifedipine

Nifedipine is a potent vasodilating drug that reduces nighttime BP and morning BP in patients with hypertension. In the recent prospective, randomized, multicenter, open-label Calcium Antagonist Controlled-Release High-Dose Therapy in Uncontrolled Refractory Hypertensive Patients (CARILLON) study, the

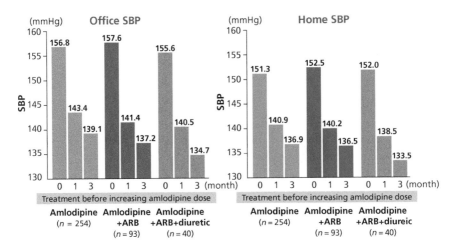

Figure 5.6 Effect of increasing the dosage of once-daily amlodipine from 5 to 10 mg in patient subgroups based on baseline medication status in 583 patients with uncontrolled hypertension in the Amlodipine Cohort study by Internet-based research for Evaluation of Efficacy (ACHIEVE) study. ARB, angiotensin receptor blocker; SBP, systolic blood pressure. *Source*: Kario et al. Curr Hypertens Rev. 2011;7:102–110 [318]. Republished with permission of Bentham Science Publishers Ltd.

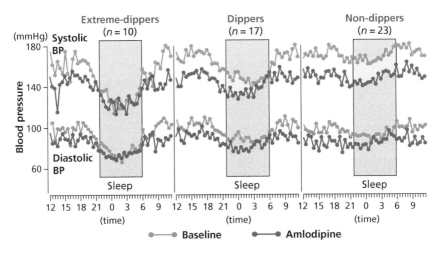

Figure 5.7 Differential blood pressure (BP)-lowering effect of amlodipine on nighttime BP in patient subgroups based on dipping status. *Source*: Kario and Shimada Am J Hypertens. 1997; 10: 261–268 [319].

ambulatory BP-lowering of nifedipine controlled release (CR) (80 mg)/ candesartan (8 mg) vs. amlodipine (10 mg)/candesartan (8 mg) was investigated in patients with uncontrolled hypertension ($n = 51$). Changes in 24-hour BP were comparable between the groups. The nifedipine group demonstrated a

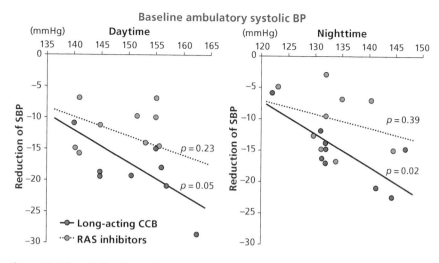

Figure 5.8 Effect of dihydropyridine calcium channel blockers on 24-hour systolic blood pressure (SBP) in Eastern Asians. BP, blood pressure; RAS, renin-angiotensin system. *Source*: Wang et al. Hypertens Res. 2011; 34: 423–430 [320].

significant decrease in the UACR, whereas the amlodipine group demonstrated a significant decrease in N-terminal pro-brain natriuretic peptide (NT-proBNP) level. Patients with higher daytime and morning surge in systolic blood pressure (SBP) at baseline had greater reductions in ambulatory BP when treated with the nifedipine combination compared with the amlodipine combination (Figure 5.9) [321].

The prospective, randomized, parallel-group, crossover effects of vasodilating vs. sympatholytic antihypertensives on sleep blood pressure in hypertensive patients with sleep apnea syndrome (VASSPS) study [231], evaluated the effects of a nighttime dose of vasodilating (nifedipine CR 40 mg) vs. sympatholytic (carvedilol 20 mg) antihypertensive agents on nighttime BP using a recently developed trigger nighttime home BP monitor (TNP) with an oxygen-triggered function that initiates BP measurement when oxygen saturation falls. The BP-lowering effects of nifedipine on the mean ($p<0.05$) and minimum ($p<0.01$) nighttime SBP readings, and morning SBP ($p<0.001$) were greater than those of carvedilol (Figure 2.73 and Table 2.6) [231]. Nighttime SBP surge (difference between the hypoxia-peak SBP measured by the oxygen-triggered function and SBP readings within 30 minutes before and after the peak SBP) was only significantly reduced by carvedilol ($p<0.05$).

Cilnidipine

Cilnidipine, a unique lipophilic L-/N-type CCB, suppresses sympathetic activity by inhibiting N-type calcium channel-associated norepinephrine release from peripheral sympathetic nerve endings. The Ambulatory Blood Pressure Control

CARILLON

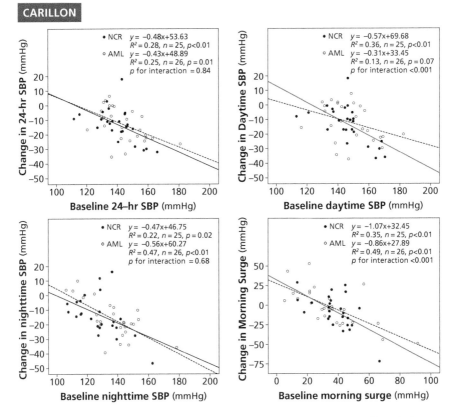

Figure 5.9 Comparison of ambulatory systolic blood pressure (SBP)-lowering effects during treatment with higher dosages of different calcium channel blockers in patients with uncontrolled hypertension in the Calcium Antagonist Controlled-Release High-Dose Therapy in Uncontrolled Refractory Hypertensive Patients (CARILLON) study. AML, amlodipine 10 mg + candesartan 8 mg; NCR, nifedipine 80 mg + candesartan 8 mg. *Source*: Mizuno et al. Blood Press. 2017; 26: 284–293 [321]. Copyright Skandinaviska Stiftelsen för Hjärt-och Kärlforskning, reprinted by permission of Taylor & Francis Ltd. www.tandfonline on behalf of Skandinaviska Stiftelsen för Hjärt-och Kärlforskning.

and Home Blood Pressure (Morning and Evening) Lowering by N-Channel Blocker Cilnidipine (ACHIEVE-ONE) trial was a large-scale clinical study of 2319 patients with hypertension treated with cilnidipine. After 12 weeks' therapy, both morning SBP and pulse rate (PR) self-measured at home reduced to a greater extent in patients with higher baseline morning SBP (−3.2 mmHg and −1.3 beats per minute [bpm] in patients with morning SBP in the first quartile; −30.9 mmHg and −3.2 bpm for those with morning SBP in the fourth quartile), and also reduced home morning PR and SBP to a greater extent in those with a higher baseline morning PR (by 0.6 bpm and −15.6 mmHg when PR was <70 bpm, and −9.7 bpm and −20.2 mmHg when PR was ≥85 bpm). When the

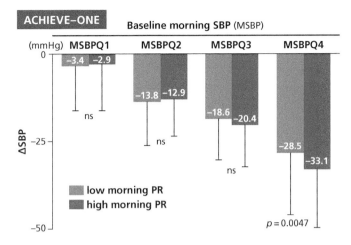

Figure 5.10 Changes in home morning systolic blood pressure (MSBP) during treatment with cilnidipine in patient subgroups based on baseline morning blood pressure and pulse rate (PR). MSBP quartile (Q) 1: <142.7 mmHg; MSBP Q2: ≥142.7 to <151.7 mmHg; MSBP Q3; ≥151.7 to ≤161.2 mmHg; MSBP Q4 ≥161.3 mmHg; low morning PR: <70 beats/min; high morning PR ≥70 beats/min. *Source*: Kario et al. J Clin Hypertens. 2013; 15: 133–142 [322].

study subjects were separated into two groups based on higher (≥70 bpm) and lower (<70 bpm) PR within each quartile of morning SBP, the highest quartile, higher PR groups had a greater reduction in morning SBP than the lower PR group (by 4.6 mmHg) (Figure 5.10) [322]. These results suggest that cilnidipine significantly reduced BP and PR in patients with morning hypertension and increased sympathetic activity.

In another study, ambulatory BP monitoring (ABPM) data were obtained from 615 patients and classified according to their nighttime dipping status as extreme dippers, dippers, non-dippers, or risers. Twelve weeks' treatment with cilnidipine significantly reduced 24-hour BP in all groups ($p < 0.001$ vs. baseline). Changes in nighttime SBP from baseline (with baseline values) were −17.9 (154.6), −11.9 (142.1), −6.6 (128.5), and 0.1 mmHg (115.8 mmHg), respectively, in risers, non-dippers, dippers, and extreme dippers. Changes from baseline in nighttime SBP reduction rate were 8.2% in risers ($p < 0.001$), but −7.0% in extreme dippers ($p < 0.001$), while no change was observed in the overall rate of nighttime SBP reduction (Figure 5.11) [323]. These results show that cilnidipine partially, but significantly, restored abnormal nighttime dipping status toward a normal dipping pattern in patients with hypertension.

Azelnidipine

Azelnidipine, another lipophilic L-/T-type CCB, restored baroreflex sensitivity and significantly lowered the heart rate to reduce morning BP compared with amlodipine [324, 325]. In a comparative ABPM study of azelnidipine 16 mg and amlodipine

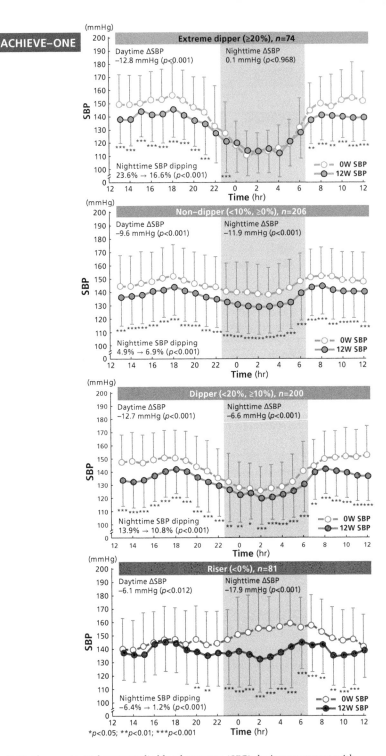

Figure 5.11 Changes in 24-hour systolic blood pressure (SBP) during treatment with cilnidipine in patient subgroups based on nighttime dipping status. *Source*: Kario et al. J Clin Hypertens. 2013; 15: 465–472 [323].

5 mg, the 24-hour BP-lowering effect, including nighttime and morning BP, was comparable between the two groups (Figure 5.12) [326]. However, 24-hour daytime and nighttime PR values were significantly suppressed in the azelnidipine group, but were increased in the amlodipine group. In our real-world observational At HOME study, office and morning home BP values were reduced to a similar extent during azelnidipine therapy, but approximately 20 mmHg for SBP and about 10 mmHg for DBP (Figure 5.13) [327].

Angiotensin-converting enzyme inhibitors

The RAS is activated in the morning and could contribute to the MBPS and the morning increase in cardiovascular risk. Long-acting angiotensin-converting enzyme (ACE) inhibitors have been reported to lower ambulatory BP without disruption of diurnal BP variation. It has been demonstrated that, in addition to circulating factors in the cardiovascular system, tissue RAS also exhibits diurnal variation, possibly in relation to a clock gene [118, 328]. In addition to reducing morning BP, ACE inhibitors may also suppress morning activation of the tissue RAS, improving protection against organ damage, and cardiovascular events in patients with hypertension.

Trandolapril is an ACE inhibitor with one of the longest-acting activity profiles, and therefore BP-lowering effects, due to its lipophilic nature [329]. The effects of bedtime vs. morning dosing of trandolapril on morning BP were studied. In the bedtime-administered group, prewakening and morning SBP levels were significantly decreased (Figure 5.14) [329]. Conversely, reductions in prewakening SBP and morning SBP did not reach statistical significance in the morning-administered group. There was no additional reduction in lowest nighttime BP in either group. Thus, bedtime administration of trandolapril appears to control morning BP without causing excessive nighttime falls in BP [329].

Angiotensin receptor blockers (ARBs)

As well as ACE inhibitors, previous large clinical trials have shown that treatment with an ARB is associated with significant suppression of organ damage and cardiovascular events [330–332]. However, different ARBs have markedly different effects on morning BP levels and the MBPS. This is due to differences in plasma half-life and the characteristics of binding to and dissociation from vascular angiotensin II receptors.

Valsartan
Valsartan is a short-acting ARB, and ideally, treatment should be given twice a day. The morning BP-lowering effect of once-daily valsartan is weaker than that of long-acting amlodipine [317].

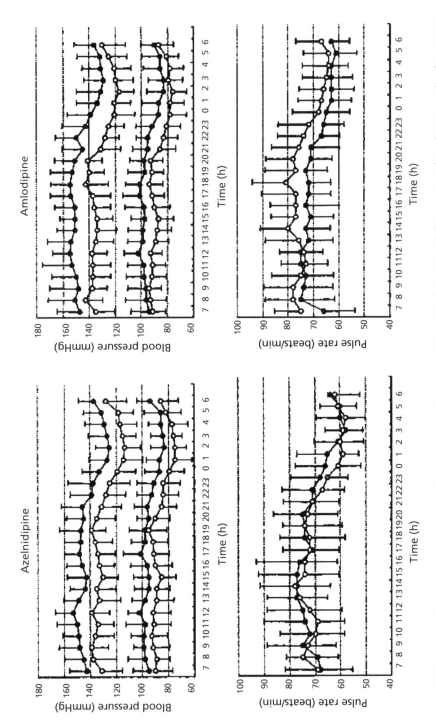

Figure 5.12 Diurnal variation of systolic and diastolic blood pressure and pulse rate before (solid circles) and after (open circles) after six weeks of treatment with azelnidipine in a six-week randomized double-blind study of 46 patients with essential hypertension. *Source:* Kuramoto et al. Hypertens Res. 2003; 26: 201–208 [326].

Objective:	**To determine the BP-and pulse rate-lowering effects of azelnidipine, a long-acting CCB, administered once daily in the morning.**
Study design:	• Open-label monitoring inmorning (At-HOME) study • *N*=4852 (mean age 64.8 years) **Inclusion:** • High SBP: ✓ Morning home SBP ≥135 mmHg ✓ Daytime office SBP ≥140 mmHg

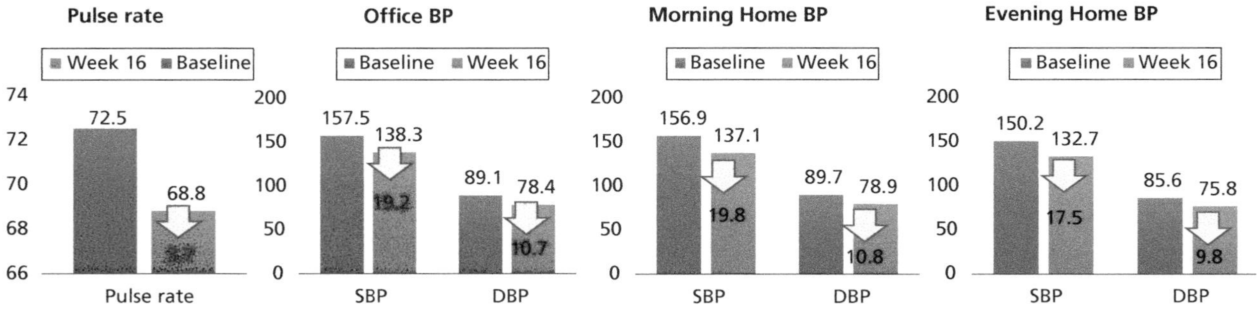
Pulse rate
Week 16
Baseline
74
72
70
68
66
72.5
68.8
Pulse rate
Office BP
Baseline
Week 16
200
150
100
50
0
157.5
138.3
19.2
89.1
78.4
10.7
SBP
DBP
Morning Home BP
Baseline
Week 16
200
150
100
50
0
156.9
137.1
19.8
89.7
78.9
10.8
SBP
DBP
Evening Home BP
Baseline
Week 16
200
150
100
50
0
150.2
132.7
17.5
85.6
75.8
9.8
SBP
DBP

Figure 5.13 Effects of azelnidipine on office and morning home blood pressure (BP), and pulse rate. At HOME (Azelnidipine Treatment for Hypertension Open-label Monitoring in the Early morning) study. CCB, calcium channel blocker; DBP, diastolic BP; SBP, systolic BP. *Source*: Created based on data from Kario et al. Drugs R D. 2013; 13: 63–73 [327].

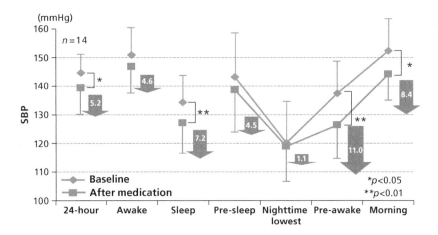

Figure 5.14 Effect of bedtime dosing of the long-acting angiotensin-converting enzyme inhibitor, trandolapril, on morning systolic blood pressure (SBP) in patients with hypertension. *Source*: Kuroda et al. Hypertens Res. 2004; 27: 15–20 [329].

Telmisartan

Telmisartan is a lipophilic ARB with the longest half-life (24 hours) of all agents in this class. A meta-analysis of the clinical efficacy of telmisartan with respect to reductions in BP in the morning hours was superior to that of short-acting nonlipophilic ARBs [333].

Candesartan

Candesartan is a specific and competitive antagonist of angiotensin-1 receptors [334]. A prospective crossover study in 73 patients with essential hypertension compared the effects of candesartan and lisinopril on ambulatory BP and early-morning BP, assessed using ABPM, and low doses of a thiazide diuretic could be added if needed [335]. The two agents had satisfactory and almost identical effects on 24-hour BP. When patients were classified into a morning surge group (the highest quartile of morning SBP surge; >36 mmHg) and a nonmorning surge group (the remaining three quartiles of morning SBP surge), candesartan was superior to lisinopril for decreasing morning BP and the MBPS [335].

The open-label, multicenter Japan Target Organ Protection (J-TOP) study was conducted in 450 patients with hypertension with self-measured home SBP >135 mmHg [223]. The results showed that bedtime dosing of candesartan titrated based on self-measured home BP was more effective for reducing albuminuria than morning dosing of an ARB in subjects with sufficiently well-controlled home BP levels both in the morning and in the evening [223]. This beneficial effect was greater in subjects with morning-dominant hypertension (morning and evening difference in home SBP of >15 mmHg) than in those with a morning and evening difference of <15 mmHg (Figure 5.15) [223]. In the J-TOP study, even though the morning BP-lowering effect was similar between the bedtime-dosing and morning-dosing groups, bedtime dosing of an ARB may be more effective for reducing albuminuria because it might suppress tissue RAS during the sleep-early morning period more potently than morning dosing [223].

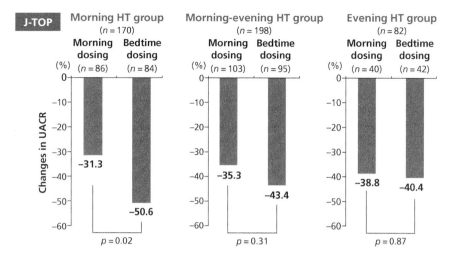

Figure 5.15 Effect of bedtime vs. morning dosing of candesartan on the urinary albumin-creatinine ratio (UACR) in patients with hypertension (HT). *Source*: Kario et al. J Hypertens. 2010; 28: 1574–1583 [223].

Olmesartan

Olmesartan is a potent ARB with persistent BP-lowering effects for 24 hours, including the nighttime and morning periods. Olmesartan can restore nighttime BP fall, as seen with diuretics and sodium restriction, possibly by enhancing daytime sodium excretion [336].

Once-daily use of olmesartan reduces morning home BP to a similar extent as office BP. The home BP-lowering effects of olmesartan were examined using data from the Home BP measurement with Olmesartan Naive patients to Establish Standard Target blood pressure (HONEST) study, a prospective observational study in patients with hypertension ($n = 21\,341$). Olmesartan reduced both office and morning home BP levels to a similar extent, indicating that the BP-lowering effect of olmesartan persists for 24 hours (Figure 5.16) [56, 337].

The BP-lowering effect of olmesartan for both morning home and office BP depends on the baseline BP level, as shown by similar slopes for the relationship between BP reduction and baseline BP (Figure 5.17) [338]. The effects of 16 weeks' treatment with olmesartan on office and morning home BP were comparable in previously treated and previously untreated patients with hypertension (Figure 5.18) [338]. When study subjects were stratified into masked hypertension, white-coat hypertension, poorly controlled hypertension, and well-controlled hypertension groups based on baseline office and morning home BP readings at 16 weeks, changes in office SBP were −1.0, −15.2, −23.1, and 1.8 mmHg, respectively, and changes in morning home SBP were −12.5, 1.0, −20.3, and 2.0 mmHg, respectively (Figure 5.19) [337]. Thus, in real-world clinical practice, olmesartan-based treatment decreased high morning home BP or office BP without excessive decreases in normal morning home BP or office BP in patient subgroups defined by the type of hypertension [339].

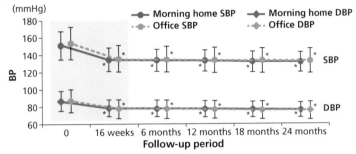

Figure 5.16 Change in office and morning home blood pressure (BP). At baseline, morning home BP was 151.2/86.9mmHg, and office BP was 153.6/87.1mmHg. Favorable BP control was maintained for two years. After two years, morning home BP was 131.5/76.3mmHg, and office BP was 132.6/75.6mmHg. DBP, diastolic BP; SBP, systolic BP. *Source*: Kario et al. Hypertension. 2014;64: 989–996 [56].

HONEST study data for patients who were not on antihypertensive medication at baseline were classified based on quartiles of baseline morning home SBP (MHSBP). In each group, patients were further classified based on baseline morning home pulse rate (MHPR). Patients with hypertension and chronic kidney disease (CKD) who had baseline MHSBP values in the fourth quartile (≥165mmHg) and a MHPR ≥70beats/minute showed a greater reduction in BP (−36.9mmHg) than those with MHPR <70bpm (−30.4mmHg) after 16weeks of olmesartan treatment. BP reductions were even greater in patients with vs. without CKD in this group (−6.6 vs. −2.2mmHg) (Figure 5.20) [340]. These data show that olmesartan was more effective in patients with hypertension who had high MHSBP and MHPR ≥70beats/minute, especially in those with CKD, suggesting that olmesartan may have enhanced BP-lowering effects by improving renal ischemia in patients with hypertension and CKD, and potential increased sympathetic nerve activity.

Azilsartan
Azilsartan, a novel ARB, has been reported to be more effective for lowering BP than other ARBs, and to have a potent antihypertensive effect over 24hours. A randomized, double-blind study of 14weeks' treatment with azilsartan (20–40mg once daily; $n = 273$) or candesartan (8–12mg once daily; $n = 275$) in Japanese patients with hypertension showed that azilsartan lowered nighttime BP in those with a dipper pattern of nighttime BP (≥10% decrease from daytime SBP) more extensively than daytime BP in non-dippers. In addition, azilsartan reduced the MBPS to a greater extent in those with exaggerated MBPS, reduced daytime SBP to a greater extent than nighttime SBP, and decreased daytime SBP to a significantly greater extent than candesartan (Figure 5.21) [341]. Thus, once-daily azilsartan improved non-dipping nighttime SBP to a greater extent than candesartan in this patient group.

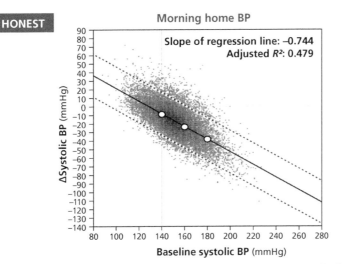

HONEST

Morning home BP

Slope of regression line: –0.744
Adjusted R^2: 0.479

Baseline BP (mmHg)	Predicted reduction (mmHg)	95% prediction interval (mmHg)	Predictive value after 16 weeks (mmHg)	Baseline dose of olmesartan (mg/day, mean ± SD)
140	–8.4	–33.5 to 16.8	131.6 (106.5 to 156.8)	18.1 ± 7.3
160	–23.2	–48.3 to 1.9	136.8 (111.7 to 161.9)	18.1 ± 6.7
180	–38.1	–63.2 to –13.0	141.9 (116.8 to 167.0)	18.9 ± 6.6

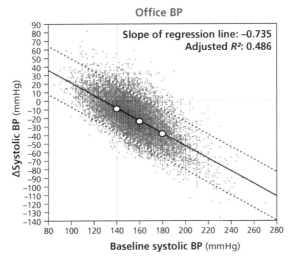

Office BP

Slope of regression line: –0.735
Adjusted R^2: 0.486

Baseline BP (mmHg)	Predicted reduction (mmHg)	95% prediction interval (mmHg)	Predictive value after 16 weeks (mmHg)	Baseline dose of olmesartan (mg/day, mean ± SD)
140	–8.4	–36.6 to 20.0	131.6 (103.4 to 160.0)	18.2 ± 7.3
160	–23.1	–51.3 to 5.1	136.9 (108.7 to 165.1)	18.1 ± 6.9
180	–37.8	–66.0 to –9.6	142.2 (114.0 to 170.4)	18.3 ± 6.5

Figure 5.17 Changes from baseline in systolic blood pressure (BP) after 16 weeks of olmesartan-based treatment. SD, standard deviation. *Source*: Kario et al. Hypertens Res. 2016;39: 334–341 [338].

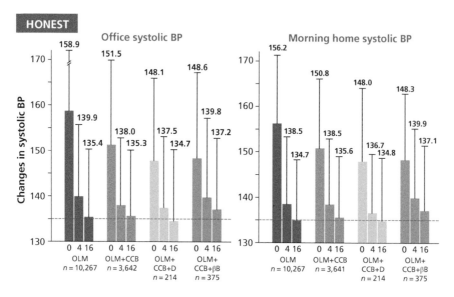

Figure 5.18 Change in clinic and morning home blood pressure (BP) after 16 weeks of olmesartan (OLM) monotherapy or combination therapy (excluding patients who switched antihypertensive treatment). ßB, beta-blocker; CCB, calcium channel blocker; D, diuretic. *Source*: Kario et al. Hypertens Res. 2016;39: 334–341 [338].

We also compared the efficacy of azilsartan and candesartan for controlling morning SBP surges in patients with and without BP surges at baseline. In the morning surge group ($n = 147$; sleep-trough BP surge ≥35 mmHg), azilsartan significantly reduced both the sleep-trough surge and the prewakening surge at week 14 compared with candesartan (least squares mean between-group differences of −5.8 [$p = 0.0395$] and −5.7 mmHg [$p = 0.0228$], respectively) (Figure 5.22) [342]. This shows that once-daily azilsartan improved the sleep-trough surge and pre-wakening surge to a greater extent than candesartan in Japanese patients with hypertension.

There are several characteristics of azilsartan that could account for its better 24-hour BP-lowering profiles compared with valsartan, including (1) higher affinity for, and slower dissociation from, angiotensin II type-1 receptors; (2) a longer half-life of around 13 hours; and (3) increased lipophilicity.

In the multicenter, randomized, open-label, parallel Azilsartan Circadian and Sleep Pressure – the 1st (ACS1) study, the nighttime BP-lowering effect of azilsartan 20 mg was weaker than that of amlodipine 5 mg, especially in older patients with hypertension [343]. In a post hoc analysis, azilsartan significantly reduced DBP compared with amlodipine in male patients aged <60 years, but amlodipine was significantly more effective than azilsartan at lowering SBP in female patients aged ≥60 years. In both younger and older patients with hypertension, shorter duration of hypertension history was significantly associated with greater 24-hour SBP reduction during therapy (Table 5.4) [344].

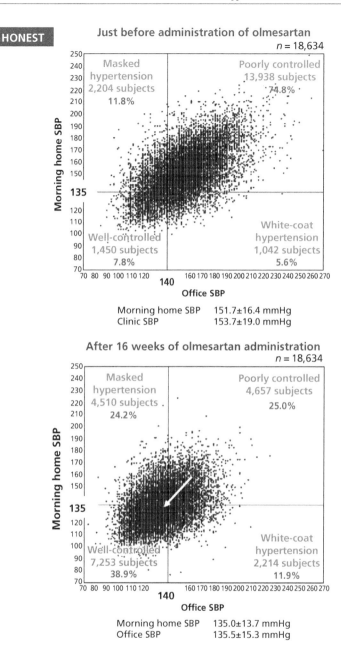

Figure 5.19 Change in office and morning home blood pressure (BP) after 16 weeks of olmesartan treatment in patient groups based on the type of hypertension. SBP, systolic BP. *Source*: Kario et al. J Hum Hypertens. 2013;27: 721–728 [337].

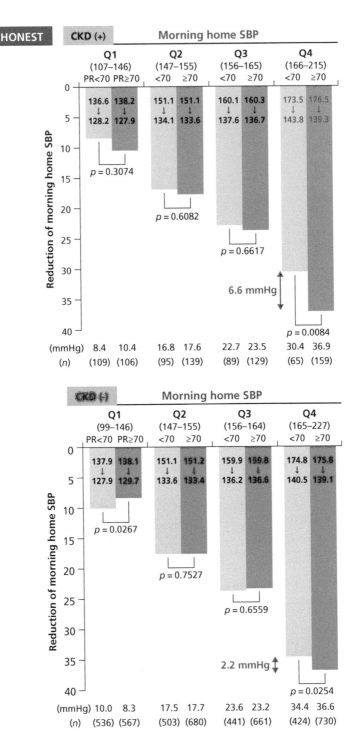

Figure 5.20 Change in morning home systolic blood pressure (SBP) after 16 weeks of olmesartan treatment in patient subgroups based on quartiles of baseline morning SBP and pulse rate (PR), in patients with or without coexisting chronic kidney disease. *Source*: Kario et al. J Clin Hypertens. 2014;16:442–450 [339].

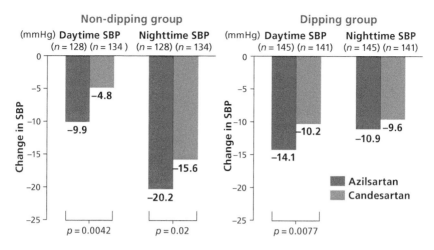

Figure 5.21 Differential effect of azilsartan on 24-hour ambulatory systolic blood pressure (SBP) in patients with a dipper or non-dipper profile of nighttime blood pressure. *Source*: Rakugi et al. Blood Press. 2013;22 Supl 1:22–28 [341]. Copyright Sk-andinaviska Stiftelsen för Hjärt-och Kärlforskning, reprinted by permission of Taylor & Francis Ltd. www. tandfonline on behalf of Skandinaviska Stiftelsen för Hjärt-och Kärlforskning.

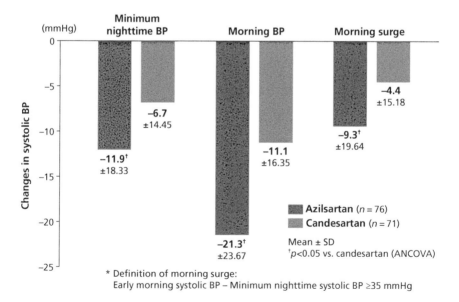

Figure 5.22 Azilsartan reduces morning BP preferentially in patients with morning surge. Of the hypertensive patients randomized into 16-week azilsartan treatment (20 mg for 8 weeks followed by an increased dose of 40 mg) and candesartan treatment groups (8 mg for 8 weeks followed by an increased dose of 12 mg), 147 patients whose morning surge was confirmed by ambulatory BP monitoring at weeks 0 and 14 were examined (double-blind controlled study). *Source*: Rakugi et al. Blood Press Monit. 2014; 19: 164–169 [342].

Table 5.4 Variables affecting reduction in 24-hour systolic blood pressure (SBP) during treatment with azilsartan. ACS1 study.

Multivariate analysis in patients younger than 60 years		
	24-hour SBP	
Variable	ß	p-value
Azilsartan		
Intercept	12.31	0.2472
Baseline SBP	−0.18	0.0103
BMI ≥25 kg/m²	4.45	0.0208
Smoker	4.53	0.0451
Duration of hypertension <5 y	−4.86	0.0425
Drinking	ND	ND
Amlodipine		
Intercept	43.39	<0.0001
Baseline SBP	−0.42	<0.0001
Complication of type 2 diabetes mellitus	7.06	0.0028
Male	5.72	0.0010
Duration of hypertension <5 y	ND	ND
BMI ≥25 kg/m²	ND	ND
Multivariate analysis in patients older than 60 years		
	24-hour SBP	
Variable	ß	p-value
Azilsartan		
Intercept	35.60	0.0042
Baseline SBP	−0.31	0.0002
Smoker	7.25	0.0068
Duration of hypertension <5 y	−4.90	0.0189
BMI ≥25 kg/m²	ND	ND
Amlodipine		
Intercept	48.31	<0.0001
Baseline SBP	−0.47	<0.0001
Male	4.91	0.0004
BMI ≥25 kg/m²	3.68	0.0076

BMI, body mass index; ND, not detectable; y, years.
Source: Kario et al. J Clin Hypertens. 2016; 18: 672–678 [344].

Diuretics

Diuretics are associated with a sustained BP-lowering effect, and they have well-established effectiveness for the prevention of cardiovascular events, especially heart failure (Figure 5.3) [285], even in elderly patients with hypertension. The mechanism of action of diuretics means that these agents provide specific reduction of nighttime BP. When morning hypertension is treated using diuretics,

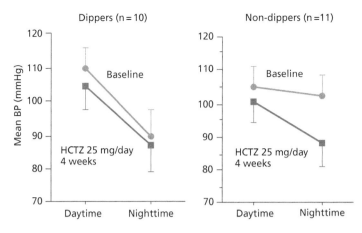

Figure 5.23 Differential blood pressure (BP)-lowering effect of diuretics in dippers vs. non-dippers. HCTZ, hydrochlorothiazide. *Source*: Uzu and Kimura Circulation. 1999; 100: 1635–1638 [345]

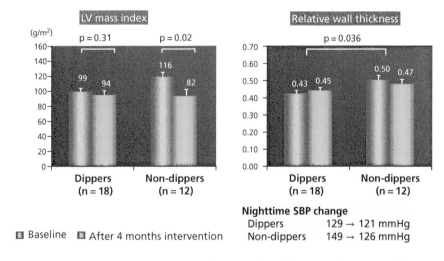

Figure 5.24 Effect of salt restriction+indapamide 1–2 mg/day on left ventricular (LV) remodelling (JMS Cardiovascular center, $n = 30$). SBP, systolic blood pressure. *Source*: Ishikawa et al. Blood Press Monit. 2011; 16(4):172–9 [346].

patients with a non-dipper profile shift toward becoming dippers, while the dipping pattern of those with a dipper profile remains unchanged or nighttime BP is reduced to a greater extent (Figure 5.23) [345]. The reduction of nighttime SBP in non-dippers after four months of management using salt restriction and indapamide was associated with a significant reduction in the left ventricular mass index (LVMI) (Figure 5.24) [346]. These effects persist or are greater when diuretics are used in combination with RAS inhibitors because RAS inhibitors increase salt sensitivity.

Alpha-adrenergic blockers and beta-adrenergic blockers

Alpha-adrenergic and alpha/beta-adrenergic blockers are effective in reducing MBPS in patients with hypertension. In particular, nighttime dosing of alpha-adrenergic blockers results in peak BP-lowering effect in the mornings, providing greater BP reductions during overnight and early morning hours. In the hypertension and lipid trial (HALT), bedtime administration of the alpha-1 blocker doxazosin predominantly reduced morning BP [11, 347]. In another study, morning BP and MBPS were reduced compared with ambulatory BP values in other periods in patients with hypertension taking doxazosin at bedtime (Figure 5.25) [89].

The alpha-adrenergic MBPS has been defined as that which is reduced by doxazosin. Alpha-adrenergic MBPS was closely associated with multiple silent cerebral infarcts (SCIs), independent of age, MBPS, 24-hour SBP, and other cofactors (odds ratio [OR] per 10-mmHg increase in MBPS, 1.96; $p = 0.006$). Figure 1.49 shows the scatter plots of MBPS and alpha-adrenergic MBPS, showing that the slope of the regression lines was significantly different patients with vs. without multiple SCIs [89]. This indicates that MBPS, particularly that which is dependent on alpha-adrenergic activity, is closely associated with advanced silent hypertensive cerebrovascular disease in elderly patients.

An open-label, multicenter trial, the Japan Morning Surge-1 (JMS-1) study of 611 medicated patients with morning hypertension (self-measured morning SBP >135 mmHg), demonstrated that bedtime dosing of doxazosin added to baseline antihypertensive medication significantly reduced morning BP and albuminuria [348]. In this study, reductions in the UACR paralleled those in morning BP. However, decreases in UACR were independent of the magnitude of reduction in morning BP. In addition, bedtime dosing of doxazosin improved the homeostatic model assessment (HOMA) index—a measure of insulin resistance—independently of the reduction in morning BP [349]. In the JMS-1 study, doxazosin significantly

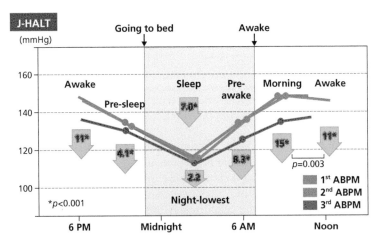

Figure 5.25 Effect of bedtime dosing of doxazosin 24-hour blood pressure in the Japan Hypertension and Lipid Trial (J-HALT; $n = 98$). The first and second ambulatory blood pressure monitoring (ABPM) periods occurred at baseline, and the third was performed after doxazosin therapy. *Source*: Kario et al. Am J Hypertens. 2004;17:668–675 [89].

Esaxerenone (CS - 3150)

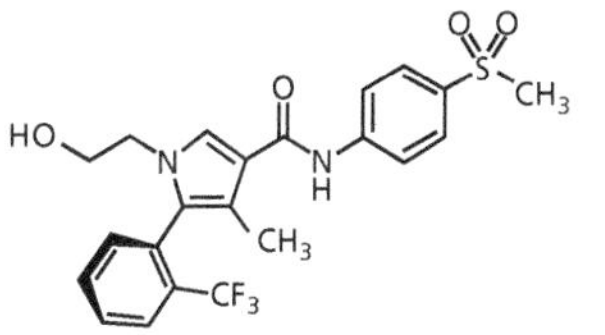

Oral, non-steroidal, selective mineralocorticoid receptor (MR) blocker

	Spironolactone	Eplerenone	Esaxerenone
Chemical structure	Steroid	Steroid	Non-steroid
In vitro MR antagonism (IC$_{50}$ in MR reporter assays*)	66nM	970nM	3.7nM
Antagonism of steroid hormone receptors (excluding MR) (IC$_{50}$ in reporter assays*)	GR : 2,600 nM PR : 640 nM AR : 180 nM	GR : 36,000 nM PR : 42,000 nM AR : 7,400 nM	GR : >5,000 nM PR : >5,000 nM AR : >5,000 nM
Agonistic effects on steroid hormone receptors (reporter assays*)	MR,PR,AR	—	—
In vivo suppression of blood pressure (BP) increase (Dahl rat)	100mg/kg	100mg/kg	0.5mg/kg
Elimination half-life (T$_{1/2}$) (healthy adults)	11.6 hr	5.00 hr	18.6 hr

*Considered concentration range : spironolactone (2.56 pM - 5µM), eplerenone (51.2 pM - 100µM), esaxerenone (2.56 pM - 5µM).

Figure 5.26 Characteristics of esaxerenone compared with spironolactone and eplerenone. IC50, 50% inhibitory concentration. *Source*: Arai et al. Eur J Pharmacol. 2015; 761: 226–234 [351]; Spironolactone package insert; Eplerenone package insert; Esaxerenone package insert.

restored orthostatic hypertension and the reduction in orthostatic BP increase was significantly associated with the reduction in UACR, independently of sitting office and home BP (Figure 2.28) [213].

There is no evidence that beta-adrenergic blockers specifically reduce MBPS. Bedtime dosing of metoprolol, a pure beta-blocker, was inferior to carvedilol, a vasodilating beta-blocker with partial alpha-adrenergic blocking activity, for reducing morning BP [79]. In addition, bedtime dosing of carvedilol effectively reduced both nighttime BP surge and nighttime heart rate in patients with hypertension and obstructive sleep apnea syndrome (OSAS) (Table 2.6) [231]. Overall, the cardioprotective effects of beta-adrenergic blockers in patients with hypertension plus coronary artery disease (CAD) and/or heart failure have been well described [178, 253, 254].

Mineralocorticoid receptor blockers (MRB)

The novel MRB, esaxerenone, was recently approved in Japan for the treatment of hypertension. Unlike eplerenone and spironolactone, esaxerenone has a nonsteroidal structure, and is a much more potent and selective MR blocker (Figure 5.26) [350, 351]. In the phase 3, comparative, ESAX-HTN study demonstrated that the reductions in nighttime SBP were significantly greater with 2.5 and 5 mg/day esaxerenone vs. eplerenone (−2.6 and −6.4 mmHg, respectively) (Figure 5.27) [350]. Esaxerenone significantly reduced nighttime BP from baseline compared with eplerenone in non-dippers with previously uncontrolled BP (Figure 5.28). In addition, esaxerenone did not markedly alter nighttime BP in extreme-dipper patients. In older patients, decreases in nighttime BP with esaxerenone 5 mg/day were greater than those with eplerenone (Figure 5.29). Thus, esaxerenone may be an

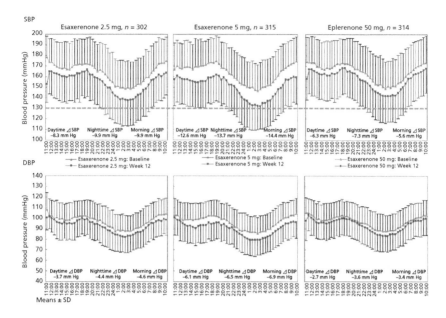

Figure 5.27 Trends in 24-hour blood pressure during treatment with esaxerenone or eplerenone. Values are mean with standard deviation. DBP, diastolic blood pressure; SBP, systolic blood pressure. *Source*: Kario et al. Am J Hypertens. 2021; 34: 540–551. [350]. Reprinted by permission of Oxford University Press.

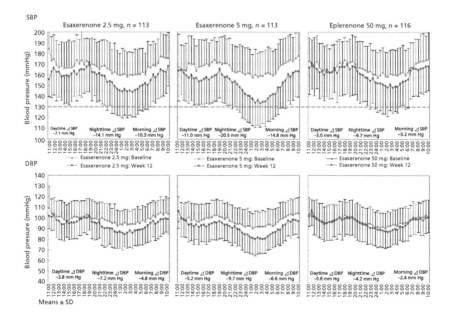

Figure 5.28 Ambulatory blood pressure trends in patients with a non-dipper pattern of nighttime blood pressure. Values are mean with standard deviation. DBP, diastolic blood pressure; SBP, systolic blood pressure. *Source*: Kario et al. Am J Hypertens. 2021; 34: 540–551. [350]. Reprinted by permission of Oxford University Press.

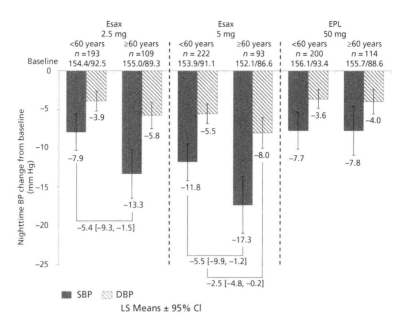

Figure 5.29 Nighttime blood pressure (BP)-lowering effect by age groups. Values are least-squares means with 95% confidence intervals (CI). DBP, diastolic BP; EPL, eplerenone; Esax, esaxerenone; SBP, systolic blood pressure. *Source*: Kario et al. Am J Hypertens. 2021; 34: 540–551. [350]. Reprinted by permission of Oxford University Press.

effective treatment option for nocturnal hypertension, especially in older patients and those with a non-dipper pattern of nighttime BP.

Angiotensin receptor-neprilysin inhibitor (ARNi)

Sacubitril/valsartan (LCZ696) is a first-in-class, angiotensin receptor-neprilysin inhibitor (ARNi) that inhibits both angiotensin type-1 (AT1) receptors and neprilysin, and has potential synergistic activity for cardiovascular protection (Figure 5.30) [274].

The recent Prospective Comparison of ARNi with ACEI to Determine Impact on Global Mortality and Morbidity in Heart Failure (PARADIGM-HF) clinical trial demonstrated that sacubitril/valsartan was superior to ACE inhibitors for improving prognosis in patients with heart failure. These results led to the drug being included in clinical practice guidelines for the management of heart failure with reduced ejection fraction (HFrEF) [247]. In addition, sacubitril/valsartan is also likely to be a useful antihypertensive agent [271].

An ABPM study showed that sacubitril/valsartan effectively reduced 24-hour BP, including nighttime BP, in both Western and Asian patients with hypertension [269, 270]. In the first randomized, double-blind, placebo-controlled study of sacubitril/valsartan in Asia, patients with hypertension (n = 389) were randomized to receive sacubitril/valsartan 100 (n = 100), 200 (n = 101) or 400 mg (n = 96), or placebo (n = 92) for eight weeks [270]. Significant reductions in 24-hour daytime and nighttime ambulatory BP were seen in patients receiving any dose of sacubitril/

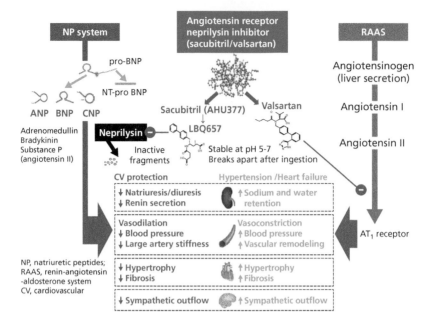

Figure 5.30 Mechanisms for the effects of sacubitril/valsartan on the cardiovascular system. ANP, atrial natriuretic peptide; AT1, angiotensin type 1; BNP, B-type natriuretic peptide; CNP, C-type natriuretic peptide; CV, cardiovascular; NP, neuropeptide; NT-pro BNP, amino terminal pro B-type natriuretic peptide; pro BNP, pro B-type natriuretic peptide; RAAS, renin-angiotensin-aldosterone system. *Source*: Kario. Curr Cardiol Rep. 2018;20:5 [274]. Reprinted with permission from Springer Nature.

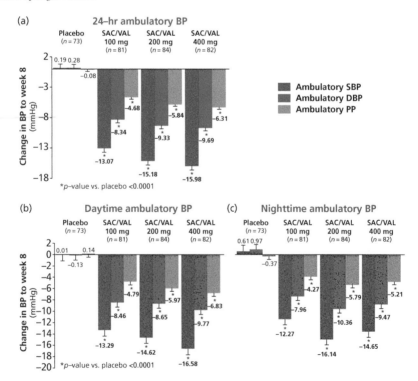

Figure 5.31 Effect of sacubitril/valsartan (SAC/VAL) on 24-hour blood pressure (BP) in Asia patients with hypertension. DBP, diastolic BP; PP, pulse pressure; SBP, systolic BP. *Source*: Kario et al. Hypertension. 2014; 63: 698–705 [270].

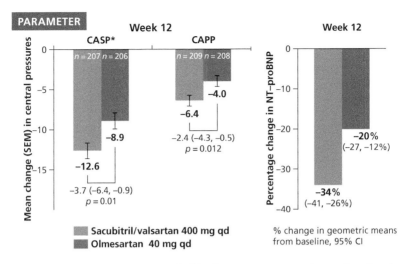

Figure 5.32 Change in central aortic systolic blood pressure (CASP) and central aortic pulse pressure (CAPP), and plasma N-terminal pro-brain natriuretic peptide (NT-proBNP) levels after 12 weeks of treatment with sacubitril/valsartan vs. olmesartan in elderly patients with isolated systolic hypertension from the Comparison of Angiotensin Receptor Neprilysin Inhibitor With Angiotensin Receptor Blocker Measuring Arterial Stiffness in the Elderly (PARAMETER) study (n = 545, age ≥60 years, systolic blood pressure ≥150 mmHg, pulse pressure ≥60 mmHg). CI, confidence interval; qd, once daily; SEM, standard error of the mean. *Source*: Williams et al. Hypertension. 2017; 69: 411–420 [272].

valsartan vs. placebo ($p < 0.0001$) (Figure 5.31). Sacubitril/valsartan was well tolerated, and no cases of angioedema were reported. Data suggest that Asian patients with hypertension may respond particularly well to this agent [273, 352–356].

Sacubitril/valsartan significantly restores 24-hour central hemodynamics in elderly patients with hypertension. A recent mechanistic study, PARAMETER (Comparison of Angiotensin Receptor Neprilysin Inhibitor with Angiotensin Receptor Blocker Measuring Arterial Stiffness in the Elderly), demonstrated that sacubitril/valsartan was superior to ARB monotherapy for preferentially reducing central aortic systolic pressure (primary endpoint), central aortic pulse pressure (secondary endpoint) (Figure 5.32), and nighttime BP (Figure 5.33) [272]. This may be due in part to increases in levels of atrial and brain natriuretic peptides during treatment with sacubitril/valsartan, which would reduce circulating volume [272]. Therefore, sacubitril/valsartan could be effective in non-dippers with true resistant hypertension. Sacubitril/valsartan was also effective for reducing levels of NT-pro BNP (Figure 5.32) [272], as demonstrated in heart failure patients with preserved left ventricular ejection fraction (HFpEF) [357].

Aging increases arterial stiffness and salt sensitivity, and decreases renal function. Age-related increases in arterial stiffness cause systolic hypertension with increased pulse pressure and central pressure (structural hypertension), while age-related increases in salt sensitivity cause hypertension with diminished nighttime dipping (non-dipper/riser pattern) (salt-sensitive hypertension). Structural and/or salt-sensitive hypertension phenotypes are likely to develop drug-uncontrolled (resistant) hypertension and HFpEF. Sacubitril/valsartan attenuated these age-related cardiovascular changes, resulting in effective prevention of heart failure (Figure 5.34) [274].

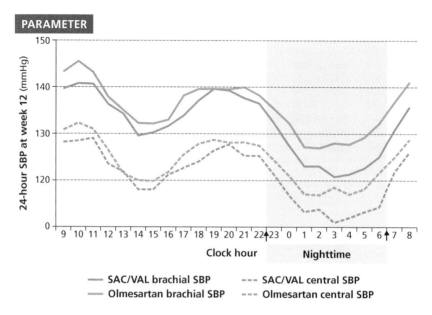

Figure 5.33 Twenty-four-hour brachial and central systolic blood pressure (SBP) after 12 weeks of treatment with sacubitril/valsartan 400 mg vs. olmesartan 40 mg in elderly patients with isolated systolic hypertension from the Comparison of Angiotensin Receptor Neprilysin Inhibitor with Angiotensin Receptor Blocker Measuring Arterial Stiffness in the Elderly (PARAMETER) study (*n* = 454, age ≥60 years, systolic blood pressure ≥150 mmHg, pulse pressure ≥60 mmHg). *Source*: Williams et al. Hypertension. 2017; 69: 411–420 [272].

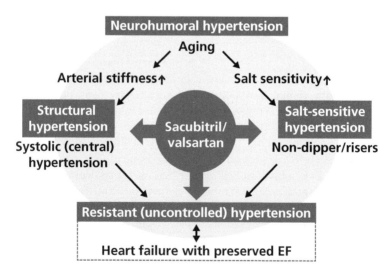

Figure 5.34 Age-related continuum from hypertension to heart failure, and intervention points for sacubitril/valsartan. EF, ejection fraction. *Source*: Kario. Curr Cardiol Rep. 2018; 20:5 [274]. Reprinted with permission from Springer Nature.

Table 5.5 Five hypertension phenotypes targeted by sacubitril/valsartan.

1. Elderly hypertension (structural hypertension with increased pulse pressure ≥60 mmHg)
2. Central hypertension (central systolic BP ≥130 mmHg)
3. Nocturnal hypertension (salt-sensitive, non-dipper/riser)
4. Drug-resistant (uncontrolled) hypertension
5. Asian hypertension (higher salt sensitivity and higher salt intake)

BP, blood pressure.
Source: Kario. Curr Cardiol Rep. 2018; 20: 5 [274]. Reprinted with permission from Springer Nature.

Considering these mechanisms, sacubitril/valsartan may be an attractive therapeutic agent to treat the elderly with age-related hypertension phenotypes such as uncontrolled (resistant) hypertension manifesting as systolic (central) hypertension (structural hypertension) and/or nocturnal hypertension (salt-sensitive hypertension) (Table 5.5). These are high-risk hypertension phenotypes that are susceptible to the development of HFpEF and CKD.

Endothelin receptor antagonists (ERA)

Endothelin-1 (ET-1) had a number of important vascular effects (Figure 5.35) [358], and also influences cell proliferation and extracellular matrix synthesis, as well as contributing to water and electrolyte homeostasis via direct effects on the

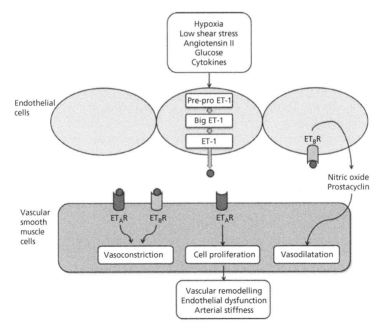

Figure 5.35 Vascular effects of endothelin-1 (ET-1); ETAR, endothelin A receptor; ETBR, endothelin B receptor. *Source*: Reprinted with permission from Moorhouse et al. Curr Hypertens Rep. 2013; 15, 489–496 [358].

kidney [359]. Data from a meta-analysis showed that treatment with an ERA was associated with significant reductions in 24-hour SBP and DBP compared with placebo (−7.65 and −5.92 mmHg, respectively), without any significant effect on all-cause mortality (relative risk 1.45, 95% CI 0.84–2.52) [360].

ERAs are not currently used extensively in clinical practice, but research is primarily focused on the use of this class of agents for the treatment of resistant hypertension [361], and on the development of new agents with a better tolerability profile (Figure 5.36) [362].

Combination therapy, including single pill combinations

First-line therapy

It is reasonable to take an age-related approach to the management of patients with hypertension. Younger patients with hypertension often present with obesity and multiple metabolic risk factors, driven by increased activity of the sympathetic nervous system and RAS (metabolic neurohumoral hypertension). In contrast, isolated systolic hypertension is common in older patients with hypertension, who usually have arterial stiffness of the large and small arteries (structural hypertension), and salt-sensitivity.

On this basis, it is reasonable to initiate antihypertensive therapy for younger patients with a RAS inhibitor, especially those with metabolic risk factors, while a CCB would be a good choice for older patients, particularly those with characteristics indicating structural hypertension (Figure 5.37). The British Hypertension Society includes recommendations for first-line therapy based on age (and ethnicity) (Figure 5.38) [363].

Key hypertension guidelines now recommend that antihypertensive therapy should be initiated with a dual combination of agents to facilitate early and complete achievement of target BP [178, 253, 254, 364]. Initiation of antihypertensive therapy with two agents that have different (and complementary) mechanisms of action has been shown to facilitate more rapid and effective achievement of target BP, often with fewer adverse events, compared with doubling the dosage of antihypertensive monotherapy [365, 366]. Regimens that include fewer pills, such as single-pill combinations (SPCs), are preferred because these have consistently been associated with better adherence and higher rates of BP control [367, 368].

Second-line therapy

When choosing add-on antihypertensive therapy to facilitate achievement of BP control, it may be practical to consider the BP variability profile, including the arterial stiffness type (characterized by increased BP variability, such as excess MBPS, and day-by-day and visit-to-visit BP variability) and the volume retention type (characterized by a non-dipper or riser nighttime BP pattern) (Figure 5.39) [267].

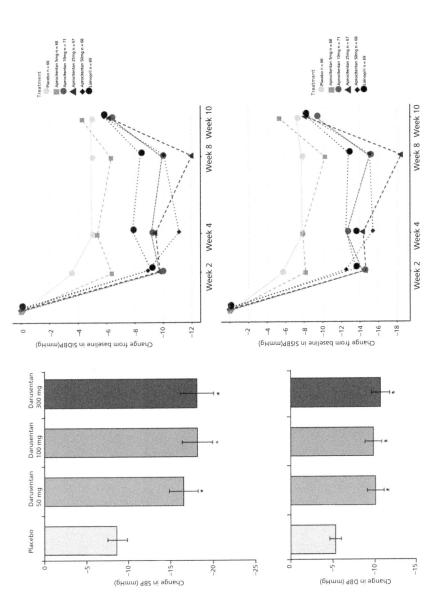

Figure 5.36 Effects of darusentan (an endothelin A receptor antagonist) on sitting office blood pressure (BP) in patients with resistant hypertension (left), and of the new dual endothelin A-endothelin B receptor antagonist aprocitentan on unattended office BP in patients with essential hypertension (right). DBP, diastolic BP; SBP, systolic BP; SiDBP, sitting DBP; SiSBP, sitting SBP. *$p < 0.001$ vs. placebo. *Source:* Reprinted from Weber et al. Lancet. 2009; 374(9699): 1423–1431 [361]. Copyright (2009), with permission from Elsevier; and Verweij et al. Hypertension. 2020; 75: 956–965 [362].

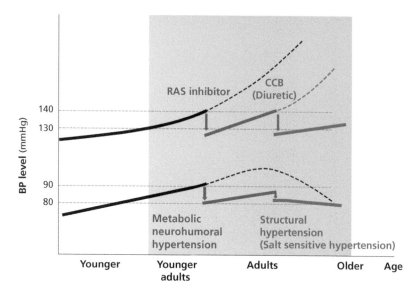

Figure 5.37 Age-related antihypertensive medication strategy. BP, blood pressure; CCB, calcium channel blocker; RAS, renin-angiotensin system. *Source*: Kario. Essential Manual on Perfect 24-Hour Blood Pressure Management from Morning to Nocturnal Hypertension: Up-to-date for Anticipation Medicine. Wiley, 2018: 1–309 [24].

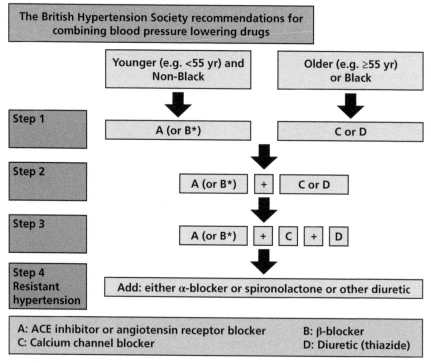

*Combination therapy involving B and D induce more new onset diabetes compared with other combination therapies. Adapted from Brown MJ et al.
Better blood pressure control: how to combine drugs. *J Hum Hypertens* 2003; 17: 81-86.

Figure 5.38 Age-based strategy for antihypertensive therapy. *Combination therapy involving ß-blockers and diuretics is associated with more new-onset diabetes than other combinations. *Source*: Williams et al. BMJ 2004; 328: 634–40 [363].

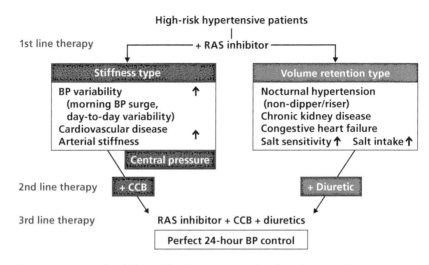

Figure 5.39 Home and ambulatory blood pressure (BP)-based combination therapy strategies for high-risk patients with hypertension. CCB, calcium channel blocker; RAS, renin-angiotensin system. *Source*: Kario J Am Soc Hypertens. 2010; 4: 215–218 [267].

Arterial stiffness type

For elderly patients with an arterial stiffness hypertension phenotype, a long-acting CCB in combination with a RAS inhibitor is the most effective approach to reducing BP and BP variability. The higher the baseline BP, the greater the BP-lowering effect expected during treatment with a CCB. This is the case even when a CCB is given in combination with a RAS inhibitor and is more pronounced at higher CCB dosages. When given at maximum dosage, a long-acting CCB minimizes the exaggerated MBPS because these agents decrease the highest morning BP more effectively than agents from other drug classes without reducing the lowest nighttime BP. Use of a CCB in combination with an ARB is an effective combination for reducing BP variability (Figure 5.40) [268].

Volume retention type

The non-dipping of nighttime BP is closely associated with increased circulating volume retention. Diuretics are the most effective class of antihypertensives for changing a non-dipping nighttime BP to a dipping pattern. This property of diuretics is augmented when used in combination with RAS inhibitors. Given that salt sensitivity is already increased in patients with hypertension receiving RAS inhibitors, the addition of low doses of diuretics may be sufficient to reduce nighttime BP. Particularly in Asians, who have increased salt sensitivity and high salt intake, a small dose of diuretics in combination with a RAS inhibitor is effective for reducing 24-hour BP, especially nighttime BP [157]. Sacubitril/valsartan and SGLT2 inhibitors are effective for this patient group (Figure 5.40) [268]. For patients with heart disease (CAD, heart failure), a beta-blocker combined with a RAS inhibitor is currently recommended.

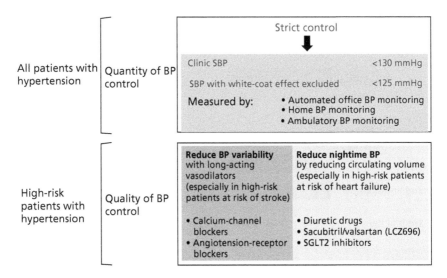

Figure 5.40 Precision medicine for the management of hypertension. Strict blood pressure (BP) control should be recommended for all patients with hypertension, while the management of high-risk patients should also take BP variability and nighttime BP into account. SBP, systolic BP; SGLT2, sodium-glucose co-transport 2. *Source*: Kari o. Nat Rev Cardiol. 2016; 13: 125–126 [268].

Clinical trials of antihypertensive combination therapy

J-CORE (olmesartan + azelnidipine vs. olmesartan + HCTZ)

The Japan-Combined Treatment with Olmesartan and a Calcium Channel Blocker vs. Olmesartan and Diuretics Randomized Efficacy (J-CORE) study investigated the effects of an ARB–CCB combination vs. an ARB–diuretic combination on central pressure and the ambulatory BP profile [128]. The combination of olmesartan + azelnidipine reduced central aortic pressure and aortic PWV to a significantly greater extent than olmesartan + hydrochlorothiazide (HCTZ), despite similar reductions in brachial BP in the two groups [146, 369] (Figure 5.41). In addition, olmesartan + azelnidipine reduced morning home SBP variability more effectively than olmesartan + HCTZ, although mean home SBP was reduced to a similar extent in both groups (Figure 5.42) [128]. This reduction in home BP variability was correlated with the reduction in PWV.

Despite similar reductions in brachial office and 24-hour BP in the two treatment groups, nighttime BP was preferentially reduced patients treated with olmesartan + HCTZ, while daytime BP was preferentially reduced in those receiving olmesartan + azelnidipine. This resulted in more significant reduction of nighttime BP dipping and the UACR in patients treated with olmesartan + HCTZ compared with olmesartan + azelnidipine (Figure 5.43) [370].

In another study, addition of a low dose of HCTZ (6.25 mg/day) to candesartan therapy reduced nighttime BP to a significantly greater extent than daytime BP (Figure 5.44) [371].

Jichi eplerenone treatment (JET) (eplerenone add-on)

In the Jichi Eplerenone Treatment (JET) study, add-on therapy with the MRB eplerenone reduced nighttime BP more extensively than daytime BP in patients with uncontrolled hypertension treated with an ARB (Figure 5.45) [372].

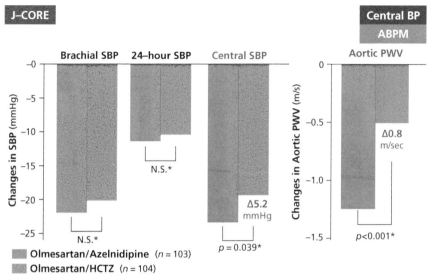

*ANCOVA (Adjusted for age, sex, BMI, previous antihypertensive medication and each baseline value)

Figure 5.41 Change in brachial, ambulatory, and central systolic blood pressure (SBP) in the Japan-Combined Treatment with Olmesartan and a Calcium Channel Blocker vs. Olmesartan and Diuretics Randomized Efficacy (J-CORE) study. ANCOVA, analysis of covariance; BMI, body mass index; BP, blood pressure; HCTZ, hydrochlorothiazide; PWV, pulse wave velocity. *Source*: Created based on data from Matsui et al. Hypertension. 2009; 54: 716–723 [369].

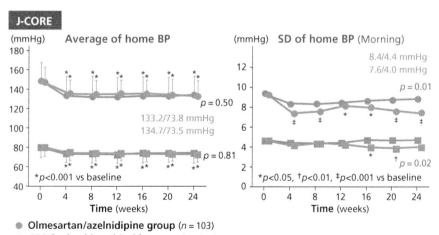

Figure 5.42 Differential effects of an angiotensin receptor blocker combined with a calcium channel blocker or a diuretic on average home blood pressure (BP), and the standard deviation (SD) of morning home BP in patients with hypertension from the Japan-Combined Treatment with Olmesartan and a Calcium Channel Blocker vs. Olmesartan and Diuretics Randomized Efficacy (J-CORE) study. ARB, angiotensin receptor blocker. *Source*: Matsui et al. Hypertension. 2012; 59: 1132–1138 [128].

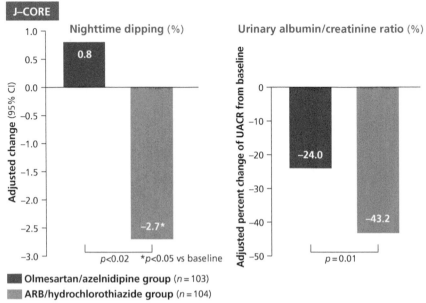

Figure 5.43 Changes in nighttime blood pressure dipping and the urinary albumin-creatinine ratio in the Japan-Combined Treatment with Olmesartan and a Calcium Channel Blocker vs. Olmesartan and Diuretics Randomized Efficacy (J-CORE) study. ARB, angiotensin receptor blocker; ANCOVA, analysis of covariance; BMI, body mass index; HCTZ, hydrochlorothiazide. *Source*: Matsui et al. Am J Hypertens. 2011; 24: 466–473 [370].

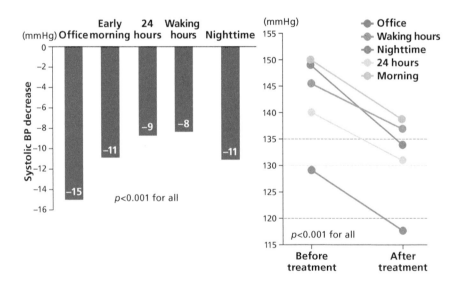

Figure 5.44 Effects of candesartan and hydrochlorothiazide (HCTZ) on 24-hour blood pressure (BP) in 40 patients with hypertension. *Source*: Eguchi et al. Blood Press Monit. 2010; 15: 308–311 [371].

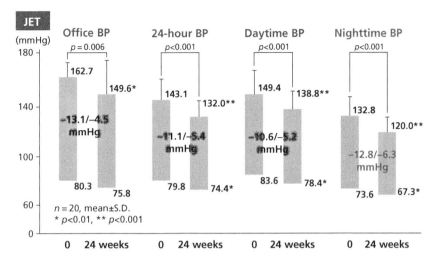

Figure 5.45 Changes in office and 24-hour blood pressure (BP) after add-on therapy with eplerenone in patients with uncontrolled hypertension receiving an angiotensin receptor blocker. SD, standard deviation. *Source*: Yano et al. J Renin Angiotensin Aldosterone Syst. 2011; 12: 340–347 [372].

ALPHABET study (losartan + HCTZ vs. high-dose amlodipine)

The open-label, multicenter ALPHABET trial investigated the effects of a losartan/ HCTZ SPC and high-dose amlodipine monotherapy [373]. After eight weeks, the effects of losartan/HCTZ and high-dose amlodipine on office, home, and ambulatory (24-hour, daytime, and nighttime) BP and BNP levels were similar, whereas reductions in the UACR were greater in the losartan/HCTZ group (Figure 5.46) [373].

In a prospective, randomized, multicenter, open-label ABPM study, 105 elderly patients with uncontrolled hypertension treated with amlodipine 5 mg/day were randomly allocated to treatment with aliskiren 150–300 mg/ amlodipine 5 mg (n = 53) or high-dose amlodipine (10 mg) (n = 52). After 16 weeks' treatment, reductions in mean 24-hour, daytime and nighttime BP values, and brachial-ankle pulse wave velocity (baPWV), were similar in the two treatment groups [374]. UACR decreased to a significantly greater extent in the aliskiren/amlodipine group compared with high-dose amlodipine. In addition, brachial flow-mediated dilation (FMD) improved significantly in the aliskiren/amlodipine group (from 2.6% to 3.7%, p = 0.001) but not in the high-dose amlodipine group; nitroglycerin-mediated vasodilation (NMD) did not change from baseline in either group [375]. Aliskiren/amlodipine was significantly less effective than high-dose amlodipine for reducing early morning BP (p = 0.002) and the MBPS (p = 0.001) (Figure 5.47) [374].

ACROBAT study (morning vs. bedtime dosing of amlodipine + telmisartan)

ACROBAT was a multicenter, prospective, randomized, open-label clinical trial that investigated differences in ambulatory and home BP after three months of treatment with telmisartan 40 mg/amlodipine 5 mg SPC given in

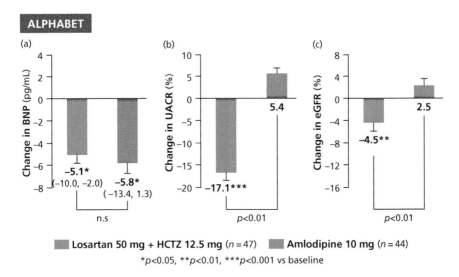

Figure 5.46 Changes in brain natriuretic peptide (BNP), urinary albumin-creatinine ratio (UACR), and estimated glomerular filtration rate (eGFR) associated with strict blood pressure control in patients with hypertension treated with losartan/hydrochlorothiazide (HCTZ) or high-dose amlodipine. n.s., not statistically significant. *Source*: Fukutomi et al. J Am Soc Hypertens. 2012; 6: 73–82 [373].

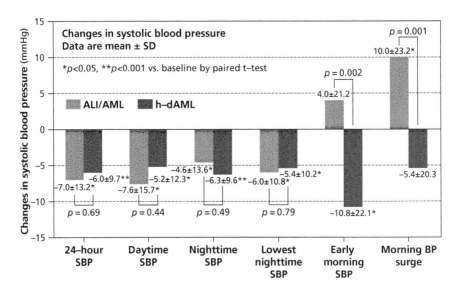

Figure 5.47 Changes in ambulatory blood pressure during 16 weeks of therapy with aliskiren/ amlodipine (ALI/AML) or high-dose amlodipine (h-dAML). SBP, systolic blood pressure; SD, standard deviation. *Source*: Mizuno et al. J Clin Hypertens. 2016; 18: 70–78 [374].

the morning or at bedtime in patients with hypertension and paroxysmal atrial fibrillation [376]. During treatment, office, home, 24-hour, nighttime, pre-wakening, and morning BP were significantly reduced, and antihypertensive effects were similar, regardless of the timing of drug administration. The SD of

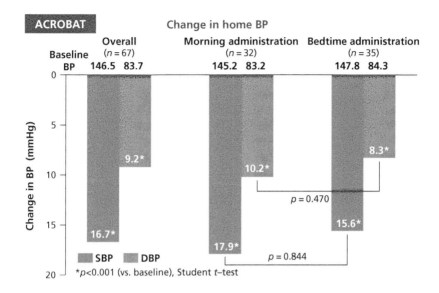

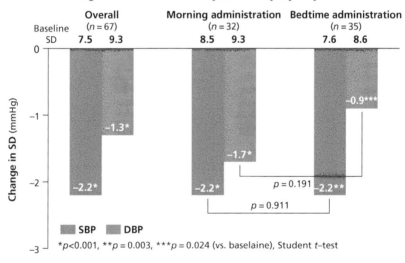

Figure 5.48 Effects of different timing of administration of telmisartan/amlodipine on home blood pressure (BP) in patients with hypertension and paroxysmal atrial fibrillation in the ARB and CCB Longest Combination Treatment on Ambulatory and Home BP in Hypertension with Atrial Fibrillation Multicenter Study on Time of Dosing (ACROBAT) study. DBP, diastolic BP, SBP, systolic BP; SD, standard deviation. *Source*: Based on data from Kario et al. J Clin Hypertens. 2016; 18: 1036–1044 [376].

day-by-day home SBP and maximum home SBP were also significantly reduced to a similar extent in the two treatment groups (Figure 5.48) [376]. These findings suggest that the antihypertensive efficacy of the telmisartan/ amlodipine SPC persists for 24 hours, regardless of when treatment is administered.

CPET study (morning vs. bedtime dosing of valsartan + amlodipine on 24-hour central BP)

The effects of morning and bedtime administration of valsartan/amlodipine combination therapy (80/5 mg) on nighttime brachial and central BP measured by ABPM in patients with hypertension were compared in the ChronotheraPy for ambulatory cEnTral pressure (CPET) study, a 16-week prospective, multi-center, randomized, open-label, crossover, noninferiority clinical trial [377]. Twenty-three patients (mean age 68.0 years) were studied. Differences in night-time brachial SBP and nighttime central SBP between morning and bedtime administration of valsartan/amlodipine were −3.2 (95% CI −0.68, 0.4) and −4.0 mmHg (95% CI −7.6, −0.4 mmHg), respectively (Figure 5.49). The upper limit of the 95% CI for change in both nighttime brachial and central SBP was below the predefined margin of 3.0 mmHg, confirming the noninferiority of morning administration to bedtime administration of valsartan/amlodipine combination therapy [377].

Taken together, the results of the ACROBAT and CPET studies show that combination therapies including at least one long-acting drug have BP-lowering effects that persist throughout a 24-hour period.

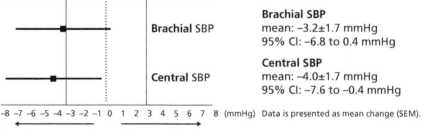

CPET
- Hypertensive patients (*n* = 23, mean 68.0 years)
- A 16-week prospective, randomised, open–label, **crossover**, non–inferiority clinical trial
- Valsartan/amlodipine combination (80/5 mg): morning vs. bedtime administration
  → the effect on nighttime brachial and central SBP measured by **24–hr ABPM (Mobil-O-Graph)**

Difference in the changes of nighttime brachial and central SBP from baseline
Non-inferiority with a margin = **3.0 mmHg**

Brachial SBP

Central SBP

Brachial SBP
mean: −3.2±1.7 mmHg
95% CI: −6.8 to 0.4 mmHg

Central SBP
mean: −4.0±1.7 mmHg
95% CI: −7.6 to −0.4 mmHg

−8 −7 −6 −5 −4 −3 −2 −1 0 1 2 3 4 5 6 7 8 (mmHg) Data is presented as mean change (SEM).

Morning administration Bedtime administration
better better

The upper limit of the 95% CI: below the margin in both nighttime brachial and central SBP
→ non-inferiority of morning administration to the bedtime administration

Figure 5.49 Change in brachial and central systolic blood pressure (SBP) with morning or nighttime dosing of valsartan amlodipine in the ChronotheraPy for ambulatory cEnTral pressure (CPET) study. ABPM, ambulatory blood pressure monitoring; CI, confidence interval; SEM, standard error of the mean. *Source*: Fujiwara et al. J Clin Hypertens. 2017; 19: 1319–1326 [377].

NOCTURNE study (irbesartan + amlodipine vs. irbesartan + trichlormethiazide on nighttime home BP)

The NOCTURNE study, a multicenter randomized controlled trial using a recently developed information and communication technology (ICT)-based nighttime home blood pressure monitoring (HBPM) device, was performed to compare the nighttime home BP-lowering effects of different ARB-based combination therapies in 411 Japanese patients with nocturnal hypertension. Patients with nighttime BP ≥120/70 mmHg at baseline while receiving ARB therapy (irbesartan 100 mg/day) were enrolled (Figure 5.50) [227]. The ARB/CCB combination therapy (irbesartan 100 mg + Amlodipine 5 mg) was associated with a significantly greater reduction in nighttime home SBP (primary endpoint) than the ARB/diuretic combination (daily irbesartan 100 mg + trichlormethiazide 1 mg) (−14.4 vs. −10.5 mmHg, respectively; $p<0.0001$) (Figure 5.51) [227], independent of urinary sodium excretion and/or nighttime BP dipping status. The change in nighttime home SBP was comparable among post hoc -defined subgroups with higher salt sensitivity (patients with diabetes or CKD, and the elderly) (Figure 5.52) [227]. Both combinations significantly reduced the UACR and NT-proBNP levels, but the reduction in NT-proBNP was greater in the ARB/CCB group (Figure 5.53) [227]. This was the first randomized controlled trial to demonstrate the feasibility of clinical assessment of nighttime BP using ICT-nighttime HBPM.

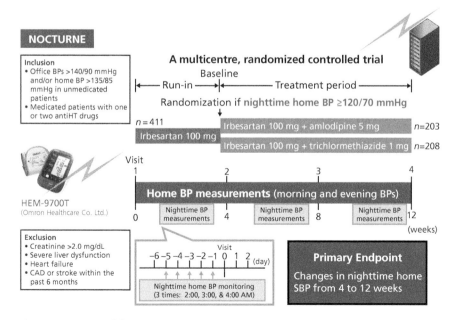

Figure 5.50 Design of the NOCTURNE study. BP, blood pressure; CAD, coronary artery disease; HT, hypertension; SBP, systolic blood pressure. *Source*: Kario et al. Circ J. 2017; 81: 948–957 [227].

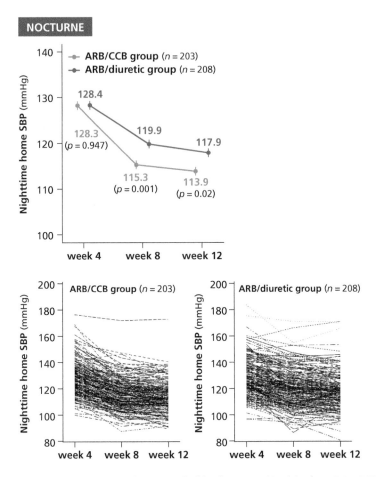

Figure 5.51 Changes in nighttime home systolic blood pressure (SBP) in the NOCTURNE study. ARB, angiotensin receptor blocker; CCB, calcium channel blocker. *Source*: Kario et al. Circ J. 2017; 81: 948–957 [227].

SUNLIGHT (valsartan + cilnidipine vs. valsartan + HCTZ on nighttime home BP)

The SUNLIGHT (Study on Uncontrolled Morning Surge for N-type CCB and Low Dose of HCTZ, Using the Internet Thorough Blood Pressure Data Transmission System) study was an eight-week prospective, multicenter, randomized, open-label clinical trial conducted in 129 patients with morning hypertension (≥135/85 mmHg self-measured using an ICT-based HBPM device) [228]. The hypothesis tested was that a valsartan/cilnidipine combination would suppress the morning home BP surge more effectively than a valsartan/HCTZ combination. Nighttime and morning SBP were significantly reduced from baseline in both treatment groups ($p < 0.001$). Morning home BP surge, a new index defined as the mean morning SBP minus the mean nighttime SBP, decreased

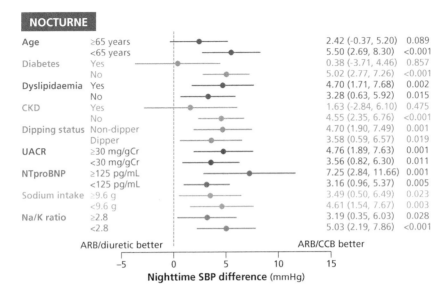

Figure 5.52 Forest plot showing the nighttime systolic blood pressure (SBP)-lowering effects of combination therapy with an angiotensin receptor blocker (ARB)/diuretic vs. an ARB/calcium channel blocker (CCB) in post hoc defined patient subgroups in the NOCTURNE study. Sodium intake was estimated based on urinary sodium and creatinine concentrations. CKD, chronic kidney disease (estimated glomerular filtration rate <60 mL/min/1.73 m^2); Na/K ratio, urinary sodium/potassium ratio; NT-proBNP, N-terminal pro B-type natriuretic peptide; UACR, urinary albumin-creatinine ratio). *Source*: Kario et al. Circ J. 2017; 81: 948–957 [227].

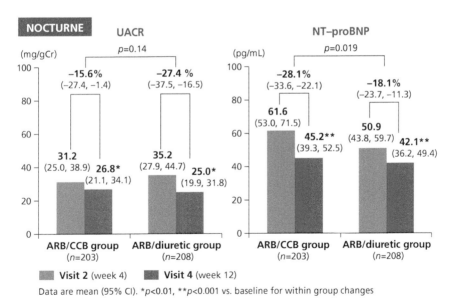

Figure 5.53 Changes in the urinary albumin-creatinine ratio (UACR) and N-terminal pro-brain natriuretic peptide (NT-proBNP) levels in the NOCTURNE study. ARB, angiotensin receptor blocker; CCB, calcium channel blocker; CI, confidence interval. *Source*: Kario et al. Circ J. 2017; 81: 948–957 [227].

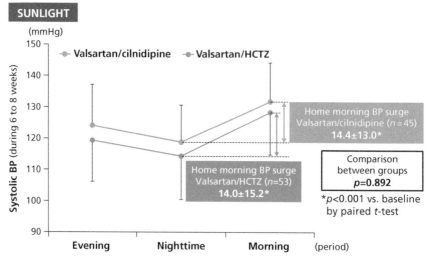

Data is presented as mean change ± SD.
p-value refers to comparison of home morning BP surge between valsartan/cilnidipine combination and valsartan/HCTZ combination.

Figure 5.54 Comparison of the morning systolic blood pressure (BP) surge at the end of the treatment period in patients treated with valsartan/cilnidipine vs. valsartan/hydrochlorothiazide (HCTZ). SD, standard deviation. *Source*: Fujiwara et al. J Clin Hypertens. 2018; 20: 159–167 [228].

significantly from baseline in both groups ($p < 0.001$), without any significant difference between groups: -14.4 vs. -14.0 mmHg ($p = 0.892$) (Figure 5.54) [228]. Achieved morning and nighttime SBP levels in the valsartan/cilnidipine combination group were about 132 and 119 mmHg, respectively (Figure 5.55) [228].

HOPE-Combi survey (cilnidipine + valsartan)

The home BP control by a single-pill combination of cilnidipine (an L-/N-type CCB) and valsartan (HOPE-Combi) survey is a multicenter, postmarketing, prospective observational study of a cilnidipine 10 mg/valsartan 80 mg SPC in patients with uncontrolled hypertension ($n = 1036$, mean age 67.5 years, 54.2% male) (Figure 5.56) [378]. The effects of treatment on MHSBP and morning home pulse pressure (MHPP) were investigated in 1036 patients with hypertension over 12 months. MHSBP decreased from baseline by 14.0 mmHg ($p < 0.01$), MHPP decreased by 6.6 mmHg ($p < 0.01$), and MHPR decreased by 2.1 beats/minute ($p < 0.01$). A more progressive and greater decrease in MHSBP (-17.2 vs. -10.3 mmHg, $p < 0.01$) and MHPP (-7.6 vs. -4.9 mmHg, $p < 0.01$) was observed in patients with higher vs. lower MHPR (≥ 70 vs. <70 beats/minute). In particular, in patients with a wide MHPP (≥ 70 mmHg), the MHPP reduction was greater in patients with higher MHPR than in those with lower MHPR (-17.9 vs. -13.6 mmHg, $p < 0.01$). These results suggest that the cilnidipine/valsartan SPC, which possesses the unique sympatholytic characteristics of an L-/N-type CCB, was particularly effective in patients with uncontrolled hypertension and sympathetic hyperactivity [378].

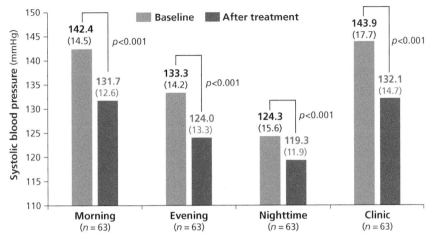

Figure 5.55 Change in home systolic blood pressures in the valsartan/cilnidipine combination arm of the SUNLIGHT study. DBP, diastolic blood pressure; ICT, information and communication technology; SBP, systolic blood pressure. *Source*: Fujiwara et al. J Clin Hypertens. 2018; 20: 159–167 [228].

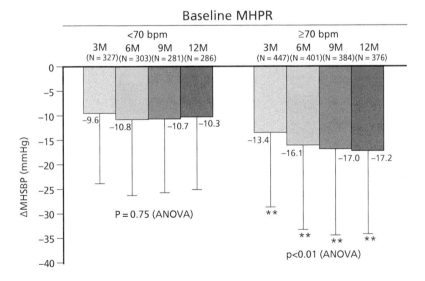

Figure 5.56 Changes in morning home systolic blood pressure (MHSBP) in patient subgroups based on baseline morning home pulse rate (MHPR; <70 vs. ≥70 beats/min [bpm]). ANOVA, analysis of variance; M, months. *Source*: Created based on data from Kario et al. J Clin Hypertens. 2020; 22: 457–464 [378].

Management of resistant hypertension

Third-line therapy

For patients with uncontrolled hypertension who cannot achieve target BP on therapy with a RAS inhibitor + CCB or RAS inhibitor + diuretic, triple combination therapy consisting of a CCB, RAS inhibitor, and a diuretic should be started (Figure 5.39) [267]. When BP control cannot be achieved with a triple combination therapy regimen that includes a diuretic, drug-resistant hypertension is diagnosed, and alternative approaches to BP control should be considered (Figure 5.57) [157]. In addition, where resistant hypertension is suspected, causes of secondary hypertension need to be excluded (Table 5.6) [178]. The most common of these are obstructive sleep apnea, primary aldosteronism, renal artery stenosis, drugs, and renal parenchymal disease (Figure 5.58) [379]. ABPM is recommended to exclude white-coat hypertension and diagnose true resistant hypertension.

For patients with true resistant hypertension, lifestyle and medication changes should be considered. Strict salt restriction would be very effective for Asian patients with resistant hypertension [380], because even mild obesity and high salt intake are important risk factors for resistant hypertension in Asians with high

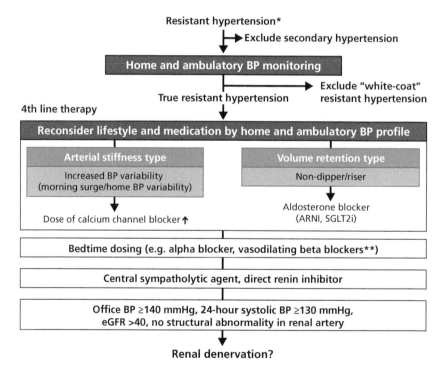

Figure 5.57 Management of resistant hypertension based on home and ambulatory blood pressure (BP) monitoring. ARNi, angiotensin receptor-neprilysin inhibitor; eGFR, estimated glomerular filtration rate (in mL/min/1.732); SGLT2i, sodium-glucose cotransport 2 inhibitor. *During treatment with a calcium channel blocker, renin-angiotensin system inhibitor and diuretic; **Carvedilol and nebivolol (not available in Japan). *Source*: Modified from Kario. Hypertension. 2013; 36: 478–484 [157].

Table 5.6 Causes of secondary hypertension.

Common causes
Renal parenchymal disease
Renovascular disease
Primary aldosteronism
Obstructive sleep apnoea
Drug or alcohol induced
Uncommon causes
Pheochromocytoma/paraganglioma
Cushing's syndrome
Hypothyroidism
Hyperthyroidism
Aortic coarctation (undiagnosed or repaired)
Primary hyperparathyroidism
Congenital adrenal hyperplasia
Mineralocorticoid excess syndromes other than primary aldosteronism
Acromegaly

Source: Reprinted from Whelton et al. Hypertension. 2018;71:1269–1324 [178]. Copyright (2017), with permission from Elsevier.

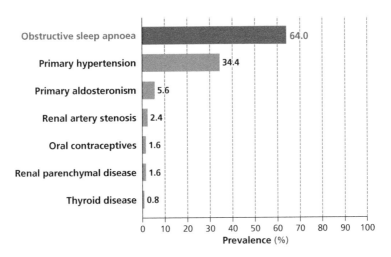

Figure 5.58 Prevalence and causes of secondary hypertension associated with resistant hypertension (n = 125). *Source*: Pedrosa et al. Hypertension. 2011; 58: 811–817 [379].

salt sensitivity. In one study, salt restriction changed nighttime BP dipping status from non-dipper to dipper [381].

Fourth-line therapy

There are several options for controlling resistant hypertension based on the BP variability profile. However, an increase in the dose of a RAS inhibitor is usually ineffective for reducing BP, while increasing the diuretic dosage worsens the glucometabolic profile and increases uric acid levels. Thus, an increase in the CCB dose is recommended, especially for patients with an arterial stiffness hypertension phenotype (Figure 5.57) [157].

MRBs are preferred as fourth-line therapy, especially in patients with a volume-retention type of hypertension, because these agents reduce circulating volume without impairing glucose metabolism. Low-dose spironolactone clearly reduced BP in subjects with resistant hypertension [382]. Eplerenone has been shown to predominantly reduce nighttime BP compared with daytime BP in patients with uncontrolled hypertension already being treated with RAS inhibitors [372]. The ARNi agent sacubitril/valsartan may also be effective in non-dippers with true resistant hypertension [269, 270].

In a double-blind, placebo-controlled, crossover trial in patients with resistant hypertension (Figure 5.59) [383], patients rotated in a preassigned randomized order, through 12 weeks of once-daily treatment with spironolactone (25–50 mg), bisoprolol (5–10 mg), doxazosin modified release (4–8 mg), or placebo, in addition to their baseline BP medication. Drug dosages were doubled after six weeks of each cycle. The average reduction in home SBP during the addition of spironolactone was superior to placebo (-8.70 mmHg, $p < 0.0001$), superior to the mean of the other two active treatments (doxazosin and bisoprolol; -4.26; $p < 0.0001$), and superior to all other treatments individually (-4.03 vs. doxazosin; $p < 0.0001$ and -4.48 vs. bisoprolol; $p < 0.0001$). Thus, spironolactone appeared to be the most effective BP-lowering treatment in the resistant hypertension setting.

SGLT2 inhibitors

Recent large randomized clinical trials have shown that inhibitors of SGLT2 significantly reduce the rate of adverse cardiovascular outcomes (especially heart failure) and preserve renal function in patients with type 2 diabetes at high

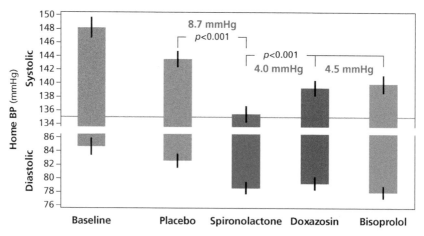

Aldosterone blocker was the most effective in patients with resistant hypertension medicated with A + C + D drugs

Figure 5.59 Home systolic and diastolic blood pressure (BP) during add-on treatment with different agents in patients with resistant hypertension already receiving calcium channel blocker (C), renin-angiotensin system inhibitor (A) and diuretic (D). *Source*: Williams et al. Lancet. 2015; 386: 2059–2068 [383].

cardiovascular risk [277, 278, 384]. Several potential novel pathways associated with the cardiovascular effects of SGLT2 inhibitors have been suggested by clinical and mechanistic studies [385]. In addition to bodyweight reduction, risk factors such as glycemia, BP, insulinemia, and oxidative stress are reported to be improved by SGLT2 inhibition [385]. However, the improvement of these factors does not completely explain the beneficial effects of SGLT2 inhibitors. A recent studies have shown that SGLT2 inhibitors significantly reduces 24-hour ambulatory BP, with significant reductions in both daytime and nighttime BP (Figure 5.60) [275, 386–391]. It has been suggested that control of nocturnal hypertension might be an efficient hemodynamic mechanism underlying the beneficial effects of SGLT2 inhibitors on the rate of heart failure in patients with diabetes [275, 385].

Figure 5.61 details the time-course of the hemodynamic consequences of SGLT2 inhibition in a 41-year-old male with diabetes, resistant hypertension, obstructive sleep apnea, and shortness of breath who was newly initiated on the SGLT2 inhibitor canagliflozin [275]. The patient had been previously treated with an ARB, a CCB, thiazides, and a dipeptidyl peptidase-4 inhibitor (candesartan 8 mg, hydrochlorothiazide 6.25 mg, and sitagliptin 25 mg). ABPM showed markedly elevated 24-hour, daytime, and nighttime BP levels at baseline, and simultaneous nighttime pulse oximetry revealed mild/moderate sleep apnea, with an oxygen desaturation index (ODI) of 12.7/h (Figure 5.61) [275]. After treatment with canagliflozin 100 mg/day for 2 months, the patient's 24-hour BP was significantly reduced, the ODI decreased markedly to 2.6/h, glycosylated hemoglobin fell from 7.3% to 6.5%, and body weight decreased by 3.1 kg. Of note, nighttime BP decreased to much greater extent than daytime BP (by 14% vs. 3%). Six months after canagliflozin initiation, daytime BP was 5% lower than at baseline, and nighttime BP remained 12% lower compared with baseline. Serial cardiac magnetic resonance imaging showed a decrease in LV end-diastolic volume and stroke volume at two months after initiation of canagliflozin, but these parameters had returned to baseline values at six months (Figure 5.62) [275]. Despite the transient nature of these hemodynamic changes, LV mass was consistently and progressively reduced (by 5% and 15% at 2 and 6 months, respectively), along with increased distensibility of the ascending aorta (indexed as the % increase in cross-sectional area and the % increase in area per 1 mmHg of central pulse pressure) (Figure 5.63) [275].

Figure 5.64 conceptualizes the impact of nocturnal hypertension on heart failure and suggests a decrease in nocturnal LV strain as a possible synergistic mechanism of SGLT2 inhibitor-associated improvement [275]. The initial effect of an SGLT2 inhibitor is a reduction in LV preload due to a decrease in circulating volume (which resulted in a mean 3% increment in hematocrit sustained throughout the three years of treatment with empagliflozin in the EMPA-REG OUTCOME trial) [278]. In addition, a decrease in LV mass with amelioration of aortic stiffness reduces LV afterload. The impact of higher BP on wall stress is stronger during sleep because the supine position increases venous return from the lower body (LV wall stress being determined by both LV pressure and LV diameter; i.e., LaPlace Law). Thus, the nighttime BP-lowering effect of SGLT2 inhibition would be synergistic with the reduction in circulating volume. In addition, the fluid shift from the lower body to the upper body during sleep worsens obstructive sleep apnea by increasing intrathoracic pressure. The effect of SGLT2 inhibition to contract

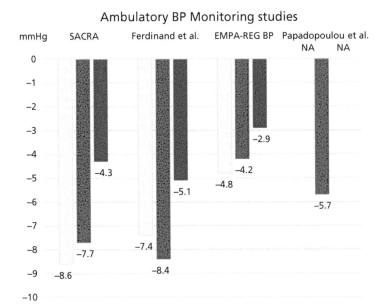

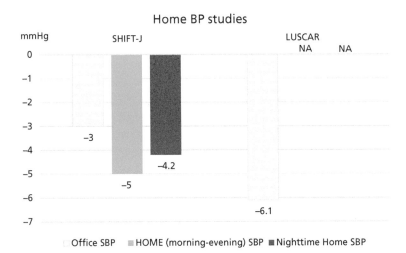

Figure 5.60 Placebo-subtracted BP change from baseline after SGLT2i treatment. SACRA [392], Empagliflozin 10 mg/d vs. placebo. Ferdinand et al. [388], Empagliflozin 10–25 mg/d vs. placebo. Papadopoulou et al. [389], Dapagliflozin 10 mg/d vs. placebo. SHIFT-J [390], Canagliflozin 100 mg/d. LUSCAR [391], Luseogliflozin 2.5 mg/d. BP, blood pressure; SBP, systolic blood pressure. *Source*: Kario et al. Circulation. 2021;143: 1750–1753 [387].

extracellular fluid volume reduces intrathoracic pressure. Better control of nocturnal hypertension acts synergistically with fluid offload to decrease nighttime LV strain. In the longer term, this may lead to protection against both heart failure and renal failure, especially in diabetic patients with obstructive sleep apnea and/or individuals with salt-sensitivity augmented by RAS inhibitors.

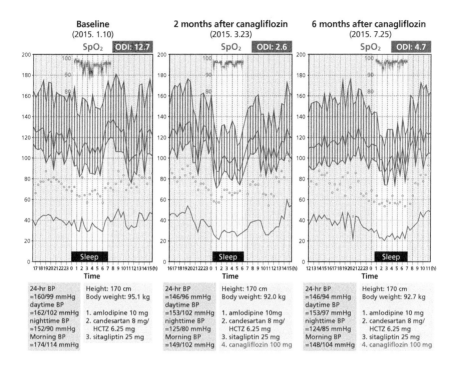

Baseline (2015. 1.10)	2 months after canagliflozin (2015. 3.23)	6 months after canagliflozin (2015. 7.25)

| 24-hr BP =160/99 mmHg daytime BP =162/102 mmHg nighttime BP =152/90 mmHg Morning BP =174/114 mmHg | Height: 170 cm Body weight: 95.1 kg 1. amlodipine 10 mg 2. candesartan 8 mg/ HCTZ 6.25 mg 3. sitagliptin 25 mg | 24-hr BP =146/96 mmHg daytime BP =153/102 mmHg nighttime BP =125/80 mmHg Morning BP =149/102 mmHg | Height: 170 cm Body weight: 92.0 kg 1. amlodipine 10mg 2. candesartan 8 mg/ HCTZ 6.25 mg 3. sitagliptin 25 mg 4. canagliflozin 100 mg | 24-hr BP =146/94 mmHg daytime BP =153/97 mmHg nighttime BP =124/85 mmHg Morning BP =148/104 mmHg | Height: 170 cm Body weight: 92.7 kg 1. amlodipine 10 mg 2. candesartan 8 mg/ HCTZ 6.25 mg 3. sitagliptin 25 mg 4. canagliflozin 100 mg |

Figure 5.61 Nocturnal hypertension in a patient with diabetes as a potential target of sodium-glucose cotransporter 2 inhibition. Change in the ambulatory 24-hour blood pressure (BP) profile during treatment with canagliflozin 100 mg/day for six months in a patient with diabetes, resistant hypertension, and obstructive sleep apnea. Ambulatory blood pressure monitoring was performed at baseline and after two and six months of canagliflozin therapy. HCTZ, hydrochlorothiazide; ODI, oxygen desaturation index; SpO$_2$, oxygen saturation. *Source*: Kario et al. J Clin Hypertens. 2018; 20: 424–428 [275].

As a result of improved aortic stiffness, SGLT2 inhibitors may also be effective agents for treating systemic hemodynamic atherothrombotic syndrome (SHATS). Clinical trials investigating the effects of SGLT2 inhibitor therapy on BP variability and arterial stiffness in patients with diabetes and hypertension would be of great interest.

SACRA study

The multicenter, double-blind Sodium-Glucose Cotransporter 2 inhibitor and Angiotensin Receptor Blocker Combination Therapy in Patients with Diabetes and Uncontrolled Nocturnal Hypertension (SACRA) study investigated the effects of adding emplagliflozin 10 mg/day or placebo to stable antihypertensive therapy [392]. Significant reductions in 24-hour, daytime and nighttime SBP with empagliflozin vs. placebo were documented using ABPM, and morning home SBP was also significantly reduced in the empagliflozin group compared with placebo (Figure 5.65). Glycemic control also improved slightly, and there was a small but significant reduction in body weight in patients receiving empagliflozin vs. placebo, while uric acid levels and the estimated glomerular filtration rate were significantly reduced in the empagliflozin group compared with placebo recipients (Figure 5.66). Additional beneficial effects during empagliflozin therapy included significant reductions in the UACR and

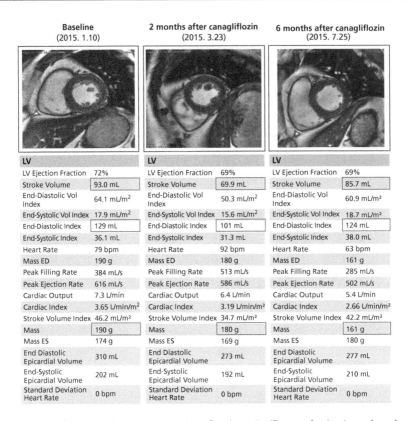

	Baseline (2015. 1.10)		2 months after canagliflozin (2015. 3.23)		6 months after canagliflozin (2015. 7.25)
LV		**LV**		**LV**	
LV Ejection Fraction	72%	LV Ejection Fraction	69%	LV Ejection Fraction	69%
Stroke Volume	93.0 mL	Stroke Volume	69.9 mL	Stroke Volume	85.7 mL
End-Diastolic Vol Index	64.1 mL/m²	End-Diastolic Vol Index	50.3 mL/m²	End-Diastolic Vol Index	60.9 mL/m²
End-Systolic Vol Index	17.9 mL/m²	End-Systolic Vol Index	15.6 mL/m²	End-Systolic Vol Index	18.7 mL/m²
End-Diastolic Index	129 mL	End-Diastolic Index	101 mL	End-Diastolic Index	124 mL
End-Systolic Index	36.1 mL	End-Systolic Index	31.3 mL	End-Systolic Index	38.0 mL
Heart Rate	79 bpm	Heart Rate	92 bpm	Heart Rate	63 bpm
Mass ED	190 g	Mass ED	180 g	Mass ED	161 g
Peak Filling Rate	384 mL/s	Peak Filling Rate	513 mL/s	Peak Filling Rate	285 mL/s
Peak Ejection Rate	616 mL/s	Peak Ejection Rate	586 mL/s	Peak Ejection Rate	502 mL/s
Cardiac Output	7.3 L/min	Cardiac Output	6.4 L/min	Cardiac Output	5.4 L/min
Cardiac Index	3.65 L/min/m²	Cardiac Index	3.19 L/min/m²	Cardiac Index	2.66 L/min/m²
Stroke Volume Index	46.2 mL/m²	Stroke Volume Index	34.7 mL/m²	Stroke Volume Index	42.2 mL/m²
Mass	190 g	Mass	180 g	Mass	161 g
Mass ES	174 g	Mass ES	169 g	Mass ES	180 g
End Diastolic Epicardial Volume	310 mL	End Diastolic Epicardial Volume	273 mL	End Diastolic Epicardial Volume	277 mL
End-Systolic Epicardial Volume	202 mL	End-Systolic Epicardial Volume	192 mL	End-Systolic Epicardial Volume	210 mL
Standard Deviation Heart Rate	0 bpm	Standard Deviation Heart Rate	0 bpm	Standard Deviation Heart Rate	0 bpm

Figure 5.62 Cardiac magnetic resonance imaging showing a significant reduction in stroke volume and end-diastolic volume after two months' treatment with canagliflozin 100 mg/day, with a return to baseline at six months after treatment initiation. Left ventricular mass was progressively reduced at two and six months. *Source*: Kario et al. J Clin Hypertens. 2018; 20: 424–428 [275].

NT-proBNP level compared with placebo (Figure 5.67). The addition of empagliflozin to the therapeutic regimen of elderly patients with diabetes was associated with similar significant reductions in 24-h ambulatory, daytime, morning home, and clinic BP to those that occurred in younger patients based on a post-hoc analysis of SACRA data [393]. Interestingly, the effects of empagliflozin on ambulatory BP appear to be greatest in Asian patients and those of Black ethnicity (Figure 5.68) [385].

SHIFT-J study

The effects of adding the SGLT2 inhibitor canagliflozin 100 mg/day compared with intensified antihyperglycemic therapy in patients with poorly controlled type 2 diabetes mellitus and nighttime BP on existing therapy were evaluated in the eight-week, randomized, open-label SHIFT-J study [390]. Reductions in morning home SBP from baseline to week four and evening home SBP from baseline to week eight were significantly greater in the canagliflozin group than in the control group; other between-group differences in office and home BP parameters did not reach statistical significance (Figure 5.69). Change from baseline in NT-proBNP levels was significantly greater in patients treated with canagliflozin compared with intensification of antihyperglycemic therapy (Figure 5.70).

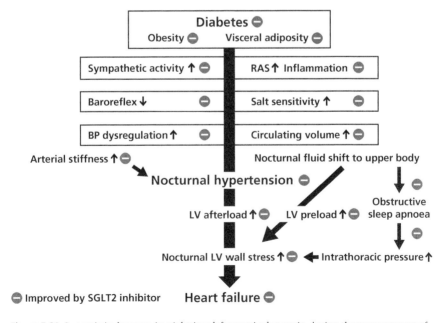

Baseline (2015. 1.10)	2 months after canagliflozin (2015. 3.23)	6 months after canagliflozin (2015. 7.25)
Ascending aorta	**Ascending aorta**	**Ascending aorta**
cross-sectional area	cross-sectional area	cross-sectional area
Max: 983 mm² Min: 902 mm²	Max: 976 mm² Min: 895 mm²	Max: 938 mm² Min: 855 mm²
* 8.98%, ** 0.243%/mmHg	* 9.05%, ** 0.251%/mmHg	* 9.708%, ** 0.303%/mmHg

* (Max – Min) /Min×100
** [(Max – Min) / Min×100] / (central SBP*** – central DBP ***)
***Central SBP and DBP are calculated by SphygmoCor.

Figure 5.63 Aortic magnetic resonance imaging showing percentage change in ascending aorta cross-sectional area during treatment with canagliflozin 100 mg/day. DBP, diastolic blood pressure; SBP, systolic blood pressure. *Source*: Kario et al. J Clin Hypertens. 2018; 20: 424–428 [275].

Figure 5.64 Synergistic decrease in nighttime left ventricular strain during the management of nocturnal hypertension with reduced fluid retention as a possible mechanism for sodium-glucose cotransporter 2 (SGLT2) inhibitor-associated cardiovascular protection in patients with diabetes mellitus. BP, blood pressure; LV, left ventricle; RAS, renin-angiotensin system. *Source*: Kario et al. J Clin Hypertens. 2018; 20: 424–428 [275].

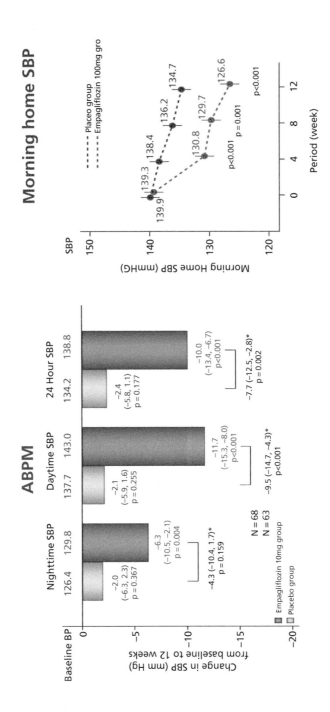

Figure 5.65 Effects of empagliflozin on systolic blood pressure (SBP) in patients with diabetes and uncontrolled nocturnal hypertension ($n = 131$). ABPM, ambulatory blood pressure monitoring. *Source:* Kario et al. Circulation. 2019; 139: 2089–2097 [392].

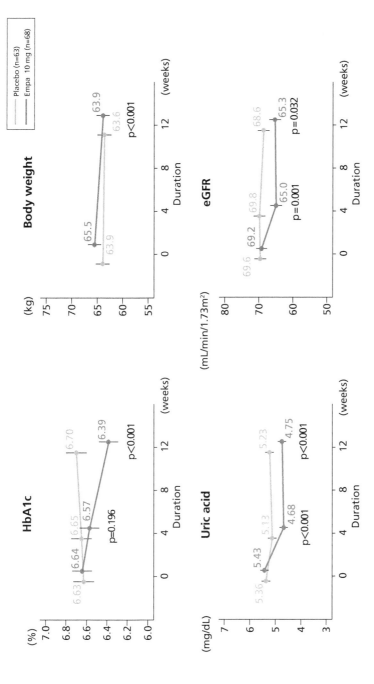

Figure 5.66 Change from baseline in glycosylated hemoglobin (HbA1c), body weight, uric acid, and estimated glomerular filtration rate (eGFR). Points and bar represent the least-square mean and standard error using the mixed-effects model with repeated measures adjusted for age and sex; *p*-values are for the between-group differences in the change from baseline. Empa, empagliflozin. *Source:* Kario et al. Circulation. 2019, 139: 2089–2097 [392].

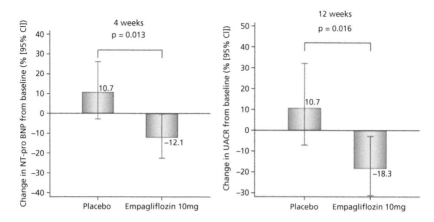

Figure 5.67 Change from baseline in the N-terminal pro-brain natriuretic peptide (NT-proBNP) level and the urinary albumin-creatinine ratio (UACR). Bar and line represent the least-square mean and 95% confidence interval using a mixed-effects model with repeated measures adjusted for age and sex. Values were % change from baseline, back-transformed from natural log; p-values are for the between-group difference change from baseline. *Source*: Kario. Circulation. 2019, 139: 2089–2097 [392].

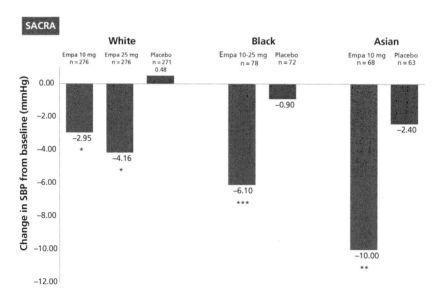

Figure 5.68 Change from baseline in 24-hour systolic blood pressure (SBP) after 12 weeks' treatment with empagliflozin (Empa) vs. placebo, by ethnic group. *$p < 0.001$, **$p < 0.01$, ***$p < 0.05$ for change from baseline with empagliflozin vs. placebo. *Source*: Kario et al. Prog Cardiovasc Dis. 2020; 63: 249–262 [385].

LUSCAR study

Luseogliflozin also reduced morning home SBP in the multicenter explorative study of beneficial effect of luseogliflozin on cardiovascular function in Japanese patients with type 2 diabetes mellitus (LUSCAR) study, and this reduction was independent of baseline BP and BP control status (Figure 5.71) [391].

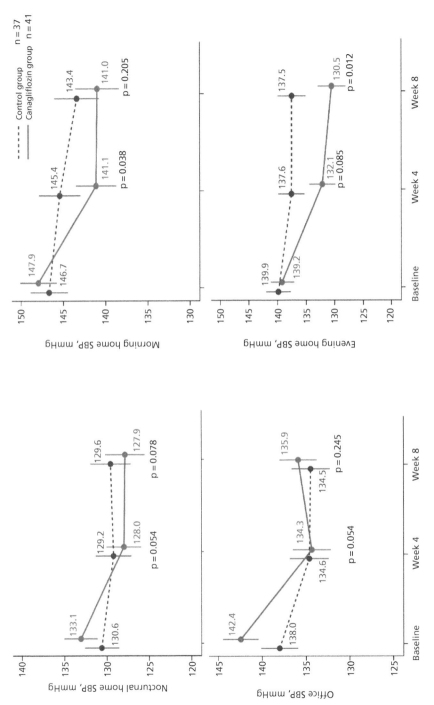

Figure 5.69 Change in office and home systolic blood pressure (SBP) with the addition of canagliflozin 100 mg/day or intensification of antihyperglycemic therapy in patients with poorly controlled type 2 diabetes and nocturnal blood pressure. Each point represents mean ± standard error in a mixed-effects model repeated measures analysis, adjusted for age and sex. *p*-values are for the between-group difference in change from baseline. *Source:* Kario et al. J Clin Hypertens. 2018; 20: 1527–1535 [390].

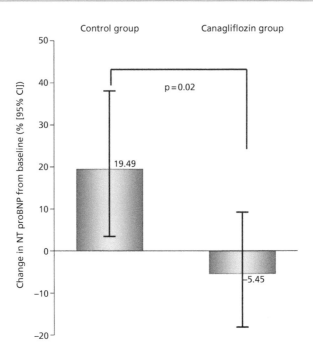

Figure 5.70 Change from baseline in N-terminal pro B-type natriuretic peptide (NT-proBNP) levels. Natural-log transformation was used for NT-proBNP levels; *p*-value is for the difference between the control and canagliflozin groups for the change from baseline to week eight with a mixed-effects model repeated measures analysis, adjusted for age and sex. Bars show 95% confidence intervals. *Source*: Created based on data from Kario et al. J Clin Hypertens (Greenwich). 2018; 20: 1527–1535 [390].

Summary

Based on currently available data, the BP-lowering effects of SGLT2i appear to be multifactorial and are likely to include the following: hemodynamic mechanisms secondary to volume depletion caused by diuresis and natriuresis; conversion of a salt-sensitive BP phenotype to a nonsalt sensitive one due to osmotic diuresis (loop diuretic-like effect); decreased arterial stiffness; reduced body weight; decreased uric acid levels; inhibition of sympathetic nervous system activity; and metabolic fuel switching (ketogenic) activity (Figure 5.72) [385]. These beneficial effects of SGLT2 inhibitors on important parameters such as body weight, serum glucose levels, and the 24-hour BP profile, these agents could potentially be introduced at earlier stages of elevated BP (e.g. prehypertension) and/or impaired glucose tolerance (Figure 5.73) [385]. This would be consistent with recommendations in the 2016 European Society of Cardiology guidelines for the prevention of cardiovascular disease, which state that introduction of an SGLT2 inhibitor should be considered early in the clinical course to reduce all-cause and cardiovascular mortality in patients with type 2 diabetes and cardiovascular disease [394].

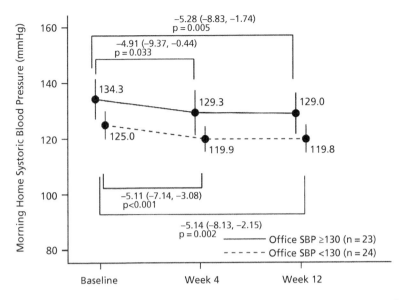

Figure 5.71 Changes in morning home systolic blood pressure (SBP) during treatment with luseogliflozin in patient subgroups based on office SBP control status at baseline. *Source*: Kario et al. J Clin Hypertens (Greenwich). 2020 Sep; 22(9):1585–1593 [391].

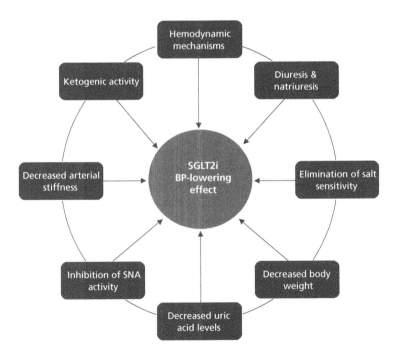

Figure 5.72 Potential mechanisms contributing to the blood pressure-lowering effects of sodium-glucose cotransporter 2 inhibitors (SGLT2i). SNA, sympathetic nervous system. *Source*: Kario et al. Prog Cardiovasc Dis. 2020; 63(3): 249–262 [385].

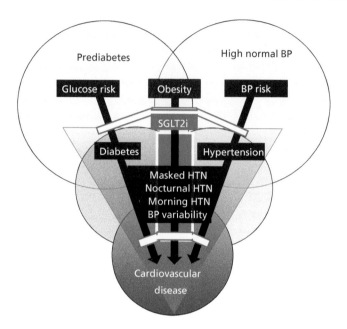

Figure 5.73 Multiple potential mechanisms of action by which sodium-glucose cotransporter 2 inhibitors (SGLT2i) could prevent the negative cardiovascular consequences of increased blood glucose and blood pressure (BP). HTN, hypertension. *Source*: Kario et al. Prog Cardiovasc Dis. 2020;63(3):249–262 [385].

Other BP-lowering therapies

Hypnotics

Clock gene abnormality and inappropriate secretion of melatonin (MT) may contribute to nocturnal hypertension. The administration of ramelteon, a selective MT1/MT2 melatonin-receptor agonist used for insomnia treatment, reduces nighttime BP and restores the circadian rhythm of BP in patients with insomnia and isolated uncontrolled nocturnal hypertension (Figure 5.74) [284]. In addition, administration of ramelteon shifts the dipping of nighttime BP from the non-dippers/riser type to the dipper type. The orexin receptor antagonist, suvorexant, also decreases 24-hour ambulatory BP levels, especially nighttime BP and nighttime BP variability in patients with uncontrolled nocturnal hypertension and insomnia (Figure 5.75).

XOR inhibitor

Xanthine oxidoreductase (XOR) inhibitors are used in the management of patients with hyperuricemia (with or without gout), but may also have beneficial effects on arterial properties such as PWV and flow-mediated dilatation suggesting a potential cardioprotective role [395]. In the Beneficial Effect by Xanthine Oxidase Inhibitor on Endothelial Function Beyond Uric Acid (BEYOND-UA) study, the XOR inhibitors febuxostat and topiroxostat both significantly reduced morning home SBP from baseline over 24 weeks of therapy in patients with hyperuricemia and hypertension (Figure 5.76) [338, 396].

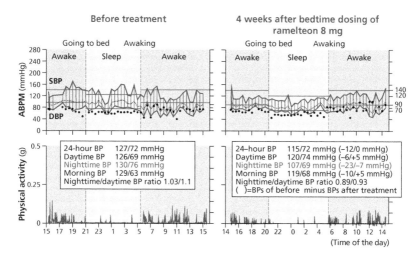

Figure 5.74 Effect of the melatonin agonist, ramelteon, in a 59-year-old woman with insomnia and uncontrolled nocturnal hypertension (current treatment regimen also included candesartan 8 mg/day, hydrochlorothiazide 6.25 mg/day, and amlodipine 10 mg/day). ABPM, ambulatory blood pressure; BP, blood pressure. *Source:* Kario. J Am Soc Hypertens. 2011; 5: 354–358 [284].

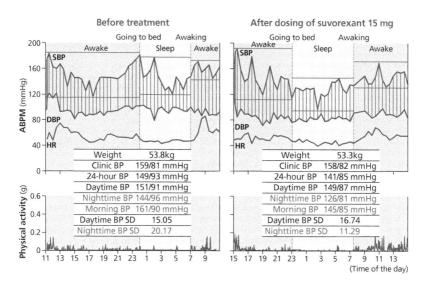

Figure 5.75 Effect of suvorexant on 24-hour blood pressure (BP) and BP variability in a 71-year-old male with insomnia and uncontrolled nocturnal hypertension. ABPM, ambulatory blood pressure monitoring; HR, heart rate; SD, standard deviation. *Source*: Kario. Essential Manual on Perfect 24-Hour Blood Pressure Management from Morning to Nocturnal Hypertension: Up-to-date for Anticipation Medicine. Wiley, 2018: 1–309 [24].

Herbal medication

There may also be a role for complementary therapy options based on the results of a randomized placebo-controlled trial of a Chinese herbal formula in patients with masked hypertension (office BP <140/90 mmHg, daytime ambulatory

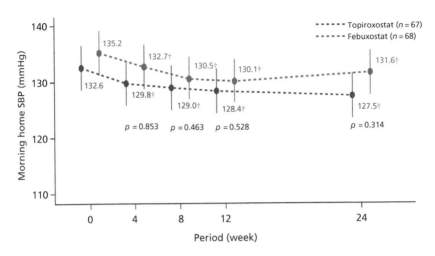

Figure 5.76 Changes from baseline in morning home systolic blood pressure (SBP). Points and bar represent the least-squares mean and 95% confidence interval using a mixed-effects model with repeated measures adjusted for sex and age; *p*-values are for the between-group difference change from baseline. *p <0.05 for change from baseline; †*p* <0.01 for change from baseline. *Source*: Kario et al. J Clin Hypertens. 2021; 23: 334–344 [396].

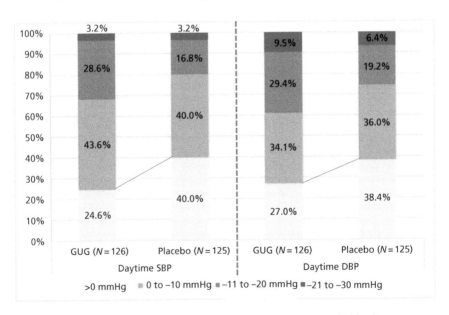

Figure 5.77 Changes in daytime systolic blood pressure (SBP) and diastolic blood pressure (DBP) after four weeks of treatment with a Chinese herbal formula (gastrodia-uncaria granules; GUG or placebo in patients with masked hypertension. *Source*: Created based on data from Zhang et al. Circulation. 2020; 142: 1821–1830 [397].

BP 135–150/85–95 mmHg) [397]. Patients were randomized to four weeks of treatment with gastrodia-uncaria granules (GUG) or placebo. There was a significant reduction in ambulatory daytime BP in the GUG vs. placebo group at the end of the study (−2.52/−1.79 mmHg; *p* ≤0.025 (Figure 5.77) [397].

CHAPTER 6

Renal denervation

Unsolved issues in the treatment of hypertension and the era for renal denervation

Despite the availability of a large number and variety of antihypertensive drugs, hypertension remains uncontrolled in up to 60% of patients receiving dual antihypertensive therapy [398]. Furthermore, about 10–15% of patients with hypertension have resistant disease, defined as a lack of blood pressure (BP) control despite treatment with optimal dosages of three or more antihypertensive agents from different drug classes or the need for treatment with ≥4 drugs to achieve BP control [399, 400]. The proportion of treated patients achieving BP control is even lower when the lower BP targets mandated in the latest hypertension guidelines are used [178, 364]. Prescription of an adequate number of antihypertensive agents at optimal dosages and adherence to prescribed therapy are essential to ensure the effectiveness of drug therapy [401]. However, fewer than half of all patients are adherent with antihypertensive therapy one year after starting treatment [402, 403]. When serum or urinary drug levels are used as a measure of drug usage, 25–65% of patients with apparent treatment-resistant hypertension are actually nonadherent to therapy [404–407].

Another weakness of medical treatment includes difficulty in controlling nighttime BP and the morning blood pressure surge (MBPS). Even if the office BP is well controlled, poorly controlled early morning and nocturnal hypertension, plus increased BP variability, increases the risk of cardiovascular disease [190, 221, 192].

Renal denervation is a new treatment approach that requires a single treatment, overcoming adherence issues, and partially blocks the renal sympathetic nervous system to reduce BP throughout the 24-period to reduce cardiovascular risk. Denervation techniques currently under clinical investigation include radiofrequency, ultrasonic, and chemical ablation with alcohol, all of which are executed through transcatheter access to the renal artery. The first denervation technique was designed to deliver low-level radiofrequency energy through the wall of the renal artery and is now improved to the spiral form with multielectrodes (Symplicity™ Spyral catheter-based renal sympathetic denervation system) (Figure 6.1).

Essential Manual of 24-Hour Blood Pressure Management: From Morning to Nocturnal Hypertension,
Second Edition. Kazuomi Kario.
© 2022 John Wiley & Sons Ltd. Published 2022 by John Wiley & Sons Ltd.

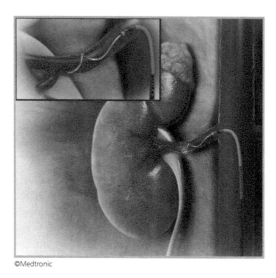

©Medtronic

Figure 6.1 Catheter-based renal denervation (Symplicity Spyral™). *Source:* Medtronic plc. ©Medtronic. Reproduced with permission.

Hypothesis of perfect 24-hour BP control by renal denervation

There is significant bidirectional interaction between the brain and kidney through the efferent and afferent sympathetic nervous system, resulting in the regulation of BP (Figure 6.2) [408]. As the mechanism of renal denervation, efferent denervation reduces renal catecholamine production and beta-1 adrenergic renin

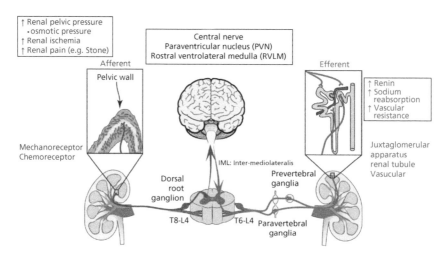

Figure 6.2 Renal sympathetic nerve anatomy and activity. *Source:* Osborn and Foss Compr Physiol. 2017; 7: 263–320 [408].

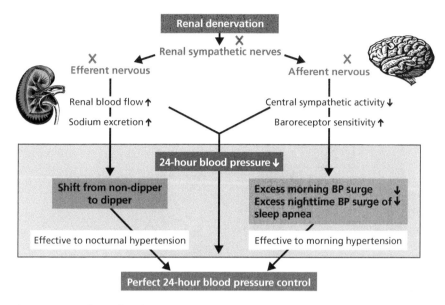

Figure 6.3 Hypothesis of perfect 24-hour blood pressure (BP) control by renal denervation in resistant hypertension. *Source:* Kario. Hypertens Res. 2013; 36: 478–484 [157].

production. These changes increase renal blood flow and reduce circulating volume, thus explaining the shift from non-dipping to dipping of nighttime BP in patients with resistant hypertension. In addition, afferent denervation decreases central sympathetic activity in response to increased baroreceptor sensitivity, thus potentially explaining the reduced variability in BP (including MBPS) and reduction in 24-hour BP, resulting from decreases in peripheral resistance and cardiac workload. It is hypothesized that renal denervation could achieve perfect 24-hour ambulatory BP control consisting of a strict reduction in the 24-hour BP level, a dipper pattern of nighttime BP, and an adequate morning BP surge (Figure 6.3). In addition, renal denervation inhibits neprilysin activity, resulting in increased circulating natriuretic peptides. This reduces myocardial fibrosis and improves left ventricular (LV) function in the setting of heart failure (HF) (Figure 6.4) [409].

History

Surgical sympathectomy was being performed on patients with hypertension prior to the 1950s, but widespread use was limited by side effects such as perioperative complications and postoperative postural hypotension [411]. Figure 6.5 shows the Clinical trial history of renal denervation (RDN) [410]. In 2009, the first hypothesis-testing SYMPLICITY HTN-1 trial reported a significant antihypertensive effect in drug-resistant hypertension using minimally invasive radiofrequency transcatheter renal denervation [412]. In this study, 12-month postprocedural decreases in systolic (SBP) and diastolic blood pressure (DBP) in patients with drug-resistant

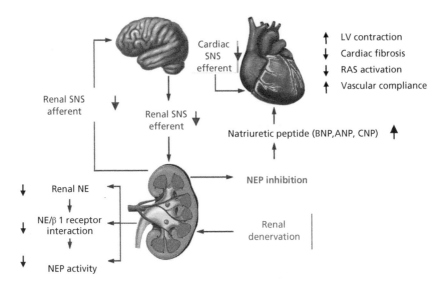

Figure 6.4 Renal denervation for heart failure. ANP, atrial natriuretic peptide; BNP, Brain natriuretic peptide; CNP, C-type natriuretic peptide; LV, left ventricular; NE, norepinephrine; NEP, neprilysin; RAS, renin-angiotensin system; SNS, sympathetic nervous system. *Source:* Reprinted from Polhemus et al. J Am Coll Cardiol. 2017; 70: 2139–2153 [409], Copyright (2017), with permission from Elsevier.

hypertension prescribed ≥3 antihypertensive medications (including diuretics) were −27 and −17 mmHg (n = 9) [412].

The subsequent SYMPLICITY HTN-2 (HTN-2) trial, published in 2010, included 106 patients with treatment-resistant hypertension randomized to pharmacotherapy plus renal denervation (52 patients) or conventional pharmacotherapy (54 patients) [413]. At six months, between-group differences in the SBP/DBP change from baseline with renal denervation vs. control were −33/−11 mmHg. Twenty-four-hour mean BP in a subset of patients was also significantly decreased in the renal denervation group, although reductions were smaller than those for office BP (between-group difference of about −8/−6 mmHg at 6 months).

The SYMPLICITY HTN-J study was initiated in Japan in 2012. Renal denervation was performed in patients with treatment-resistant hypertension using the first-generation, single-electrode radiofrequency (RF) Symplicity "Flex" catheter (Medtronic) and found to be highly effective upon initial investigation (Figure 6.6). However, in 2014, the SYMPLICITY HTN-3 (HTN-3) trial with a sham-controlled comparison group found no significant difference in BP-lowering level between the renal denervation and sham group [414]. Subsequently, several renal denervation trials, including the SYMPLICITY HTN-J study, were stopped. However, we found that renal denervation tended to reduce 24-hour SBP compared with the sham group (−6.2 mmHg, p = 0.087) (Figure 6.7) [415], and that reductions in BP increased over time in the renal denervation group (Figure 6.8) [416]. Furthermore, subsequent pooled analysis combining data from the SYMLICITY HTN-3 trial and interim analysis data from SYMPLICITY HTN-J found that renal denervation

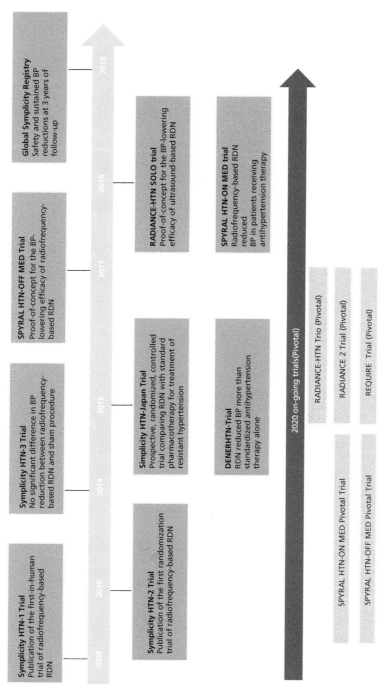

Figure 6.5 Clinical trial history of renal denervation (RDN). *Source:* Kario and Hettrick Cardiovascular Dis. 2021; 1: 112–127 [410].

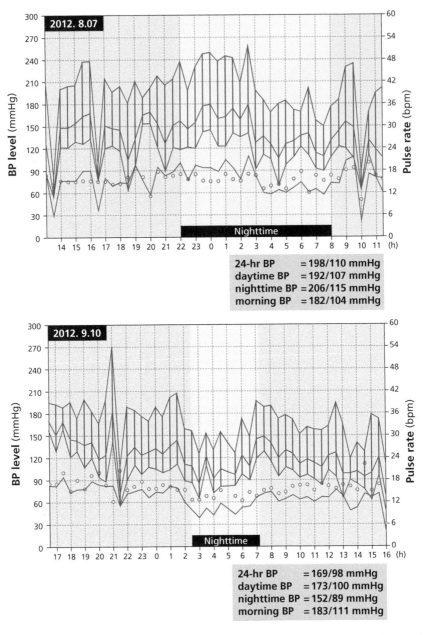

24-hr BP   = 198/110 mmHg
daytime BP   = 192/107 mmHg
nighttime BP = 206/115 mmHg
morning BP   = 182/104 mmHg

24-hr BP   = 169/98 mmHg
daytime BP   = 173/100 mmHg
nighttime BP = 152/89 mmHg
morning BP   = 183/111 mmHg

Figure 6.6 First case of renal denervation in Japan, a 38-year-old man with hypertension and diabetes (treated with a calcium channel blocker, angiotensin II receptor blocker, diuretics and a ß-blocker). BP: blood pressure. *Source:* Kario. Essential Manual on Perfect 24-Hour Blood Pressure Management from Morning to Nocturnal Hypertension: Up-to-date for Anticipation Medicine. Wiley, 2018: 1–309 [24].

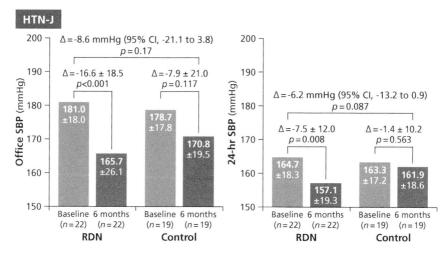

Figure 6.7 Six-month change in clinic and 24-hour ambulatory systolic blood pressure (SBP) in patients treated with renal denervation (RDN) or a sham procedure (control) in the SYMPLICITY HTN-Japan study. The proportion of patients with medication changes was 9.1% in the RDN group and 5.3% in the control group. CI, confidence interval; hr, hour. *Source:* Kario et al. Circ J. 2015; 79: 1222–1229 [415].

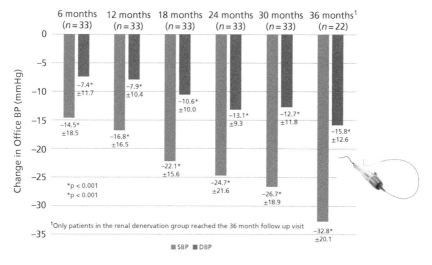

Figure 6.8 Long-term results from the SYMPLICITY HTN-Japan study showing sufficient and persistent reductions in office blood pressure (BP) in patients treated, or crossing over to, renal denervation. DBP, diastolic BP; SBP, systolic BP. *Source:* Kario et al. Circ J. 2019; 83: 622–629 [416].

clearly lowered the BP during the nighttime and early morning, when the effects of antihypertensive drugs are less likely to be seen (Figure 6.9) [281].

In 2015, the French prospective randomized DENERHTN trial reported positive results using similar techniques and the same device as the SYMPLICITY HTN trial series [417]. The trial compared RDN ($n = 53$) with standardized stepped-care

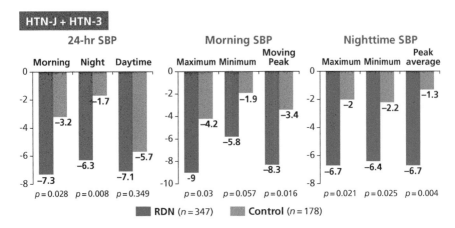

Figure 6.9 Six-month change in ambulatory blood pressure parameters after renal denervation (RDN) based on pooled data from the SYMPLICITY.HTN-Japan and - HTN-3 studies.hr, hour; SBP, systolic blood pressure. *Source:* Kario et al. Hypertension. 2015; 66: 1130–1137 [281].

antihypertensive treatment (n = 53) in patients with resistant hypertension and showed significant between-group reductions in the primary endpoint of daytime SBP at 6 months (−5.9 mmHg; p = 0.0329); levels of drug nonadherence were high (about 50%) but were similar in the two groups [418].

Advances in devices

Several renal denervation devices have been introduced clinically and, to date, serious procedure-related complications are rare.

Symplicity spyral system (radiofrequency thermal ablation)

The SPYRAL HTN clinical trial program was designed to compensate for confounding factors in the SYMPLICITY HTN-3 study, with a focus on patient selection, procedural details, and variability in patient drug nonadherence behavior [419, 420].

The first-generation radiofrequency SYMPLICITY "Flex" ablation device used in the SYMPLICITTY HTN trial series had only one electrode and required rotation and repositioning between lesions, resulting in between-operator variability. The subsequent SPYRAL HTN studies employed a second-generation spiral-shaped catheter device (Symplicity "Spyral"), which includes a four-electrode array mounted on a 4F catheter that self-expands into a helical configuration with electrodes located at 90° from each other circumferentially (Figure 6.10 upper panel) [421]. Radiofrequency energy treatment is delivered simultaneously to all four renal artery quadrants for 60 seconds. This device allows simultaneous independent ablation, and temperature and impedance monitoring, at four radially and longitudinally dispersed positions, ensuring electrode-tissue contact and reducing the risk of stenosis. More complete denervation can be achieved by performing ablations in the distal portion of the main renal artery and in the branching vessels. In an experimental study,

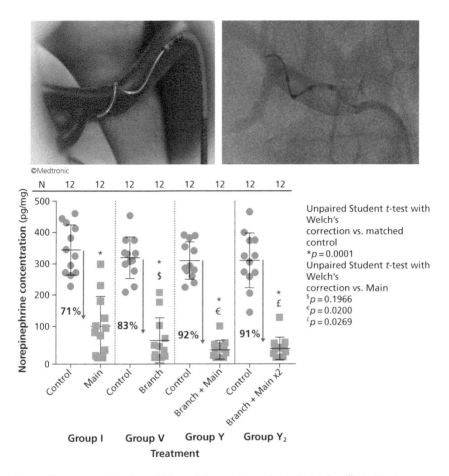

Figure 6.10 The Symplicity SpyralTM renal denervation catheter depicted in illustration (upper left panel) and under fluoroscopy (upper right panel). Upper left: The Symplicity Spyral™ catheter includes a four-electrode array mounted on a 4F catheter that self-expands into a helical configuration with electrodes located at 90° from each other circumferentially. Radiofrequency energy treatment is delivered simultaneously to all four renal artery quadrants for 60 seconds. Upper right: After guide wire withdrawal, the catheter adopts a spiral conformation in the renal artery. Lower panel: Renal norepinephrine concentration after renal denervation in the main artery (I), in the renal branches (V), and in both the main renal artery and branches (Y). The variation in response of renal norephinephrine is larger when the renal artery branches are untreated (I) or undertreated (V). Combination treatment of renal artery branches and main artery provided the best and most consistent reduction of norephinephrine (Y). *Source:* Upper figures: Kandzari et al. Am Heart J. 2016;171:82–91 [421]. Reprinted with permission from Elsevier. Lower figure: Mahfoud et al. J Am Coll Cardiol. 2015; 66(16): 1766–1775 [422].

combination renal denervation treatment of renal artery branches and the main artery provided the best and most consistent reduction in norepinephrine levels (Figure 6.10 lower panel) [422, 423]. Clinical data showed an association between incrementally greater BP reductions with distal and branch ablation compared with main artery ablation only [424, 425].

In the SPYRAL HTN OFF-MED and ON-MED studies, ablations were performed in both the main renal arteries and vessel branches using a Spyral catheter. The primary endpoint was a change in 24-hour mean SBP, measured using ambulatory BP monitoring (ABPM). These proof-of-concept trials showed impressive results, with significant differences in both office and ambulatory SBP and DBP with in the renal denervation group compared with sham control [283, 426]. In 2020, the prospectively powered SPYRAL HTN OFF-MED Pivotal trial also showed positive results, and thus finally the possibility of introducing transcatheter renal denervation into clinical practice is on the horizon [427].

Iberis® system

Clinical trials with the Iberis® multielectrode radiofrequency thermal ablation renal denervation system (TCD-16164; Terumo Corporation, Tokyo, Japan) (Figure 6.11), which includes a radiofrequency ablation catheter and generator, are currently underway in Japan and China. This system is similar to SPYRAL renal denervation device.

Paradise system (ultrasonic thermal ablation)

In the RADIANCE-HTN SOLO study, the Paradise system (ReCor) was used to perform renal denervation in patients not taking any antihypertensive medications. The Paradise device cools the renal arterial walls via a circulating fluid-filled

Iberis® Renal Denervation System
Radiofrequency ablation catheter & Generator

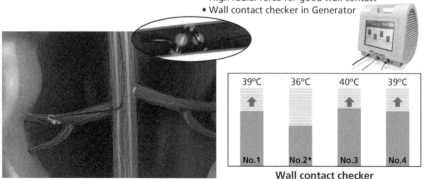

Safe deliverability	Good wall contact
• Good trackability for branch ablation	• Optimised catheter design to ablate nerves more efficiency and ease
• One size fits for 3–8 mm diameter	• Four radiofrequency electrodes for circumferential ablation
• TRI type catheter (developing now)	• High radial force for good wall contact
	• Wall contact checker in Generator

Ablation in branch artery through trans radial (TRI)

Wall contact checker
*No.2 is not good contact.

Figure 6.11 Iberis® renal denervation system. *Source*: Reproduced with permission from TERUMO CORPORATION Copyright ©Shanghai AngioCare Medical Technology Ltd, All Rights Reserved.

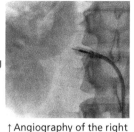

- Deeper denervation (possibly more efficient)
- No direct contact with vessel wall required for heating (possibly minimal damage on non-target tissues)

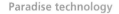

Paradise technology
Ultrasonic heating + Water cooling → Paradise thermal profile

↑Angiography of the right renal artery‡

Vessel wall   Nerve distribution
←——————10 mm——————→

Radio frequency

3 mm   59% of nerve covered

Coolant flow

6 mm

Ultrasound   1 mm   5 mm

↑Heating image on computer simulation model*

→Bench test in gel which turns white at 70°C†

79% covered

Cooled

Figure 6.12 Catheter-based ultrasound renal denervation: major differences from radiofrequency. *Source:* Reprinted from †Sakakura et al. Eurointervention. 2015;10:1230–1238 [428]. Copyright (2015), with permission from Europa Digital & Publishing; *Mauri et al. Am Heart J. 2018;195:115–129 [429]. Copyright (2018), with permission from Elsevier; ‡Mabin et al. Eurointervention. 2012; 8: 57–61 [430]. Copyright (2012), with permission from Europa Digital & Publishing.

balloon while delivering ultrasonic energy circumferentially, allowing ablation of the sympathetic nerves (Figure 6.12) [428–430]. Multiple sequential ablations are typically performed in the main vessel.

Peregrine system (trans-arterial alcohol injection)

Recently, a multicenter, open-label first-in-man study tested the efficacy and safety of the Peregrine catheter system (Ablative Solutions) that chemically denervates the sympathetic nervous system by injecting dehydrated alcohol locally into the periadventitial space of the renal artery (Figure 6.13) [431]. Forty-five patients with treatment-resistant hypertension underwent renal denervation (0.6 mL of alcohol injected into each renal artery). After six months, reductions in 24-hour SBP/DBP were −11/−7 mmHg (p < 0.001 vs baseline). No significant complications occurred, with transient microleaks observed in 42% and 49% of the left and right renal arteries, respectively, and small dissections in two cases, which did not require treatment. Evaluation of this system in a prospective, randomized, sham-controlled trial is ongoing (NCT03503773).

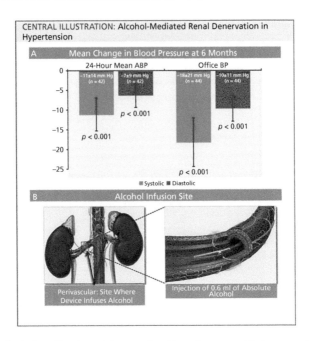

Figure 6.13 Alcohol-mediated renal denervation (Peregrine system) in hypertension. BP: blood pressure. *Source:* Reprinted from Mahfoud et al. J Am Coll Cardiol Interv. 2020; 13: 471–484 [431], Copyright (2020), with permission from Elsevier.

Other energy modalities

Various other modalities, including microwave [432], ionizing radiation [433], cryo-ablation [434, 435], and modified laparoscopic techniques [436, 437] have been studied for renal denervation application, each with specific potential clinical advantages. However, these technologies have not yet progressed beyond the preclinical or early clinical phase of research. They will require rigorous prospective clinical evaluation to determine safety and efficacy compared with established modalities such as radiofrequency ablation.

Evidence for renal denervation treatment of hypertension from Sham-controlled trials

SPYRAL trials

The SPYRAL HTN OFF-MED and ON-MED trials are multicenter international feasibility studies conducted in Europe, the United States, Australia, and Japan, using the second-generation Spyral radiofrequency ablation system [283, 426].

The SPYRAL HTN OFF-MED proof-of-concept trial included patients with hypertension not taking antihypertensive medication and showed a greater reduction from baseline in 24-hour SBP in the renal denervation versus control group at 3-month follow-up (mean difference −4.0 mmHg; p=0.0005) (Figure 6.14) [283]. Treated patients with hypertension taking 1–3 antihypertensive agents were included in the SPYRAL HTN ON-MED trial. In this proof-of-concept study, 24-hour

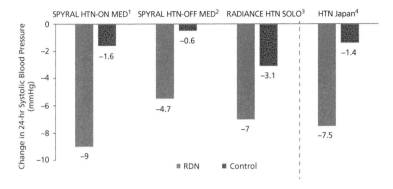

Figure 6.14 Change in 24-hour systolic blood pressure after renal denervation in four-prospective randomized controlled trials. (1) Kandzari et al. Lancet. 2018; 391: 2346–2355 [426] (six-month follow-up); (2) Böhm et al. 2020 [427] (three-month follow-up); (3) Azizi et al. Lancet. 2018; 391: 2335–2345 [438] (two-month follow-up); (4) Kario et al. Circ J. 2015; 79: 1222–9 [415] (six-month follow-up). Modified from Kario et al. Hypertension 2019, 74: 244–249 [439].

SBP decreased from baseline by –9 mmHg in the renal denervation group compared with –1.6 mmHg in the sham control group after six months' follow-up (Figure 6.14).

The results of the SPYRAL HTN OFF-MED pivotal study were released in 2020 [427]. This pivotal trial included patients from the OFF-MED feasibility study and continued the same protocol, expanding the total number of patients to 331 [427]. At three-month follow-up, the between-group difference in change from baseline for renal denervation vs. control was –6.6 mmHg for office SBP and –4.0 mmHg for 24-hour SBP (Figure 6.15) [427]. Results from the prospectively powered sham-controlled SPYRAL HTN ON-MED extension study are expected in 2021.

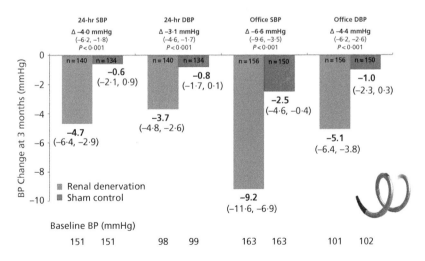

Figure 6.15 Changes in 24-hour and office systolic and diastolic blood pressure (BP) in the SPYRAL OFF-MED pivotal trial. DBP, diastolic BP; hr, hour; SBP, systolic BP. *Source:* Reprinted from Böhm et al. Lancet. 2020;395:1444–1451 [427], Copyright (2020), with permission from Elsevier.

RADIANCE-HTN SOLO study

RADIANCE-HTN SOLO was a multicenter, international, single-blind, randomized, sham-controlled trial using the Paradise (Recor Medical) balloon-tipped ultrasonic denervation catheter system in untreated patients with hypertension [440]. The renal denervation group showed a greater reduction in the primary endpoint (daytime ambulatory SBP) at two months than the sham control group (between-group difference: –6.3 mmHg) (Figure 6.16). After six months, the number of antihypertensive drugs per patient was significantly lower in the renal denervation vs. sham group (0.9±0.9 vs. 1.3±0.9; p = 0.010) (Figure 6.17).

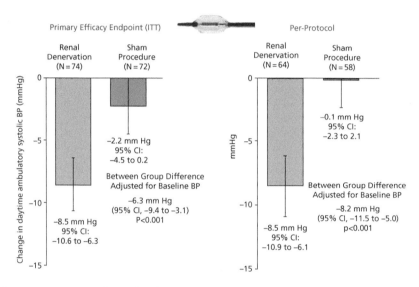

Figure 6.16 Primary endpoint data from the RADIANCE-HTN SOLO study (two-month follow-up). BP, blood pressure; CI, confidence interval; ITT, intention to treat. *Source:* Reprinted from Azizi et al. Lancet. 2018; 391: 2335–2345 [438]. Copyright (2018), with permission from Elsevier.

	RDN (n = 69)	Sham (n = 71)	P Value
# Anti-HTN Meds	0.9 ± 0.9	1.3 ± 0.9	0.010
Defined Daily Dose	1.4 ± 1.5	2.0 ± 1.8	0.018
Anti-HTN Med Load Index	0.5 ± 0.5	0.7 ± 0.6	0.014
Med Class in Patients on Meds			
CCB	73% (33/45)	83% (50/60)	0.234
RAS blockers	51% (23/45)	47% (28/60)	0.696
Diuretic	20% (9/45)	20% (12/60)	1
Beta blocker	0% (0/45)	1.7% (1/60)	1
Aldosterone antagonist	0% (0/45)	5.0% (3/60)	0.258

Figure 6.17 Medication burden at six months the RADIANCE-HTN SOLO study. CCB, calcium channel blocker; HTN, hypertension; RAS, renin-angiotensin system; RDN, renal denervation. *Source:* Azizi et al. Circulation. 2019; 139: 2542–2553 [440].

In addition, awake SBP measured by ABPM was significantly lower in the renal denervation group than in the sham group (difference adjusted for baseline BP and number of medications: –4.3 mmHg) [440]. These results suggest that renal denervation may reduce the number of subsequent doses of antihypertensive medication; thereby attenuating the impact of poor drug adherence and the need for polypharmacy.

The ongoing, international, prospective, randomized, and sham-controlled RADIANCE HTN-TRIO trial will further evaluate the efficacy of renal denervation with this device in patients with uncontrolled hypertension despite treatment with antihypertensive medication.

Evidence from Japanese populations

Individuals of Asian ethnicity are known to be relatively salt-sensitive vs. other ethnic groups, and have a higher salt intake than Westerners [441, 442]. These and other features of hypertension in Asians, including a high stroke rate, suggest that renal denervation may be particularly effective in this group [443].

Although stopped early after the unexpected neutral results of SYMPLICITY HTN-3, the SYMPLICITY HTN-J trial in Japanese patients with treatment-resistant hypertension reported a similar postprocedural 24-hour SBP value that was comparable to that in three sham-controlled trials of renal denervation Figure 6.14) [439]. This indicates that ablation of the main renal artery alone can significantly lower BP. In addition, long-term follow-up of the Japanese data showed that the antihypertensive effect of renal denervation was maintained over a three-year period (office SBP –30 mmHg) (Figure 6.8) [416].

Additional evidence for the benefit of renal denervation in patients of Asian ethnicity comes from a long-term registry-based analysis, which showed that the antihypertensive effects of renal denervation in a Korean population was superior to that of a matched Western cohort [444]. Recently, the Asian Renal Denervation Consortium published a consensus document based on the latest clinical data. They state that, in addition to SYMPLICITY HTN-J in Japan, data from South Korea and Taiwan suggest that renal denervation is effective in treating nocturnal and early morning hypertension, which is common in Asia, and that the procedure is likely to reduce BP in patients with poorly controlled hypertension, including treatment-resistant hypertension, over the long term [445]. Current clinical trial programs include studies in Japan, and Japanese patients are represented in international trials (Table 6.1).

The Global SYMPLICITY Registry (GSR)

The ongoing prospective Global SYMPLICITY Registry (GSR) is an international registry of sympathetic renal denervation in patients with poorly controlled hypertension. In the most recent update, the registry included 2747 patients and the overall reduction in 24-hour SBP at three years after renal denervation was –9.2 mmHg [446]. Similar significant reductions in 24-hour BP were reported in several high-risk patient subgroups (–10.4 mmHg in patients with treatment-resistant hypertension, –8.7 mmHg in those aged ≥65 years, –10.2 mmHg in patients with diabetes, –8.6 mmHg in those with isolated systolic hypertension,

Table 6.1 Ongoing renal denervation trials.

Product (Company)	Proof of concept trials	Pivotal trials (Sham-controlled)	Technology
Paradise (ReCor)	RADIANCE Trio (US/EU) RADIANCE Solo (US/EU)	REQUIRE (JP/KR) RADIANCE II (US/EU)	Ultrasound
Spyral (Medtronic)	SPYRAL HTN ON-MED (US/EU/JP/AUS) SPYRAL HTN OFF-MED (US/EU/JP/AUS)	SPYRAL HTN ON-MED (US/EU/JP/AUS) SPYRAL HTN OFF-MED (US/EU/AUS)	Radiofrequency
Iberis (Terumo/ AngioCare)	Iberis (JP)[a]		Radiofrequency

AUS, Australia; EU, Europe; JP, Japan; KR, Korea; US, United States.
[a] No Sham arm in Iberis trial.
Source: clinicaltrials.gov (https://www.clinicaltrials.gov/), umin clinical trials registry (https://www.umin.ac.jp/english/), industry sources.

−10.1 mmHg in patients with chronic kidney disease, and −10.0 mmHg in those with atrial fibrillation (all $p < 0.0001$ vs. baseline) [447]. Furthermore, the BP-lowering effects of renal denervation were consistent in patients with higher atherosclerotic cardiovascular disease risk scores.

Safety of the renal denervation procedure

Short- and long-term analyses from clinical trials and registries, as well as several recent meta-analyses [448–451], support the safety of the renal denervation procedure, particularly with more frequently studied radiofrequency devices. No patients in the SPYRAL HTN ON- and OFF-MED trials [283, 426] and only one patient in the RADIANCE HTN SOLO trial [438] required a renal artery stent in the 3–6 months after the renal denervation procedure. In a recent meta-analysis of 50 published trials, including 5769 subjects with 10 249 patient-years of follow-up, the pooled annual incidence rate of stent implantation after radiofrequency renal denervation was 0.20% [451]. Subanalysis of Global SYMPLICITY Registry data showed a modest decline in renal function through three years of follow-up in patients with or without chronic kidney disease [452]. Recent meta-analyses also reported minimal change in renal function after renal denervation, both in single-arm and controlled trials [448–450].

24-hour BP lowering profile for cardiovascular protection

Renal denervation reduced BP vs. sham control in both the presence and absence of concomitant drug therapy, showing that the effectiveness of the procedure is not affected by drug adherence. Renal denervation therefore provides 24-hour BP control, including at night and early in the morning when the BP-lowering effects of pharmacological therapy may be attenuated due to the timing of drug administration and pharmacokinetics [24]. Although it was initially thought that the results of the SYMPLICITY HTN-3 were neutral, an analysis focused on BP levels at night and in the early morning actually showed significant BP reductions in the renal denervation group compared with sham control [281]. The effects of renal denervation on 24-hour BP profiles in the SPYRAL HTN OFF-MED/ON-MED and RADIANCE HTN SOLO studies are shown in Figure 6.18 [427, 439, 453]. These studies all showed that renal denervation can adequately reduce not only daytime BP but also nocturnal and early morning BP, which are "blind spots" for drug

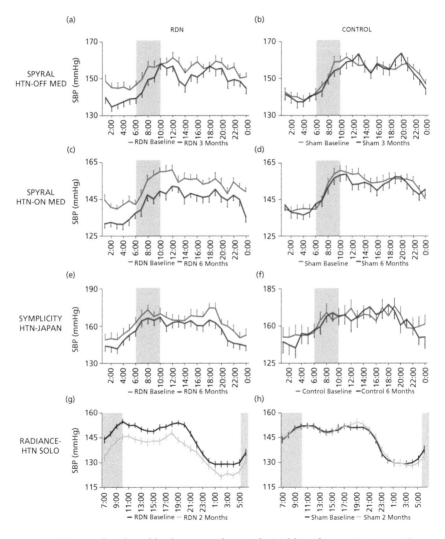

Figure 6.18 Twenty-four-hour blood pressure changes derived from four recent prospective randomized controlled trials at baseline and follow-up. (a, b) SPYRAL HTN-OFF MED [453] (3-month follow-up); (c, d) SPYRAL HTN-ON MED [426] (6-month follow-up); (e, f) SYMPLICITY HTN-Japan [415] (6-month follow-up); (g, h) RADIANCE-HTN SOLO [440] (2-month follow-up). RDN: Renal denervation. *Source:* Kario et al. Hypertension. 2019, 74: 244–249 [439].

therapy. Therefore, renal denervation could be a complementary treatment for patients whose hypertension is poorly controlled with drug therapy, especially during the high-risk nighttime and morning surge periods. In addition, the cardiovascular stress associated with the MBPS might be suppressed by renal denervation. The slope of morning surge of diastolic BP was significantly suppressed in the renal denervation group compared with sham-controlled group (Figure 6.19) [454].

Responders and clinical indications

The antihypertensive effect of renal denervation varies between individuals, with apparent responders and nonresponders [281, 283, 426, 440]. In the RADIANCE-HTN Solo study, the proportion of patients with a ≥5 mmHg reduction in BP was 66% (Figure 6.20) [438]. There are three possible reasons for interindividual variation in the antihypertensive effect of renal denervation: (1) pathophysiology – the extent to which the sympathetic nervous system contributes to elevated BP; (2) anatomy – the extent to which left and right sympathetic nerve fibers course away from the renal artery [455, 456]; and (3) operator technique (i.e. the accuracy of denervation). Identification of the best candidates for renal denervation is important due to the invasive nature of the procedure, although most randomized trials have been prospectively designed to identify responders. However, identification of individual responders may be fraught due to visit-to-visit BP variability [457]. Inclusion criteria for renal denervation trials to date have focused on the level of BP control and the number of antihypertensive drugs used. However, it would be desirable to enroll patients with increased sympathetic nerve activity, but this has not occurred to date (Figure 6.21).

A post hoc analysis of the SPYRAL HTN OFF-MED trial indicated that the BP-lowering effects of renal denervation were greater in patients with an increased heart rate measured by ABPM [458]. Sympathetic activation is also seen in patients with sleep apnea, which is characterized by nocturnal hypertension with nighttime BP surge, known as "neurogenic hypertension," secondary to apnea-related hypoxemia and arousal. Renal denervation suppresses the nocturnal surge of sleep apnea and significantly reduces nighttime BP (Figure 6.22 and Table 6.2) [282, 459] Renal denervation has also been shown to lower BP and improve apnea/hypopnea index in a randomized trial [460].

Patients with increased arterial stiffness (shown as increased pulse wave velocity) may not be responsive to RDN, because some post hoc analyses suggest that patients with isolated systolic hypertension (DBP <90 mmHg) experienced less BP reduction following renal denervation. However, a recent analysis of the Global SYMPLICITY Registry showed that reductions in this group were similar to those in other patients with hypertension after adjustment for baseline BP [461]. This could indicate that isolated systolic hypertension itself is not a sensitive predictor of increased arterial stiffness [462–464]. Thus, renal denervation may have a greater antihypertensive effect in younger patients without vascular damage than in elderly patients with increased vascular stiffness.

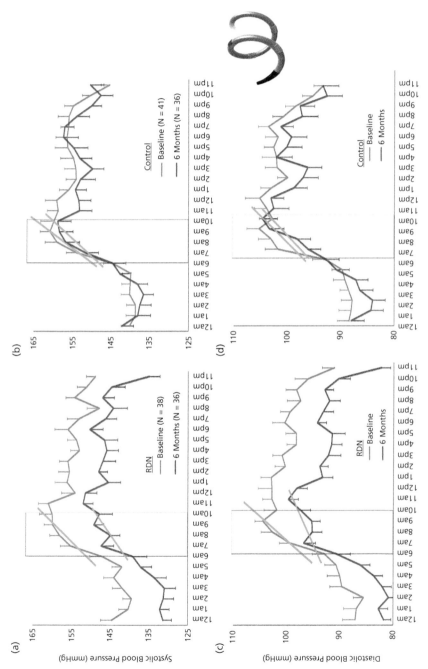

Figure 6.19 Effects of renal denervation (RDN) on the morning blood pressure surge (data from the SPYRAL HTN-ON MED trial). (a, b) Systolic blood pressure; (c, d) Diastolic blood pressure. *Source:* Kario et al. Clin Res Cardiol. 2021; 110: 725–731 [454].

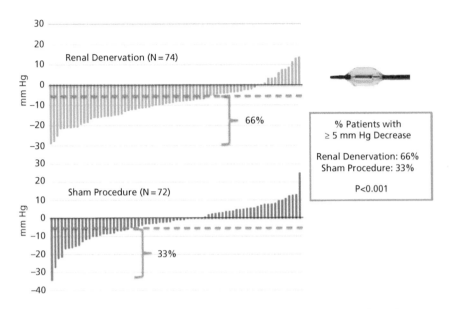

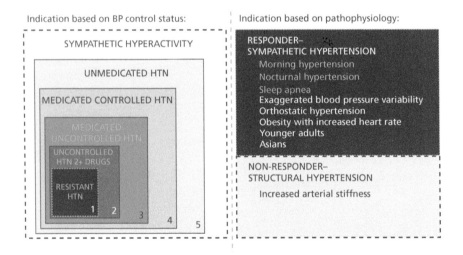

Figure 6.20 Change in daytime ambulatory systolic blood pressure at two months in the intention-to-treat population of the RADIANCE-HTN SOLO study. *Source:* Reprinted from Azizi et al. Lancet. 2018; 391: 2335–2345 [438]. Copyright (2018), with permission from Elsevier.

Figure 6.21 Possible indications for renal denervation. BP, blood pressure; HTN, Hypertension. *Source:* Kario and Hettrick Cardiovasc Dis. 2021; 1: 112–127 [410].

The most well-researched clinical indication for renal denervation is currently uncontrolled hypertension despite treatment with ≥3 antihypertensive agents, including diuretics. Renal denervation may also be effective in patients who cannot achieve BP control during treatment with one or two BP-lowering drugs. Individual circumstances such as a patient's inability or preference not to use

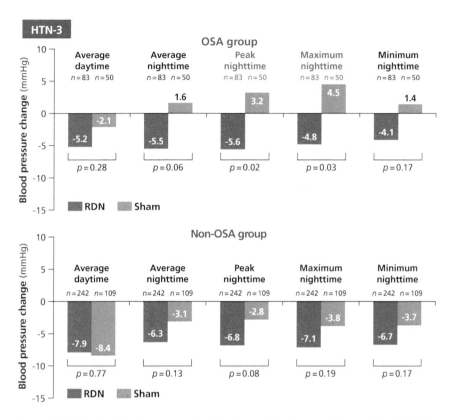

Figure 6.22 Nighttime blood pressure reduction six months after renal denervation (RDN) in patients from the SYMPLICITY HTN-3 study with or without obstructive sleep apnea (OSA). *Source:* Kario et al. Circ J. 2016; 80:1404–1412 [282].

antihypertensive medications due to adverse effects should also be considered. The need for more intensive 24-hour antihypertensive and sympathetic suppression in high-risk groups may require consideration of renal denervation, depending on comorbidities and risk factors [447]. Current European hypertension guidelines suggest that invasive procedures such as renal denervation may be considered when antihypertensive drug treatment is ineffective (Grade IIb evidence) [254].

Patient preferences should be taken into account when deciding whether to prescribe drug treatment or renal denervation after excluding secondary hypertension and confirming the presence of "true poorly controlled hypertension" by 24-hour ABPM and high cardiovascular risk. Recent scientific surveys of patient preference for renal denervation vs. additional pharmacologic therapies indicate that about 30–40% would prefer the option of a one-time invasive procedure over increased polypharmacy [465, 466].

Japanese patients with hypertension are more likely to have increased early morning BP and MBPS compared with Blacks and Whites. In addition, Asians are

Table 6.2 Changes in nighttime blood pressure (BP) parameters repeatedly measured by trigger nighttime BP monitoring after renal denervation.

n	−1 to 0 month 19 nights	0 to 1 month 22 nights	1 to 2 month 20 nights
Nighttime BP			
Fixed-interval function			
Mean SBP (mmHg)	134.2±12.2	127.7±7.2[a]	123.1±6.3[c,d]
Mean DBP (mmHg)	76.5±4.6	75.1±3.5	72.5±2.6[b,d]
Mean PR (bpm)	52.9±3.3	55.4±2.9[b]	56.5±3.1[c]
Basal nighttime SBP (mmHg)	113.3±8.8	108.5±6.6[a]	106.5±5.7[b]
Oxygen-triggered function			
Hypoxia-peak SBP (mmHg)	164.2±19.4	152.9±17.6[a]	153.5±16.1[a]
Mean SBP (mmHg)	144.1±16.8	132.3±10.4[b]	132.2±8.6[b]
Mean DBP (mmHg)	78.5±6.1	76.5±4.8	76.5±5.1
Mean PR (bpm)	52.4±3.5	54.7±2.8[a]	56.0±2.6[c]
Nighttime SBP surge (mmHg)	29.7±10.4	24.5±14.0	26.9±12.5
Morning BP			
SBP (mmHg)	169.2±15.4	160.1±8.4[a]	145.6±10.1[c,e]
DBP (mmHg)	90.1±5.9	89.7±3.6	83.0±3.5[c,e]
PR (bpm)	55.1±4.5	59.6±4.6[b]	59.4±3.4[b]
Oxygen desaturation index (per hour)	**9.2±3.3**	**11.1±4.5**	**13.0±5.6[b]**

bpm, beats/min; DBP, diastolic BP; SBP, systolic BP; PR, pulse rate.
[a] $p < 0.05$, [b] $p < 0.01$, [c] $p < 0.001$ vs. before 1 month, by t-test.
[d] $p < 0.05$, [e] $p < 0.001$, vs. after 1 month, by t-test.
Source: Kario et al. J Clin Hypertens. 2016;18:707–709 [459].

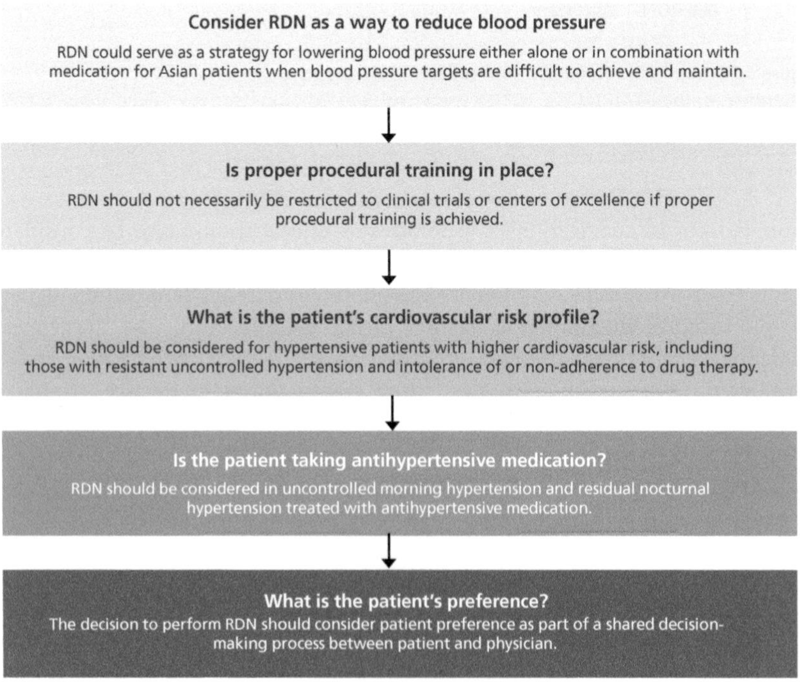

Figure 6.23 Summary of Asia Renal Denervation Consortium Consensus Panel Recommendations for the use of renal denervation (RDN) in Asia. *Source:* Kario et al. Hypertension. 2020; 75: 590–602 [468].

at least twice as sensitive to beta-blockers than Whites [467]. This suggests that Asians may be more sensitive to sympathetic fluctuations, and therefore may respond better to renal denervation [468]. The Asia Renal Denervation Consortium (ARDeC) has recommended that renal denervation should be considered not only in patients with treatment-resistant hypertension but also in those with masked hypertension, poorly controlled early morning and nocturnal hypertension, stroke, coronary artery disease, poorly controlled hypertension with a history of heart failure, poor adherence to antihypertensive medication, and a 24-hour heart rate >74 beats/min (Figure 6.23) [468].

CHAPTER 7

Blood pressure linked telemedicine and telecare

Telemedicine refers to the practice of remote data exchange between patients and healthcare professionals to facilitate the evaluation, diagnosis, and management of disease (Figure 7.1) [469]. It is used to increase patients' access to care and provide effective healthcare services at a distance. Technological advances over recent decades have dramatically increased the availability, applicability, range, and quality of telemedicine solutions. There are many potential applications for telemedicine in the management of patients with hypertension [470].

Anticipation medicine

The concept of anticipation medicine presents a unique and exciting challenge in the era of information and communication technology (ICT) and Internet of things (IoT)-based big data. In addition, video consultation as an alternative to an office visit, blood pressure (BP)-related telemedicine and telecare could help to reduce the incidence of cardiovascular events and therefore improve patient longevity (Figure 7.2) [172].

Hemodynamic biomarker-initiated anticipation medicine that can predict BP surge based on individual hemodynamic profiles and trigger early intervention using an ICT-based real-time feedback system could prevent or mitigate the onset, recurrence, and aggravation of cardiovascular events. In the context of cardiovascular disease, anticipation medicine is defined as medicine that predicts the time and place of the onset of cardiovascular events, based on a time-series of data, and provides a patient or doctor with advanced warning of potential risk factors, resulting in proactive, real-time risk reduction.

The field of individualized medicine is currently split into two distinct approaches (Figure 7.3) [156]. One is precision medicine, utilizing population-based big data such as genomic information, and the other is anticipation medicine, using individual-based big data such as time-series data. While there is a huge body of evidence on the relation between hypertension and cardiovascular disease risk based on population-based big data, there is less-available information

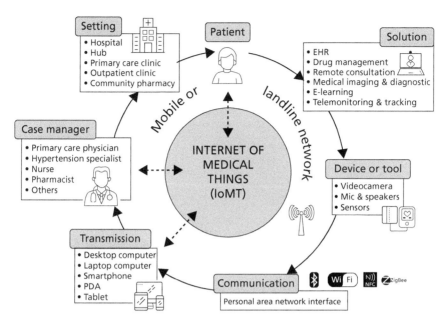

Figure 7.1 Basic telehealth services and their workflow. EHR, electronic health record; IoMT, internet of medical things; Mic, microphone; NFC, near-field communication; PDA, personal digital assistant. *Source:* Omboni Front Cardiovasc Med. 2019;6:76 [469].

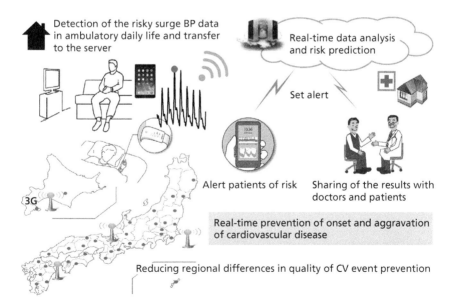

Figure 7.2 A model of information and communication technology-based real-time anticipation medicine of cardiovascular (CV) disease. BP, blood pressure. *Source:* Reprinted from Kario et al. Prog Cardiovasc Dis. 2017;60:435–449 [172], with permission from Elsevier.

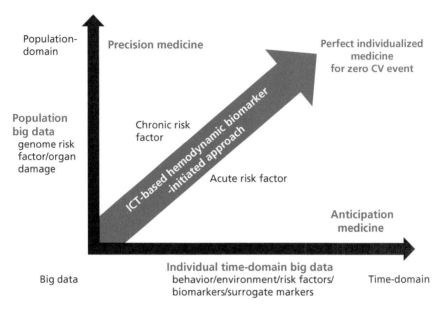

Figure 7.3 Anticipation medicine of cardiovascular (CV) disease. *Source:* Reprinted from Kario. Prog Cardiovasc Dis. 2016;59:262–281 [156], with permission from Elsevier.

on the use of anticipation medicine to predict the time and place of cardiovascular events in individual subjects using time-series data for BP and influencing factors.

Innovation technology

To establish real-time anticipation medicine, several technical innovations are needed. These include the following: (1) a wearable multisensor device to detect biological and environmental signals; (2) an ICT- and IoT-based platform for real-time big data transmission and analysis; and (3) pathophysiologic domain-interactive artificial intelligence (AI). Using these technologies, time-series big data collection with short-term intervals could be performed in the context of a prospective study (Figure 7.4) [172].

BP surge-initiated anticipation medicine, in combination with data on organ damage and psycho-behavioral, genomic, environmental, and nutritional risk factors, has the potential to achieve a perfect individualized medicine regimen for zero cardiovascular events (Figure 7.5) [156].

Wearable BP monitoring increases the number of serial BP measurements, which in turn increases the accuracy of the diagnostic and target BP levels, and increases the ability to detect various surges with different time phases (Figure 7.6) [471]. The former contributes to guideline-based medicine, and the latter contributes to anticipation medicine for the prediction of cardiovascular events.

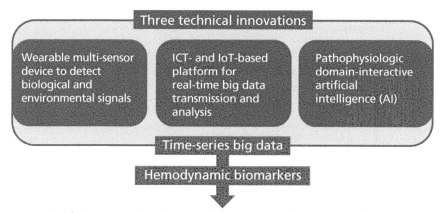

Real-time anticipation medicine for cardiovascular disease
(defined as medicine that predicts the time and place of the onset of cardiovascular events, based on the time-series of individual big data, and reduces risk proactively)

Figure 7.4 Technical innovations to establish real-time anticipation medicine for cardiovascular disease (the key biomarker of real-time anticipation medicine for cardiovascular disease is blood pressure variability). ICT, information and communication technology; IoT, internet of things. *Source:* Reprinted from Kario et al. Prog Cardiovasc Dis. 2017;60:435–449 [172], with permission from Elsevier.

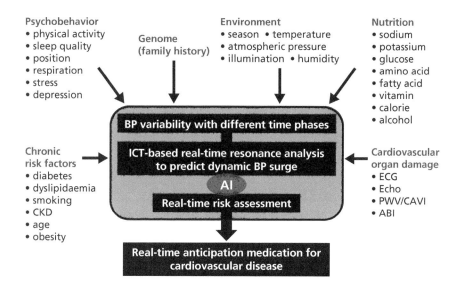

Figure 7.5 Hemodynamic biomarker-initiated anticipation medicine for preventing the onset and aggravation of cardiovascular events. ABI, ankle-brachial index; AI, artificial intelligence; BP, blood pressure; CAVI, cardio-ankle vascular index; CKD, chronic kidney disease; ECG, electrocardiography; Echo, cardiac and carotid echography; PWV, pulse wave velocity. *Source:* Reprinted from Kario. Prog Cardiovasc Dis. 2016;59:262–281 [156], with permission from Elsevier.

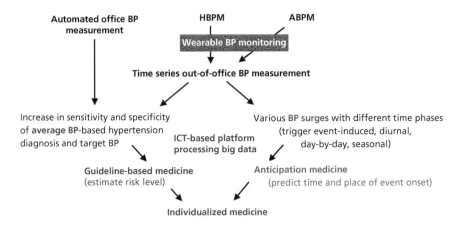

Figure 7.6 Time-series out-of-office blood-pressure (BP)-based anticipation management of hypertension. ABPM, ambulatory blood pressure monitoring; HBPM, home blood pressure monitoring; ICT, information and communication technology. *Source:* Kario et al. J Clin Hypertens(Greenwich). 2019;21:344–349 [471].

Concept of "trigger" management

The management of hypertension should move from BP control to event management. It is a shift away from focusing on the absolute BP level to focusing on BP surge. BP surge management will lead to the effective prevention of cardiovascular event onset, especially in high-risk subjects with vascular disease.

A BP surge management strategy based on the resonance hypothesis consists of the following three goals: (1) minimizing triggers of BP surge; (2) reducing the amplitude of each surge peak; and (3) avoiding the synchronization of peaks with different time phases (Figure 7.7) [172]. The aim of this strategy is to avoid the generation of a large dynamic BP surge that could trigger cardiovascular events.

In practical terms, to reduce the amplitude of morning BP surge, it is recommended that patients reduce their alcohol and salt intake at dinner. In winter, abrupt high-intensity running just after rising without adequate protection against the cold weather should be avoided to attenuate the winter morning BP surge. Regular physical exercise is recommended, especially low-intensity running, to improve cardiorespiratory fitness, which is associated with a reduction in BP variability due to a decrease in arterial stiffness and BP level [472–474].

Monotherapy or combination therapy with long-acting antihypertensives, and/or bedtime dosing, is recommended to reduce the peak of BP surge [475]. In addition, renal denervation reduces sympathetic tonus resulting in the suppression of morning and nighttime BP peaks [157, 281, 283, 476], especially in patients with obstructive sleep apnea [282, 459].

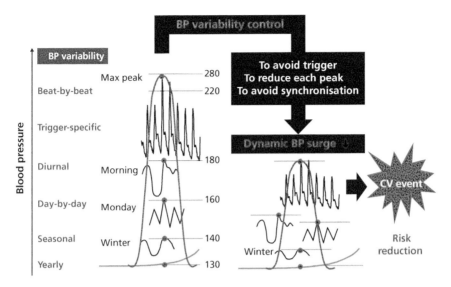

Figure 7.7 Blood pressure (BP) variability control strategy based on the synergistic resonance hypothesis, aimed at the prevention of cardiovascular (CV) event onset. *Source:* Reprinted from Kario et al. Prog Cardiovasc Dis. 2017;60:435–449 [172], with permission from Elsevier.

Multisensors and the real-time hybrid Wi-SUN/Wi-Fi transmission system

The new ICT multisensor (IMS)-ambulatory BP monitoring (ABPM) system uses new ICT/IoT-based biological and environmental signal monitoring that can simultaneously monitor the environment (temperature, illumination, and humidity) at five different locations in a house (the entryway, bedroom, bathroom, toilet, and living room) and activities measured by using wrist-type high-sensitive actigraph to identify the location of patients (Figure 7.8) [172]. Using cloud computing with an IoT gateway and bridges based on hybrid Wi-SUN, 92 LTE, and Bluetooth Low Energy (BLE) transmission systems, we can collect and store individual time-series home and ambulatory BP data, waveform data, and data on individual physical activity and environmental signals specific to different rooms in the house (Figure 7.9) [172]. The IoT bridges collect the data from the IMS-ABPM, wrist-type actigraph, and body weight scale via BLE transmission. Data are then converted to Wi-SUN transmission signal format and transmitted to the IoT gateway by a Wi-SUN multihop transmission system. The Wi-SUN system is based on IEEE 802.15.4g-based international new IoT standards 92 and certified by the Wi-SUN alliance. In the IoT gateway, the received Wi-SUN signal is also converted to LTE transmission signal format and transmitted to the cloud over a conventional LTE wide-area network. Moreover, each IoT bridge has devices for environmental monitoring such as a thermometer, illuminometer, and hygroscope. The environment-monitoring data at each IoT bridge is also transmitted to the cloud.

Housing conditions are important for the prevention of cardiovascular disease events, the onset of which exhibits significant seasonal variation with a peak in

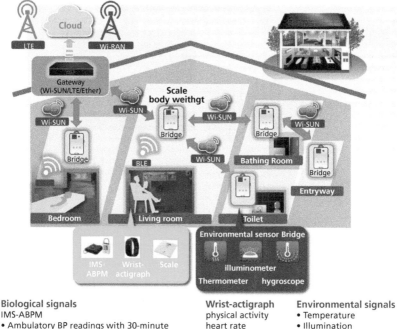

Biological signals
IMS-ABPM
- Ambulatory BP readings with 30-minute intervals (occasional)
- Home BPs (daily, morning x2, evening x2)
- Envelope of intra-cuff pressure
- Pressure waveform
- Activity, temperature, atmospheric pressure

Wrist-actigraph
physical activity
heart rate
Scale
body weight

Environmental signals
- Temperature
- Illumination
- Humidity
× 5 places
- Entryway • Bedroom
- Bathing room
- Living room
- Toilet

Figure 7.8 Multisensors and real-time and hybrid Wi-SUN/Wi-Fi transmission system of individual biological and environmental signals in the living condition. BLE, bluetooth®, BP, blood pressure; IMS-ABPM, ICT based multi-sensor ambulatory BP monitoring. *Source:* Reprinted from Kario et al. Prog Cardiovasc Dis. 2017;60:435–449 [172], Copyright (2017), with permission from Elsevier.

the winter. The death rate, especially the cardiovascular death, increases in the winter. On the other hand, data show that the winter mortality rate was higher in the north Kanto area (middle of Japan) than in Hokkaido, where winters were severely cold [Figure 2.30]. This inverse phenomenon is considered to be partly due to the increasing prevalence of energy-saving homes with good thermal insulation performance in colder countries. Our hypothesis is that heterogeneity of room temperatures within the home (i.e. different temperatures between rooms, and even within the same room) could increase the risk of cardiovascular disease events by contributing to exaggerated BP variability.

AI and anticipation models

In the Anticipate study using IMS-ABPM, mixed-model analysis of the association between daytime ambulatory systolic blood pressure (SBP) and physical activity, temperature, atmospheric pressure, and season (4699 data points obtained from

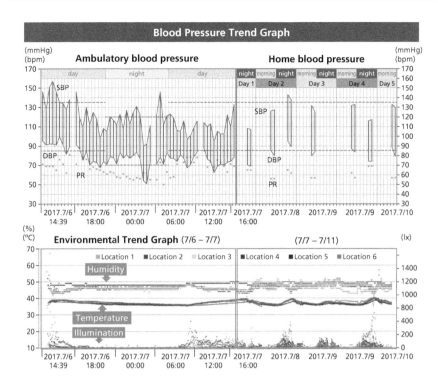

Figure 7.9 Time trend of multibioenvironmental signals from the information and communication technology multisensor (IMS)-ambulatory blood pressure monitoring (ABPM) system (IMS-ABPM) and hybrid transmission system in a 78-year-old woman with hypertension living in Tatsuno City, Hyogo, Japan. Time-trend data gathered by multisensors in the house are successfully transmitted by the hybrid Wi-SUN/Wi-Fi transmission system. bpm, beats per minute; DBP, diastolic blood pressure; PR, pulse rate; SBP, systolic blood pressure. *Source:* Reprinted from Kario et al. Prog Cardiovasc Dis. 2017;60:435–449 [172], Copyright (2017), with permission from Elsevier.

79 patients in summer and 72 patients in winter) demonstrated that a 10°C decrease in temperature was associated with a 10.4 mmHg increase in SBP (Figure 7.10) [172]. For example, SBP of 130 mmHg at rest (100 G) in an indoor setting at 25°C will increase to 151 mmHg when the conditions change to walking (1000 G) outdoors at 5°C (Figure 7.10).

In a prediction model of hypertension, AI increases the prediction accuracy for future-onset hypertension in normotensive patients [477]. Age, body mass index, the cardio-ankle vascular index (CAVI), and triglycerides were selected in this algorithm. In the recent Predict study using time series of home BP data and room temperature, AI allowed the prediction of BP levels over the coming two weeks to within approximately 6 mmHg [478] (Figures 7.11 and 7.12).

Development of wearable beat-by-beat (surge) BP monitoring

The current status and future direction of out-of-office BP monitoring are summarized in Figure 7.13. In future, wearable 24-hour BP monitoring/guided step 24-hour BP monitoring could facilitate the achievement of perfect 24-hour BP

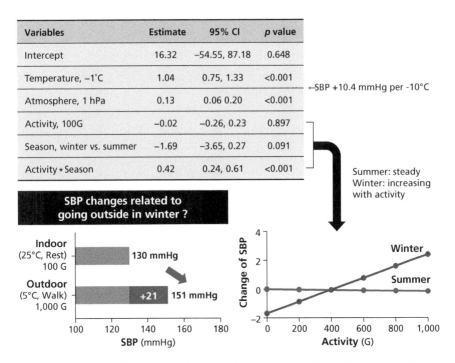

Variables	Estimate	95% CI	p value
Intercept	16.32	−54.55, 87.18	0.648
Temperature, −1°C	1.04	0.75, 1.33	<0.001
Atmosphere, 1 hPa	0.13	0.06 0.20	<0.001
Activity, 100G	−0.02	−0.26, 0.23	0.897
Season, winter vs. summer	−1.69	−3.65, 0.27	0.091
Activity * Season	0.42	0.24, 0.61	<0.001

←SBP +10.4 mmHg per -10°C

Summer: steady
Winter: increasing
with activity

SBP changes related to going outside in winter ?

Indoor (25°C, Rest) 100 G — 130 mmHg

Outdoor (5°C, Walk) 1,000 G — +21 151 mmHg

SBP (mmHg)

Change of SBP

Winter

Summer

Activity (G)

Figure 7.10 Mixed-model analysis of the association between daytime ambulatory systolic blood pressure (SBP) and physical activity, temperature, atmospheric pressure and season (4699 data obtained from 79 patients in summer and 72 patients in winter). *Source:* Reprinted from Kario et al. Prog Cardiovasc Dis. 2017;60:435–449 [172], Copyright (2017), with permission from Elsevier.

management (Figure 7.14). The research and development of continuous beat-by-beat "surge" BP monitoring has started, but it is still in the early stages [41, 172].

There are marked individual differences in the short-term dynamic BP change caused by various triggers (Figure 7.15) [479]. Wearable noninvasive beat-by-beat BP monitoring has been the dream of doctors who manage hypertension. Omron Healthcare Co., Ltd. recently publicized the prototype of a wearable surge BP monitoring (WSP) that uses recent advances in automatically controlled technology and measures absolute values of the maximum peaks of beat-by-beat pressure (Figure 7.16). The first prototype (WSP-1) has two tonometry sensor plates and the angle of the arrayed sensor plate to cover the radial artery is automatically adjusted to obtain effective applanation. This device is being tested and improved in collaboration with Omron, with the goal of developing more accurate beat-by-beat WSP (Figure 7.16) [156].

Using the WSP device, continuous beat-by-beat BP during sleep was monitored simultaneously with polysomnography (Figure 7.17). Nighttime BP and BP variability were significantly lower during Stages 2 and 3 sleep, and higher in Stage 1 and rapid eye movement (REM) sleep, and during waking hours (Figure 7.18) [235]. Three nighttime BP surges were detected, associated with REM sleep, arousal (unconscious microarousal) (Figure 7.19a), and a sleep apnea episode (Figure 7.19b) [235].

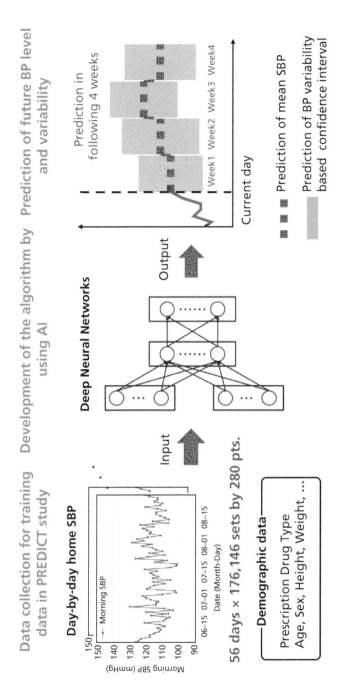

Figure 7.11 Prediction of BP variability using artificial intelligence (AI). *Source:* Presented at Joint Meeting ESH-ISH 2021 (on-air) held on April 11-14, 2021.

The algorithm could predict future BP increases by approx. 10 mmHg.

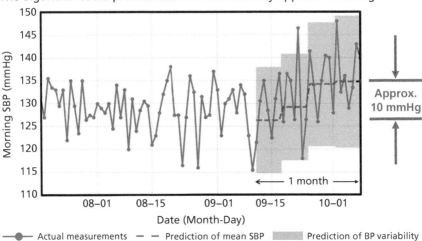

Figure 7.12 Typical case of BP prediction by the algorithm (75y, male). *Source:* Presented at Joint Meeting ESH-ISH 2021 (on-air) held on April 11-14, 2021.

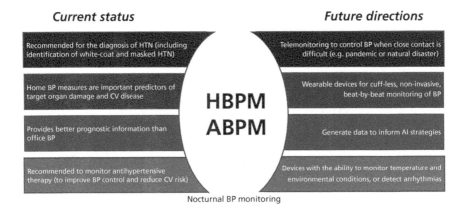

Figure 7.13 Out-of-office nocturnal blood pressure (BP) monitoring. ABPM, ambulatory blood pressure monitoring; AI, artificial intelligence; CV, cardiovascular; HBPM, home blood pressure monitoring; HTN, hypertension. *Source:* Kario. Am J Hypertens. 2021; 34: 783–794 [215]. Reprinted by permission of Oxford University Press.

The peak of sleep apnea-triggered nighttime BP surge was successfully detected by analyzing data from a newly developed tonometry-type WSP-1 device together with data obtained from a hypoxia-triggered nighttime BP monitoring. The peak SBP surge detected using beat-by-beat WSP-1 was 242 mmHg, which was higher than the hypoxia-triggered BP surge detected by trigger nighttime BP monitoring (TNP) using the oscillometric method (208 mmHg) (Figure 7.20) [235]. In a 50-year-old normotensive woman with obstructive sleep apnea (OSA), WSP-2 (the second prototype: equipped with a calibration function based on BP values

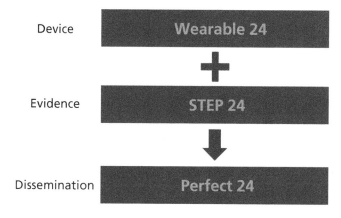

Figure 7.14 Anticipation DeVice-ApplicatioN Core Evidence Blood Pressure (ADVANCE blood pressure) program project, 2020-2035. *Source:* Kario K. Essential Manual of 24 Hour Blood Pressure Management: From Morning to Nocturnal Hypertension, Second Edition. Wiley, 2022.

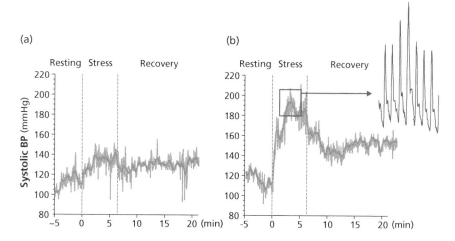

Figure 7.15 A typical case of hyperreactive blood pressure (BP) triggered by psychological distress (anger recall): (a) normal control; (b) hyperreactive case. *Source:* Kario et al. Hypertens Res. 2002;25:543–551 [479].

obtained using the oscillometric method) detected the highest peak of nighttime BP surge one day before (Day 1: baseline), and on the day of nighttime dosing of carvedilol 20 mg (Day 2: carvedilol-added). Carvedilol was associated with a reduction in the surge index (frequency of surge) from 17.2/hour to 7.4/hour. Surge peak was also decreased from 178 to 133 mmHg by the oscillometric method (Figure 7.21a), and from 184 to 137 mmHg by the continuous beat-by-beat method (Figure 7.21b) [235]. There are limitations of WSP-1/WSP-2, because the weaknesses of a tonometry BP monitoring device are that the sensor must be strictly positioned to cover the artery, and artifacts caused by movement of the wrist (which disturb effective applanation) are frequent.

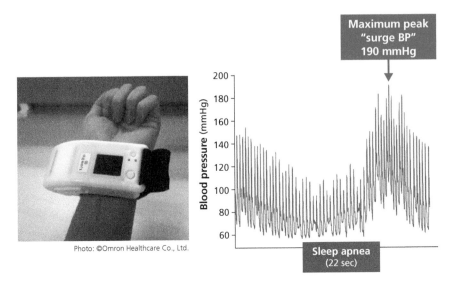

Figure 7.16 Beat-by-beat tonometry-type wearable surge blood pressure (BP) monitoring-1 (WSP-1) device and nighttime surge triggered by sleep apnea (right graph shows nighttime BP surges detected by WSP-1 in a patient with hypertension and sleep apnea). *Source:* Kario. Prog. Cardiovasc Dis. 2016;59:262–281 [156].

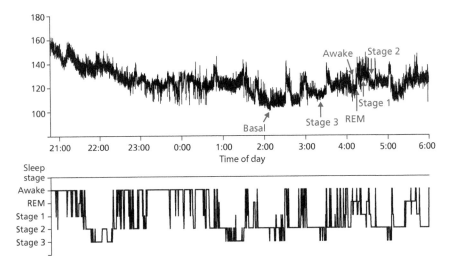

Figure 7.17 Beat-by-beat nighttime blood pressure (BP) continuously monitored by the newly developed tonometry-type wearable surge BP monitoring-1 (WSP-1) in different sleep stages defined by the simultaneous polysomnography (data from a healthy 43-year-old woman). REM: rapid eye movement. *Source:* Reprinted from Kario. Sleep and cardiovascular medicine. In: Encyclopedia of Cardiovascular Research and Medicine (Vasan R., Sawyer D., eds), Amsterdam, The Netherlands: Elsevier 2018, pp. 424–437 [235]; Copyright (2018), with permission from Elsevier.

Teams at Omron Healthcare Co., Ltd. (Mitsuo Kuwabara, Noboru Shinomiya, Shingo Yamashita, Toshikazu Shiga, Takahide Tanaka), Jichi Medical University (Kazuomi Kario, Naoko Tomitani, Satoshi Hoshide, Tomoyuki Kabutoya, Yuri Matsumoto), and Kyusyu University collaborated on research and development

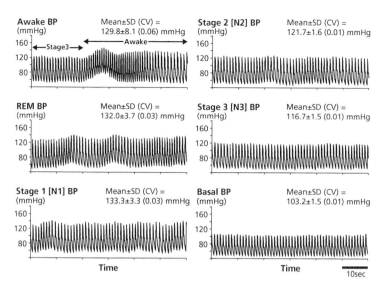

Figure 7.18 Beat-by-beat short-term nighttime blood pressure (BP) variability continuously monitored by the newly developed tonometry-type wearable surge BP monitoring-1 (WSP-1) in different sleep stages shown in Figure 7.17. BP surges during periods of wakefulness or rapid eye movement (REM) sleep were more pronounced than those during slow wave sleep (N3). The basal BP, the lowest BP, is usually found during N3 sleep. *Source:* Reprinted from Kario. Sleep and cardiovascular medicine. In: Encyclopedia of Cardiovascular Research and Medicine (Vasan R., Sawyer D., eds), Amsterdam, The Netherlands: Elsevier 2018, pp. 424–437 [235]; Copyright (2018), with permission from Elsevier.

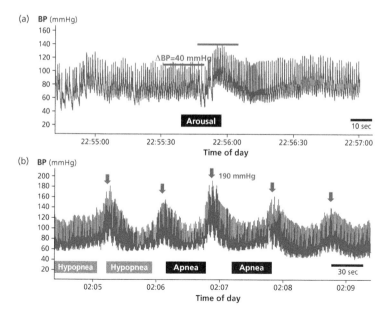

Figure 7.19 Nighttime blood pressure (BP) surges triggered by arousal (a: data from a 36-year-old healthy male) and apnea/hypopneas (b: data from a 50-year-old male with severe obstructive sleep apnea). Beat-by-beat nighttime BP was continuously monitored by the newly developed tonometry-type wearable surge BP monitoring-1 (WSP-1). *Source:* Reprinted from Kario. Sleep and cardiovascular medicine. In: Encyclopedia of Cardiovascular Research and Medicine (Vasan R., Sawyer D., eds), Amsterdam, The Netherlands: Elsevier 2018, pp. 424–437 [235]; Copyright (2018), with permission from Elsevier.

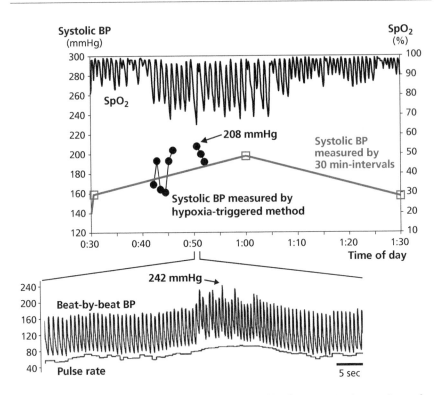

Figure 7.20 The peak of sleep apnea-triggered nighttime blood pressure (BP) surge detected by the newly developed tonometry-type wearable surge BP monitoring-1 device (data from a 53-year-old male with obstructive sleep apnea). SpO$_2$, oxygen saturation. *Source:* Reprinted from Kario. Sleep and cardiovascular medicine. In: Encyclopedia of Cardiovascular Research and Medicine (Vasan R., Sawyer D., eds), Amsterdam, The Netherlands: Elsevier 2018, pp. 424–437 [235]; Copyright (2018), with permission from Elsevier.

of new BP monitoring systems utilizing hemodynamic indices, such as the surge index and the baroreflex index (BRI) (Figure 7.22) [146].

Surge index

Surge index is the frequency of significant surge BP values detected by beat-by-beat BP monitoring and is calculated as the number of BP surges per hour. Stress events trigger short-term BP surge in the second order during stress and recovery phases (Figure 7.23a) [479]. Based on the shape of BP surge, various cardiovascular reactivity and recovery parameters fall into six categories: reactivity phase; recovery phase; amplitude; upward; downward; and whole duration (Figure 7.23b) [480].

The newly developed nighttime beat-by-beat continuous BP monitoring (tonometry method) successfully detected surge BPs corresponding to episodes of sleep apnea at baseline in patients with diabetes, hypertension, and obstructive sleep apnea (Figure 7.24a). Surge BP was suppressed during treatment with a sodium glucose cotransport-2 (SGLT2) inhibitor (Figure 7.24b). We have developed a new surge BP autodetection algorithm (Figures 7.25 and 7.26), and the

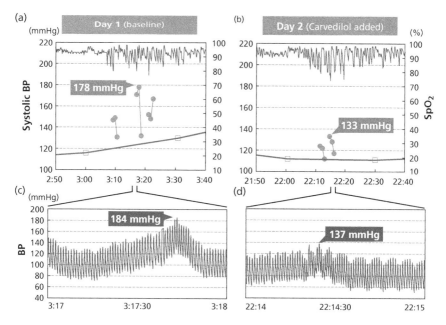

Figure 7.21 Nighttime surges in blood pressure (BP) at the time of an apnea episode in a 50-year-old normotensive woman with obstructive sleep apnea syndrome ((a, b) BPs detected by trigger nighttime BP monitoring [TNP]; closed circles represent systolic BP measured by an oxygen triggered function, (c, d) BPs monitored by wearable surge BP monitoring [WSP-2]). SpO₂, oxygen saturation. *Source:* Kario. Essential Manual on Perfect 24-Hour Blood Pressure Management from Morning to Nocturnal Hypertension: Up-to-date for Anticipation Medicine. Wiley, 2018: 1–309 [24].

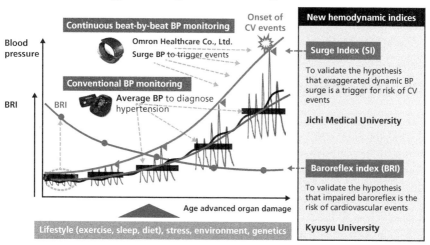

Figure 7.22 Innovation of blood pressure (BP) monitoring device and new hemodynamic indices. CV: cardiovascular. *Source:* Kario. Essential Manual on Perfect 24-Hour Blood Pressure Management from Morning to Nocturnal Hypertension: Up-to-date for Anticipation Medicine. Wiley, 2018: 1–309 [24].

(a)

(b)

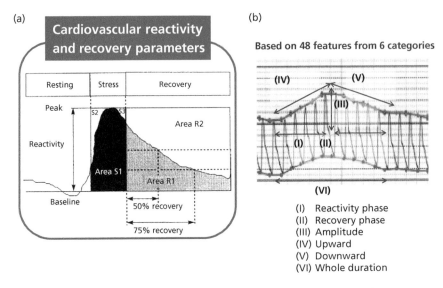

(I)   Reactivity phase
(II)   Recovery phase
(III)   Amplitude
(IV)   Upward
(V)   Downward
(VI)   Whole duration

Figure 7.23 Cardiovascular reactivity and recovery parameters. *Source:* Kario et al. Hypertens Res. 2002; 25: 543–551 [479]; Modified from Kokubo et al. Med Biol Eng Comput. 2020; 58: 1393–1404 [480].

lower panels show surge index values before and after treatment (Figure 7.27). Surge index during the entire sleep period was markedly decreased after treatment. Because whole sleep continuous beat-by-beat BP monitoring produces large volumes of data, software equipped with autodetection algorithms to detect BP variability profiles and interpret the individual BP data are needed for clinical practice. A recent study showed that beat-by-beat BP variability can persist despite best medical management (Figure 7.28) [481] and is associated with future stroke events in high-risk patients with history of transient ischemic attack and stroke (Figure 7.29) [482].

Disaster cardiovascular prevention (DCAP) network

The town of Minanisanriku was severely damaged by the Great East Japan earthquake and associated tsunami in 2011 (Figure 7.30). The DCAP network system was introduced into the major shelter in Minamisanriku town where Dr Masafumi Nishizawa had been working hard for victims since immediately after the earthquake (Figure 7.31). The DCAP network is a model for telemedicine management.

To better assess and reduce the risks for disaster-associated cardiovascular events, the web-based DCAP network (consisting of DCAP risk and prevention score assessment and self-measured BP monitoring at both a shelter and the home) was established to help survivors (Figure 7.32) [483–485]. The DCAP network system was developed using cloud-based computing on the Internet to monitor individual self-measured BP data. Disaster-induced increases in BP have

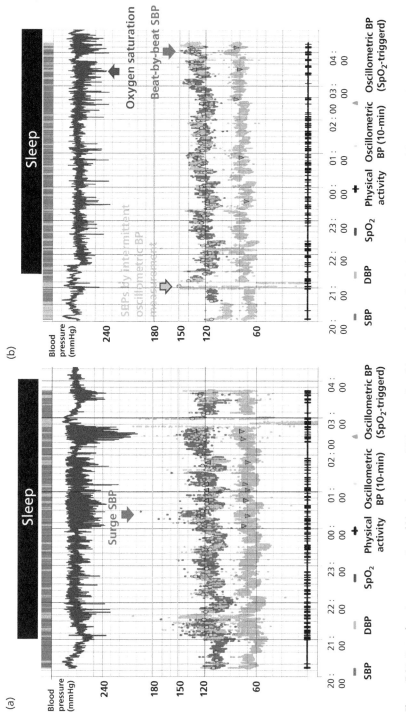

Figure 7.24 Data showing suppression of blood pressure (BP) surges trigged by apneic episodes during sleep in a 77-year-old woman with hypertension, diabetes, and obstructive sleep apnea. Sleep surge systolic (red dots) and diastolic (green dots) BP values were detected by the newly developed nocturnal beat-by-beat continuous BP monitoring (tonometry method) at baseline (treatment regimen: amlodipine 5 mg/day, aspirin 100 mg/day and sitagliptin 25 mg/day) (a) and after four weeks of add-on therapy with dapagliflozin 10 mg/day (b). *Source:* Kario. Hypertension. 2020; 76: 640–650 [221].

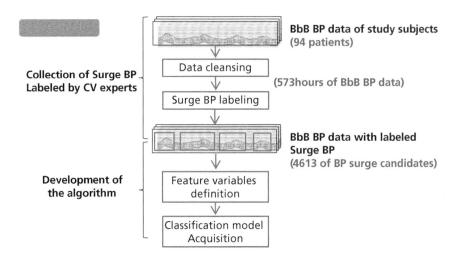

Figure 7.25 Automatic Detection Algorithm for "Surge Blood Pressure." Overall structure for algorithm development. Collected BbB BP data is given labels of surge BP by cardiovascular experts. These surge BP labels are used for development of the algorithm. BbB, beat-by-beat; BP, blood pressure; CV, cardiovascular. *Source:* Modified from Kokubo et al. Med Biol Eng Comput. 2020; 58: 1393–1404 [480]. doi: 10.1007/s11517-020-02162-4.

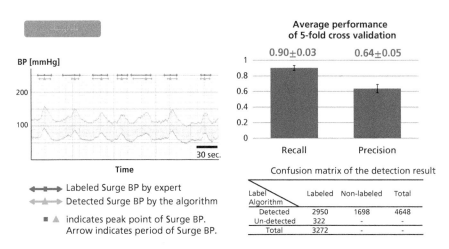

Figure 7.26 Automatic Detection Algorithm for "Surge Blood Pressure" [LEFT] Typical cases of detected surge BP by the algorithm. [RIGHT] Performance of surge BP detection. Numeric values in each cell in confusion matrix are numbers of cases. The "-" indicates uncountable. *Source:* Kokubo et al. Med Biol Eng Comput. 2020;58(6):1393–1404 [480]. doi: 10.1007/s11517-020-02162-4.

been shown to be influenced by the white-coat effect [486]. Thus, BP measurement by the disaster medical assistance team (DMAT) or unknown medical volunteers under stressful conditions in a shelter may overestimate BP, and thus self-measured BP could be considered better for guiding adequate antihypertensive medication under such conditions [487, 488]. In fact, the results showed that

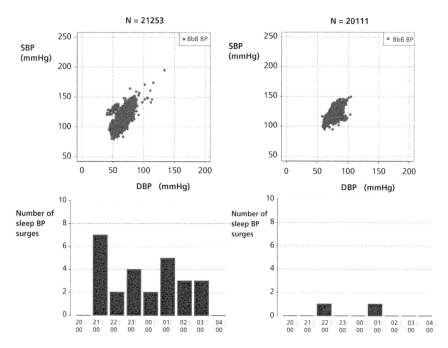

Figure 7.27 Pathological surge blood pressure (BP) detected by a new beat-by beat 'surge' BP monitoring and BP surge detection algorithm. The upper panels show the distribution of systolic blood pressure (SBP) and diastolic blood pressure (DBP) before (left) and after (right) four weeks of dapagliflozin. The lower panels show nighttime blood pressure (BP) surges detected by a newly developed surge autodetection algorithm. *Source:* Kario K. Hypertension. 2020; 76: 640–650 [221]. doi: 10.1161/HYPERTENSIONAHA.120.14742.

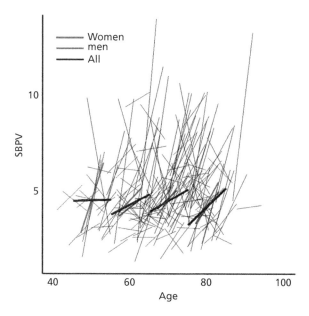

Figure 7.28 Increasing progression of beat-to-beat systolic blood pressure variability (SBPV) over five years with increasing age. Thick lines show the summary estimates within age groups (<55, 55–65, 65–75, >75). *Source:* Webb et al. Hypertension. 2021; 77: 193–201 [481].

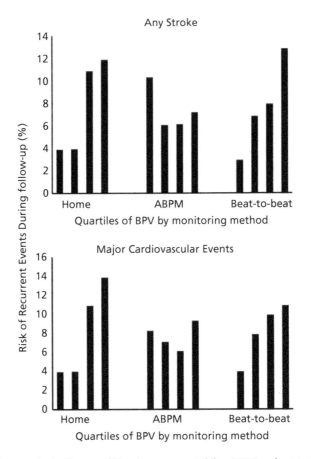

Figure 7.29 Prognostic significance of blood pressure variability (BPV) on beat-to-beat monitoring after transient ischemic attack (TIA) and stroke (n =405). Absolute risks by quartile of BPV. ABPM, ambulatory blood pressure monitoring. *Source:* Webb et al. Stroke. 2018; 49(1): 62–67 [482].

there were marked differences between volunteer-measured BP and self-measured BP in conjunction with the DCAP system (Figure 7.33) [487].

In most patients, the increases in office BP and self-measured BP were transient and BP levels returned to the preearthquake baseline levels within four weeks [486, 487, 489–491]. This characteristic of disaster-induced BP increase is important because persistent intensive antihypertensive treatment for subjects with high BP at the time of a disaster could result in excessive BP reduction, as was observed in a patient who had started treatment with antihypertensive agents just after the Great Hanshin-Awaji earthquake [488]. She was referred to the clinic because she developed dizziness three months later. Her antihypertensive medication was discontinued, and ambulatory BP was taken. This was found to be normal, and her symptoms disappeared. Thus, it is recommended that BP should be monitored, and the dose of antihypertensive medication reconsidered every two weeks during a disaster situation (Figure 7.34) [487, 488].

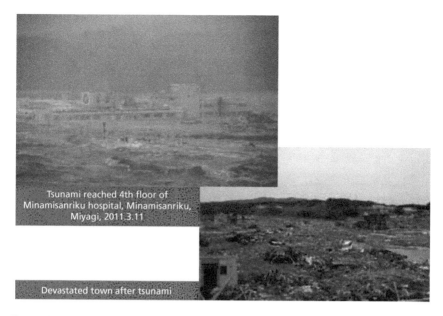

Figure 7.30 Great East Japan Earthquake 2011. *Source:* Kario. Essential Manual on Perfect 24-Hour Blood Pressure Management from Morning to Nocturnal Hypertension: Up-to-date for Anticipation Medicine. Wiley, 2018: 1–309 [24].

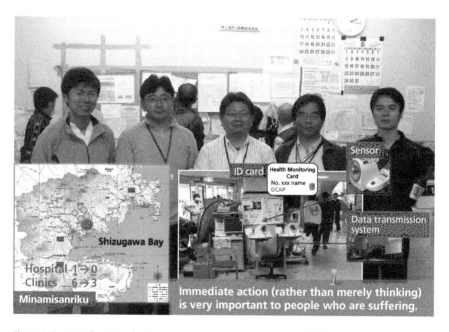

Figure 7.31 Introduction of a disaster cardiovascular prevention (DCAP) network system to the shelter in Minamisanriku area (April 29, 2011). From left: Satoshi Hoshide, Masahisa Shimpo, Masafumi Nishizawa (center), Kazuomi Kario, and Yuichiro Yano. Lower left: Shizugawa Bay; reduction in the number of hospital and clinics after the earthquake. *Source:* Kario. Essential Manual on Perfect 24-Hour Blood Pressure Management from Morning to Nocturnal Hypertension: Up-to-date for Anticipation Medicine. Wiley, 2018: 1–309 [24].

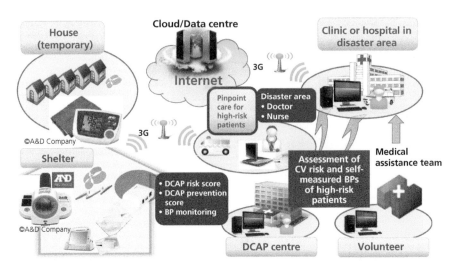

Figure 7.32 Disaster cardiovascular prevention (DCAP) network. BP, blood pressure; CV, cardiovascular. *Source:* JCS, JSH and JCC Joint Working group. Circ J. 2016; 80: 261–284 [485].

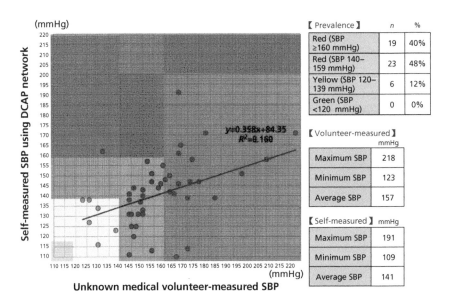

【 Prevalence 】

	n	%
Red (SBP ≥160 mmHg)	19	40%
Red (SBP 140–159 mmHg)	23	48%
Yellow (SBP 120–139 mmHg)	6	12%
Green (SBP <120 mmHg)	0	0%

【 Volunteer-measured 】 mmHg

	mmHg
Maximum SBP	218
Minimum SBP	123
Average SBP	157

【 Self-measured 】 mmHg

	mmHg
Maximum SBP	191
Minimum SBP	109
Average SBP	141

$y=0.358x+84.35$
$R^2=0.160$

Figure 7.33 Unknown medical volunteers-measured versus self-measured blood pressure (BP) using disaster cardiovascular prevention (DCAP) network (Minami-Sanriku, April 29-May 6, 2011). DBP, diastolic blood pressure; SBP, systolic blood pressure. *Source:* Kario. Circ J. 2012;76:553–562 [487].

In disaster victims, memory of the major earthquake and its damage may have augmented the pressor effect of an aftershock even though this occurred 19 months after the initial event. ABPM was used in eight patients with hypertension who lived in Minamisanriku town, the disaster area at the time of the first

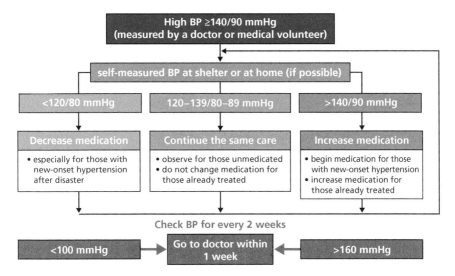

Figure 7.34 Management of disaster hypertension. BP, blood pressure. *Source:* Kario. Circ J. 2012;76:553–562 [487].

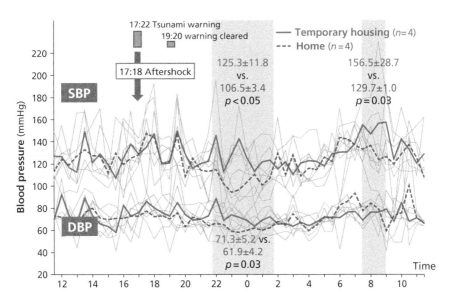

Figure 7.35 Ambulatory blood pressure monitoring (ABPM) data at the time of aftershocks (*n* = 8). DBP, diastolic blood pressure; SBP, systolic blood pressure. *Source:* Created based on data from Nishizawa et al. Am J Hypertens. 2015;28:1405–1408 [492].

major aftershock. A pressor effect of ambulatory BP was found immediately after the aftershock. A persistent pressor effect generated a non-dipper pattern of night-time BP and exaggerated morning BP surge in patients living in temporary housing (Figure 7.35) [492].

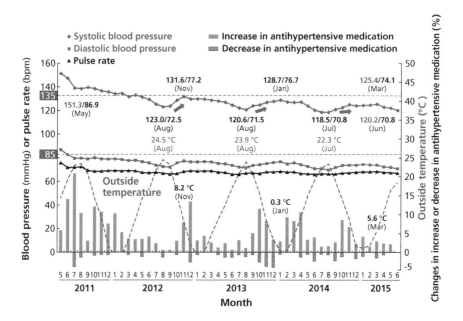

Figure 7.36 Changes in home blood pressure in disaster cardiovascular prevention (DCAP) participants (*n* = 351) after 2011 great east Japan earthquake. *Source:* Nishizawa et al. J Clin Hypertens. 2017;19:26–29 [493].

Successful anticipation model of ICT-based BP control

Successful home BP control was achieved in DCAP participants after the 2011 Great East Japan earthquake (Figure 7.36) [493]. After four years, home SBP had decreased from 151 to 125 mmHg in the winter and to 120 mmHg in the summer. This BP control status is almost identical to the ideal levels of the Systolic Blood Pressure Intervention Trial (SPRINT) [179], and less than the universal BP goal mandated in the 2017 American Heart Association/American College of Cardiology guidelines [178]. Importantly, seasonal variation had decreased to ≤5 mmHg even in patients living in the severely damaged area. In addition, the duration from the summer low to the winter peak of home BP decreased year-on-year. This may have been due to timely and appropriate titration of antihypertensive medication by anticipation of the individual seasonal variation of the previous year by serial time trend chart of BP changes.

Housing condition and age are important for winter morning BP surge. Patients with hypertension aged ≥75 years who lived in their own homes were at significant risk for the highest quintile of winter morning SBP surge (odds ratio 5.21, *p* = 0.010) (Figure 7.37) [494]. Therefore, it is essential to prepare suitable housing conditions for elderly patients with hypertension following a disaster.

Disaster hypertension

Damage resulting from natural disasters is growing worldwide. A major disaster triggers serial cardiovascular events (Figure 7.38) [487]. Increase in thrombophilic tendency and BP are the leading cause of disaster-induced cardiovascular events (e.g. stroke, cardiac events, and heart failure (Figure 7.39)) [487].

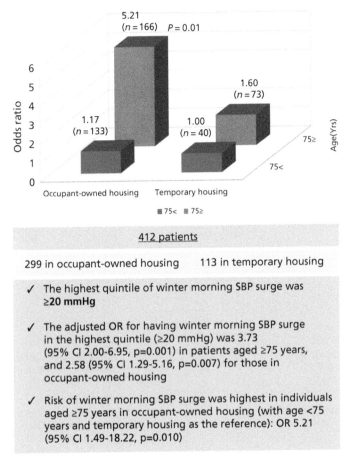

Figure 7.37 Relative risk for the highest quintile of winter morning surge in systolic blood pressure (SBP) due to differences in housing conditions and age. CI, confidence interval; OR, odds ratio. *Source:* Nishizawa et al. J Clin Hypertens (Greenwich). 2019; 21(2): 208–216 [494].

At the time of the Great Hanshin-Awaji earthquake in 1995, the author was working for the Awaji-Hokudan Public Clinic in the area near the epicenter of the earthquake and found a disaster-associated increase in BP. Patients with borderline hypertension developed uncontrolled hypertension but BP returned to previous levels after one month in the majority of patients. However, some patients, especially those with microalbuminuria, developed persistent uncontrolled disaster hypertension (Figure 7.40) [486, 489].

Based on previous experience, a disaster cardiovascular risk score was developed to identify patients who are at high risk of developing disaster-induced cardiovascular events, as well as a prevention score (Figure 7.41) [487]. As shown in the lower panel of Figure 7.36, the dose of antihypertensive medication was increased from October 2012, then the winter BP peak was suppressed during December to February (the coldest temperatures). In the following year (2013),

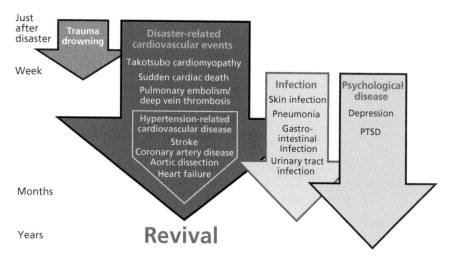

Figure 7.38 Time course of the onset of disaster-related disease. PTSD, posttraumatic stress disorder. *Source:* Kario. Circ J. 2012;76:553–562 [487].

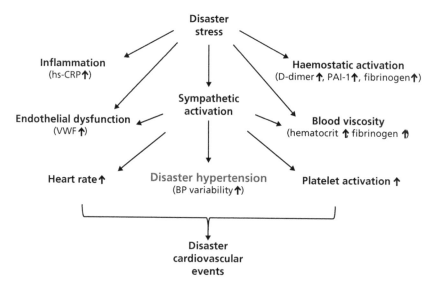

Figure 7.39 Disaster-activating cardiovascular risk factors. BP, blood pressure; hs-CRP, high-sensitivity C-reactive protein; PAI-1, plasminogen activator inhibitor-1; VWF, von Willebrand factor. *Source:* Kario. Circ J. 2012;76:553–562 [487].

drug titration was initiated in September, and the winter BP peak was again suppressed. This proactive adjustment of drug dosages can only be achieved when the doctor and patient both recognize the seasonal variation in BP from previous years. This is one of the most successful models of anticipation medicine using telemedicine and telecare.

At the time of the Great East Japan earthquake in 2011, marked, uncontrolled disaster hypertension was again found in individuals residing in temporary shelters

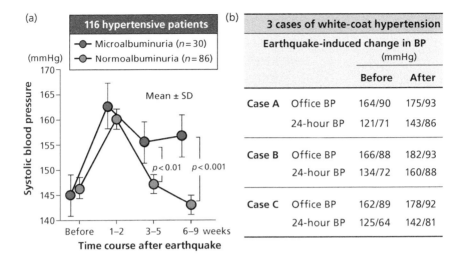

Figure 7.40 Earthquake-induced blood pressure (BP) increase (Hanshin-Awaji earthquake 1995). (a) Systolic blood pressure values (mean ± SD) after the earthquake in patients with microalbuminuria and patients with normal urinary albumin excretion (<20 μg/min). P values are for comparisons with baseline values. (b) Office and ambulatory BP in three patients with white-coat hypertension before and after earthquake. *Source:* (a) Kario et al. Am J Med. 2001;111:379–384 [486], (b) Kario et al. Lancet. 1995;345:1365 [489].

(Figure 7.42). High salt intake and increased salt sensitivity caused by disrupted circadian rhythms are suggested as the two leading causes of this disaster hypertension, via neurohumoral activation under stressful conditions [487, 490, 491] (Figure 7.43). In fact, estimated sodium intake (along with diabetes mellitus and chronic kidney disease) was found to be a significant risk factor for the presence of disaster hypertension (Table 7.1) [495, 496]

COVID-19 era

Strict lockdown and social distancing rules in place to mitigate the coronavirus disease 2019 (COVID-19) pandemic saw a surge in the use of remote health consultations, and the value of telemedicine strategies quickly became evident. In addition, the importance of effective management of noncommunicable diseases such as hypertension was highlighted by higher levels of COVID-19-related morbidity and mortality in the presence of several comorbidities [496]. Hypertension is a particularly common comorbidity in COVID-19-positive deceased patients [496].

Although early progression may be asymptomatic, severe cases of COVID-19 show rapid worsening after symptom onset, progressing to acute respiratory distress syndrome and significant disease manifestations across a range of organ systems (Figure 7.44). Hypertension was seen as a particularly relevant comorbidity in COVID-19 because the spike protein on the surface of the SARS-CoV2 virus binds to the extra-cellular domain of transmembrane angiotensin-converting enzyme-2 (ACE2) receptor to gain entry into host cells (Figure 7.45). The fact that

DCAP-AFHCHDC7 Risk Score and DCAP - SEDWITMP8 Prevention Score		✓
1 Age (A)	>75 years	☐
2 Family (F)	death or hospitalisation (partner, parents, or children)	☐
3 Housing (H)	completely destroyed	☐
4 Community (C)	completely destroyed	☐
5 Hypertension (H)	Positive (under medication, or systolic blood pressure >160 mmHg)	☐
6 Diabetes (D)	Positive	☐
7 Cardiovascular disease (C)	Positive (coronary artery disease, stroke, heart failure)	☐
	Average total score*_____	
DCAP-SEDWITMP8 Prevention Score#		
1 Sleep (S)	Sleep duration >6 hr, arousal <3 times during sleep	☐
2 Physical activity (E)	Walking >20 min/day	☐
3 Diet (D)	Reduce salt intake with high potassium intake (3 serves of green vegetable, fruit, or seaweed/day)	☐
4 Body weight (W)	change < ±2 kg	☐
5 Infection prevention (I)	regular face mask use and washing hands	☐
6 Thrombosis (T)	sufficient water intake >1,000 mL per day	☐
7 Medication (M)	continuous use of antihypertensive medication and antiplatelet agents and/or anticoagulation	☐
8 Blood pressure control (P)	<140 mmHg systolic (clinic, shelter, or self-measured)	☐
	Average total score*_____	

Figure 7.41 Disaster cardiovascular prevention (DCAP) risk score (AFHCHDC7) and prevention score (SEDWITMP8). *Total number of each risk factor as the individual risk score (0–7 points). A score of ≥4 defines a high-risk group. #Total number of each prevention factor as the individual prevention score (0–8 points); recommended prevention score is ≥6, particularly in high-risk patients. *Source:* Kario. Circ J. 2012;76:553–562 [487].

both angiotensin receptor blockers (ARBs) and ACE inhibitors, agents commonly used to treat hypertension, have been shown experimentally to increase expression of ACE2 on cell membranes [497–499], meant that there was initially concern about the potential for higher SARS-CoV2 infection rates and more severe COVID-19 disease in patients being treated with these agents. However, this does not appear to be the case [500–502]. Nevertheless, there are several mechanisms by which COVID-19 might increase cardiovascular risk (Figure 7.46).

Hypertension is a common comorbidity in COVID-19-positive deceased patients [496], making effective management of patients with these two conditions especially important. The Hypertension Cardiovascular Outcome Prevention and Evidence in Asia (HOPE Asia) Network has provided some useful guidance in this area (Table 7.2) [500]. Current recommendations for the use of out-of-office BP monitoring in hypertension management mean that this field is better placed than many to adapt to patient management during a global pandemic. This is facilitated by the availability of new ICT-based home BP monitoring devices, as

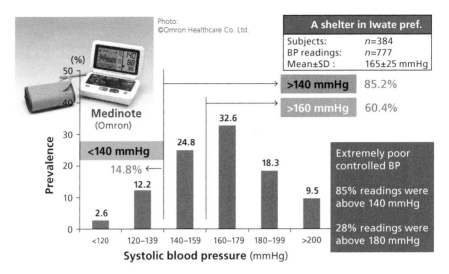

Figure 7.42 Blood pressure (BP) values recorded in individuals housed in a shelter (First Jichi Medical University Supporting Team) March 25–April 1, 2011. SD, standard deviation. *Source:* Kario. Essential Manual on Perfect 24-Hour Blood Pressure Management from Morning to Nocturnal Hypertension: Up-to-date for Anticipation Medicine. Wiley, 2018:1–309 [24].

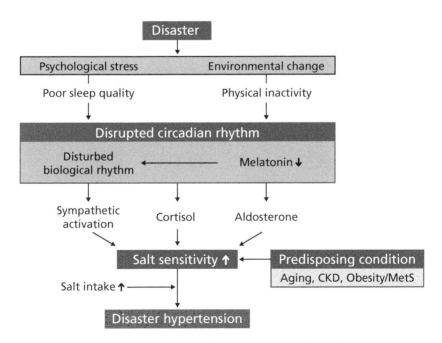

Figure 7.43 Possible mechanisms of disaster hypertension. CKD, chronic kidney disease; MetS, metabolic syndrome. *Source:* Kario. Circ J. 2012;76:553–562 [487].

Table 7.1 Sodium intake and disaster hypertension among evacuees in acute phase of the Great East Japan Earthquake.

Total population	Event/n	OR (95% CI) of sodium per 1 g increase	P for interaction
Entire group	158/272	1.16 (1.05–1.30)	NA
Subgroup of salt sensitive hypertension (SSHT)			
Low risk of SSHT	36/80	1.01 (0.83–1.24)	0.068
High risk of SSHT[a]	122/192	1.26 (1.11–1.43)	
The population without prevalent hypertension before the disaster			
Entire group	66/146	1.28 (1.08–1.51)	NA
Subgroup of salt sensitive hypertension (SSHT)			
Low risk of SSHT	18/55	0.99 (0.73–1.35)	0.030
High risk of SSHT[a]	48/91	1.51 (1.21–-1.88)	

Disaster hypertension was defined as BP ≥140/90 mmHg.
CI, confidence interval; OR, odds ratio; SSHT, salt-sensitive hypertension.
[a] Risk factors for SSHT included age ≥65 years, body mass index ≥25 kg/m^2, chronic kidney disease and diabetes.
Source: Hoshide et al. Hypertension. 2019;74(3): 564–571 [495].

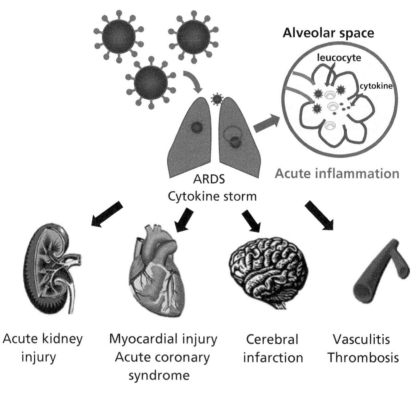

Figure 7.44 Variety of organ damage seen in patients with COVID-19. ARDS, acute respiratory distress syndrome. *Source:* Kario et al. J Clin Hypertens. 2020;22(7):1109–1119 [500].

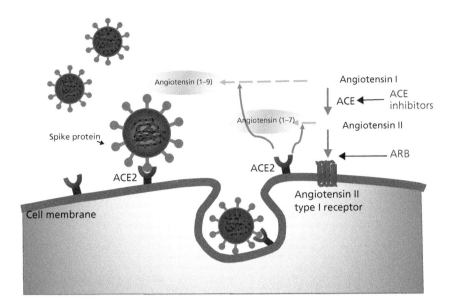

Figure 7.45 SARS-CoV-2 and the renin-angiotensin system. ACE, angiotensin-converting enzyme; ARB, angiotensin receptor blocker. *Source:* Kario et al. J Clin Hypertens. 2020;22(7): 1109–1119 [500].

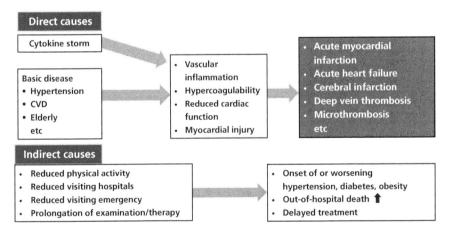

Figure 7.46 COVID-19 and cardiovascular disease. (Drawing by Hoshide S and Kario K). *Source:* Kario K. Essential Manual of 24 Hour Blood Pressure Management: From Morning to Nocturnal Hypertension, Second Edition. Wiley, 2022.

previously applied in a postdisaster setting. This will ensure that patients with hypertension have well-controlled BP despite not being able to have face-to-face physician visits. Maintaining well-controlled BP has the potential to mitigate the negative effects of hypertension on prognosis in patients with COVID-19 [500].

Table 7.2 Clinical practice guidance for the management of hypertension in the COVID-19 era.

COVID-19 and Comorbidities: Assessment and Management

- Patients with hypertension, especially older individuals and those with other known risk factors, are at increased risk of developing severe symptoms during COVID-19 infection
- High-risk patients, such as those with hypertension, are more likely to develop cardiac injury during COVID-19 infection
- Diabetes mellitus should be carefully managed, and these patients need to be closely monitored for the development of myocardial injury and arteriovenous thrombosis
- Consider determining levels of key biomarkers, especially troponin and D-dimer, to get a complete clinical picture and information about prognosis in patients with COVID-19
- Oxygen saturation should be determined at presentation; if oxygen saturation is <94% then COVID-19 should be considered as severe
- COVID-19 progression and cardiovascular status can be monitored by measuring blood pressure and taking the patient's temperature
- Antihypertensive therapy with ACE inhibitors or ARBs in patients with COVID-19 should be carefully continued, with careful monitoring to detect hypotension and kidney injury
- Unmedicated older COVID-19 patients whose only comorbidity is hypertension can be treated with calcium channel blockers
- Physicians should be aware of physical manifestations of stress (e.g., cardiovascular events), even in individuals not infected with COVID-19 (especially those with pre-existing hypertension)

Source: Kario et al. J Clin Hypertens. 2020; 22: 1109–1119 [500].

CHAPTER 8
Asia perspectives

There are significant ethnic differences in cardiovascular-renal demographics around the world, and hypertension is one of the most powerful risk factors associated with these demographic differences. Both compared with other regions and within Asia, there are significant country-specific, regional, and ethnic differences in blood pressure (BP) control status. To achieve effective protection against cardiovascular-renal events in Asia, it is important that Asian characteristics of hypertension-related cardiovascular-renal disease are identified and addressed.

What is the HOPE Asia Network?

The Hypertension, brain, cardiovascular and renal Outcome Prevention and Evidence in Asia (HOPE Asia) Network was officially established in 2018 [503]. Its mission is to improve the management of hypertension and organ protection with the ultimate goal of achieving zero cardiovascular events in Asia. Activity is based on three initiatives: (1) the examination and analysis of existing evidence related to hypertension; (2) formation of a consensus regarding hot clinical topics in hypertension; and (3) conducting Asia-wide clinical studies in hypertension. Two additional goals were added in 2020: to disseminate evidence and to foster young researchers (Figure 8.1) [504, 505].

The HOPE Asia Network is proud to be a member organization of the World Hypertension League (WHL) and looks forward to contributing actively to the WHL's mission of confronting the global epidemic of hypertension and the high burden of premature death and disability that results from this condition [506–508]. Since November 2019, the HOPE Asia Network has also been an affiliated society of the International Society of Hypertension (ISH).

Groups of Asian hypertension researchers (e.g. the Asia BP@Home investigators and the COME Asia-MHDG [Characteristics on the ManagEment of Hypertension in the Asia-Morning Hypertension Discussion Group]) have studied the characteristics of hypertension and cardiovascular-renal disease in Asian populations [270, 320, 442, 443, 475, 509]. Collaboration between these groups was instrumental in

Essential Manual of 24-Hour Blood Pressure Management: From Morning to Nocturnal Hypertension,
Second Edition. Kazuomi Kario.
© 2022 John Wiley & Sons Ltd. Published 2022 by John Wiley & Sons Ltd.

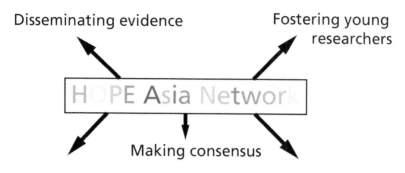

Figure 8.1 Missions of the Hypertension, brain, cardiovascular and renal Outcome Prevention and Evidence in Asia (HOPE Asia) Network. *Source:* Kario. J Clin Hypertens. 2018; 20: 212–214 [503] and Kario and Wang. JACC Asia. 2021; 1: 121–124 [505].

forming the HOPE Asia Network. In a previous survey of awareness of hypertension management in Asia, 87% of all physicians who responded said that they did take the Asian lifestyle and Asian-specific characteristics of hypertension into consideration, and 92% recognized the need for an Asian-specific guideline for the management of hypertension (Figures 8.2 and 8.3) [510].

HOPE Asia Network resources and up-to-date information relating to hypertension management in Asian countries can be found at the group's website: https://www.hope-asia-network.com.

HOPE Asia Network achievements

The first HOPE Asia Network project determined the current status and evidence relating to home BP in 12 Asian countries based on a search of the medical literature [511]. Subsequently, several meetings were held with the purpose of achieving a consensus on home BP-guided clinical management of hypertension in Asia [184, 512], and on locally based recommendations for ambulatory BP monitoring (ABPM) [512, 513].

Research by the HOPE Asia Network showed that there are marked differences in the current prevalence and awareness of hypertension, the proportions of patients with treated and controlled hypertension (Figure 8.4) [148, 511], and in the usage of common antihypertensive drugs between countries in Asia (Figure 8.5) [504]. The group is also active in research and review in the hypertension field, especially concerning clinically important "hot topics" relating to the management of hypertension and the prevention of cardiovascular-renal disease in Asia. These efforts have been supported by the *Journal of Clinical Hypertension*, which published the first "Asia Special Issue" in March 2020 [185, 261, 287, 378, 477, 504, 514–537]. This was repeated in March 2021 [513, 538–571], and will be supported by the journal on ongoing basis.

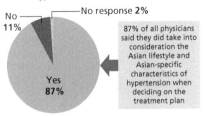

Q1. When you treat hypertensive patients, do you consider the Asian lifestyle and characteristics of hypertension?

No response 2%

No 11%

Yes 87%

87% of all physicians said they did take into consideration the Asian lifestyle and Asian-specific characteristics of hypertension when deciding on the treatment plan

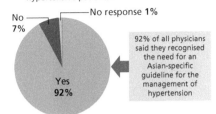

Q2. Do you think we need an Asian-specific guideline for the management of hypertensive patients?

No response 1%

No 7%

Yes 92%

92% of all physicians said they recognised the need for an Asian-specific guideline for the management of hypertension

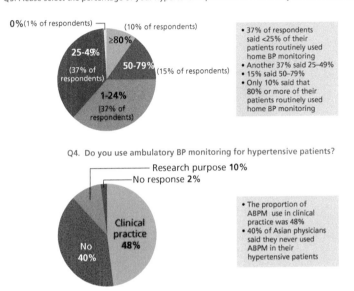

Q3. Please select the percentage of your hypertensive patients who routinely undertake home BP monit

0%(1% of respondents)

(10% of respondents)

≥80%

25-49% (37% of respondents)

50-79% (15% of respondents)

1-24% (37% of respondents)

- 37% of respondents said <25% of their patients routinely used home BP monitoring
- Another 37% said 25–49%
- 15% said 50–79%
- Only 10% said that 80% or more of their patients routinely used home BP monitoring

Q4. Do you use ambulatory BP monitoring for hypertensive patients?

Research purpose 10%
No response 2%

Clinical practice 48%

No 40%

- The proportion of ABPM use in clinical practice was 48%
- 40% of Asian physicians said they never used ABPM in their hypertensive patients

Figure 8.2 Asian physicians' knowledge of hypertension management. A total of 133 physicians attending conferences in Asia over the period March to May 2014 responded to the questionnaire. Physicians were from China ($n = 33$), Taiwan ($n = 29$), Indonesia ($n = 8$), Thailand ($n = 7$), Vietnam ($n = 7$), Myanmar ($n = 7$), Pakistan ($n = 1$), Korea ($n = 3$), Philippines ($n = 3$), Malaysia ($n = 1$), Egypt ($n = 1$), Hong Kong ($n = 1$), Saudi Arabia ($n = 1$), and unknown ($n = 28$). ABPM, ambulatory blood pressure monitoring; BP, blood pressure. *Source:* Hoshide et al. Curr Hypertens Rev. 2016;12:164–168 [510]. Republished with permission of Bentham Science Publishers Ltd.

The initial focus of the HOPE Asia Network has been on home BP values because we consider that a home BP-guided approach is the most effective and practical in clinical practice. Accordingly, HOPE Asia Network expert panel consensus recommendations for home blood pressure monitoring (HBPM) in Asia have been published, focusing on the practical usage of HBPM (Table 8.1) [183].

Specific research activity by the HOPE Asia Network includes the Asia BP@ Home study, which investigated the current status of home BP control in different Asian countries [521, 572, 573]. This is the first HBPM study to use the same device and monitoring schedule across all countries and study centers.

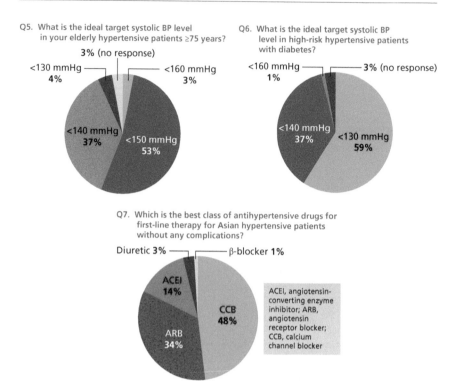

Q5. What is the ideal target systolic BP level in your elderly hypertensive patients ≥75 years?

3% (no response)
<130 mmHg 4%
<160 mmHg 3%
<140 mmHg 37%
<150 mmHg 53%

Q6. What is the ideal target systolic BP level in high-risk hypertensive patients with diabetes?

<160 mmHg 1%
3% (no response)
<140 mmHg 37%
<130 mmHg 59%

Q7. Which is the best class of antihypertensive drugs for first-line therapy for Asian hypertensive patients without any complications?

Diuretic 3%
β-blocker 1%
ACEI 14%
CCB 48%
ARB 34%

ACEI, angiotensin-converting enzyme inhibitor; ARB, angiotensin receptor blocker; CCB, calcium channel blocker

Figure 8.3 Asian physicians' knowledge of hypertension management ($n = 133$). BP, blood pressure. *Source:* Hoshide et al. Curr Hypertens Rev. 2016;12:164–168 [510]. Republished with permission of Bentham Science Publishers Ltd.

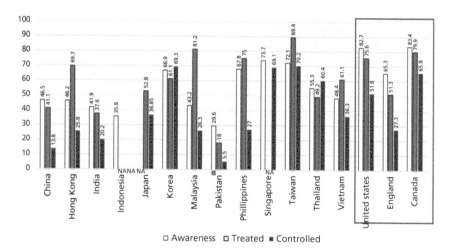

□ Awareness □ Treated ■ Controlled

Figure 8.4 Awareness, treatment, and control rate of hypertension in Asian countries. NA, data not available. *Source:* Kario and Wang. Hypertension. 2018; 71: 979–984 [148].

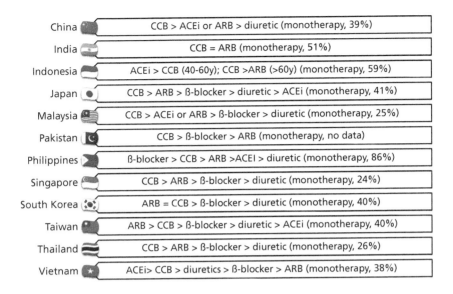

Figure 8.5 Usage of antihypertensives and proportion of monotherapy by country. ACEi, angiotensin-converting enzyme inhibitor; ARB, angiotensin receptor blocker; CCB, calcium channel blocker. *Source:* Kario et al. J Clin Hypertens. 2020;22:331–343 [504].

Characteristics of cardiovascular disease in Asia

It is well established that the characteristics of hypertension and its related diseases are markedly different in Asians compared with Caucasians and Blacks (Table 8.2) [138, 155, 179]. Several factors contribute to hypertension and cardiovascular disease in Asia (Figure 8.6) [504, 505]. For example, the phenotypes of cardiovascular disease, stroke, and heart failure that are closely associated with high BP are more common in Asia (Figure 8.7) [574]. In the recent prospective, Home blood pressure measurement with Olmesartan Naive patients to Establish Standard Target blood pressure (HONEST) study in an Asian population, the incidence of stroke in treated patients with hypertension was around 2.8-times higher than that of myocardial infarction (2.92 vs. 1.03 per 1000 person-years) (Table 8.3) [56]. The incidence of coronary artery disease (composite of myocardial infarction and angina pectoris with intervention) (2.80 per 1000 person-years) was almost comparable to that of stroke. Furthermore, the slope of the association between BP and cardiovascular events is steeper in Asians compared with Western populations (Figures 8.8 and 8.9) [575, 576]. Thus, the impact of 24-hour hypertension control would be greater in Asians [138, 169, 179].

Obesity and salt intake in Asia

The impact of obesity on high BP may be different between Asian and Caucasian individuals. Asians are likely to develop high BP even in the presence of mild obesity. Looking at the risk of elevated BP/stage 1 hypertension (previously known as prehypertension), the impact of a body mass index (BMI) of 25 kg/m²

Table 8.1 Summary of recommendations for home blood pressure (BP) monitoring in Asia.

Recommendations	Class of recommendation	Level of evidence
1. HBPM is an accurate adjunct for diagnosing hypertension when a validated device is used and the measurement is performed correctly	I	B
2. Method of measuring home BP: • Sitting BP after 2 min of rest • Wearing light clothes while taking the reading is allowed • At least 2 readings, with a 1-min interval, twice daily, for at least 3 days, but preferably 7 days • Morning: within 1 h after waking, after urination, before breakfast, and before drug intake • Evening: before going to bed • Elevated BP is shown by a mean reading of ≥ 135/85 mmHg	I	B
3a. HBPM is a better predictor of cardiovascular outcome than office BP. When there is a discrepancy of diagnosis between office and home BP, a home BP-based diagnosis should have priority and, when possible, be confirmed by ABPM.	I	B
3b. Morning hypertension is a better predictor of prognosis than clinic BP	I	B
4. Antihypertensive treatment strategies should target a home BP level of <135/85 mmHg	I	B
Strict antihypertensive treatment targeting a home systolic BP level of <125 mmHg may have benefit in high-risk Asian hypertensive patients, especially those with diabetes or chronic kidney disease, and/or cardiovascular disease	IIa	B
5a. The diagnosis and treatment of hypertension should still be guided by office BP readings where HBPM is not readily available. However, HBPM can improve compliance when combined with active intervention, and thus improve BP control compared with current standard care alone	I	B
5b. Self-monitoring and self-titration may be feasible if carefully monitored by healthcare professionals and help to improve blood pressure control. However, local policies must be adhered to as self-titration is not recommended in certain countries	IIb	B
6. Titration should be based on targeting a mean home BP of <135/85 mmHg. However, in case of high morning BP and normal evening BP, uptitration of drug treatment should be considered even if mean home BP is <135/85 mmHg. HBPM may aid chronotherapy of hypertension by helping identify those patients who experience isolated morning hypertension	IIa	B
7. HBPM may be incorporated into local clinical hypertension guidelines	IIa	C
8. Information and communication technology (ICT)-based HBPM may be beneficial, especially for patients who live in remote Asian geographical locations. The expert panel agreed that that telemonitoring of home BP, which requires active participation by patients, may have an important role in clinical practice in the near future in Asia	IIb	B

Table 8.1 (Continued)

Recommendations	Class of recommendation	Level of evidence
9. A validated brachial BP measuring oscillometric device should be used for meaning home BP	I	C
Where this is not feasible, the brachial BP measuring oscillometric device of choice should be calibrated every 6–12 months	IIb	C

Classes of recommendations:
Class I: evidence and/or general agreement that a given treatment or procedure is beneficial, useful, effective (is recommended/is indicated);
Class IIa: weight of evidence/opinions is in favour of usefulness/efficacy (should be considered);
Class IIb: usefulness/efficacy is less well established by evidence/opinion (may be considered);
Class III: evidence or general agreement that the given treatment or procedure is not useful/effective, and in some cases may be harmful (is not recommended).
Levels of evidence:
A: data derived from multiple randomised clinical trials or meta-analyses;
B: data derived from a single randomised clinical trial or large nonrandomised studies;
C: consensus of opinion of the experts and/or small studies, retrospective studies, registries.
BP, blood pressure; HBPM, home BP monitoring.
Source: Park et al. J Hum Hypertens. 2018; 32: 249–258 [183].

Table 8.2 Characteristics of hypertension in Asia.

1. Stroke, especially hemorrhagic stroke, more common than myocardial infarction
2. Steeper association between blood pressure and cardiovascular disease
3. Higher salt intake with higher salt sensitivity
4. Obesity and metabolic syndrome epidemic
5. Morning and nocturnal hypertension more common

Source: Modified from Kario et al. Hypertens Res. 2013;36:478–484 [157].

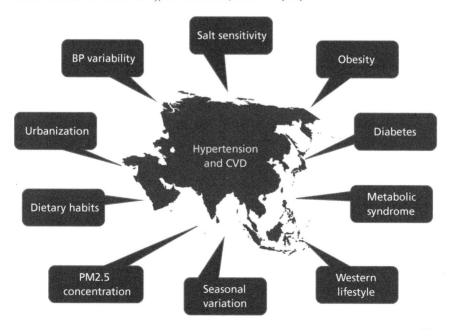

Figure 8.6 Factors contributing to hypertension and cardiovascular disease in Asia. *Source:* **317** Kario et al. Hypertens Res. 2013;36:478–484 [157].

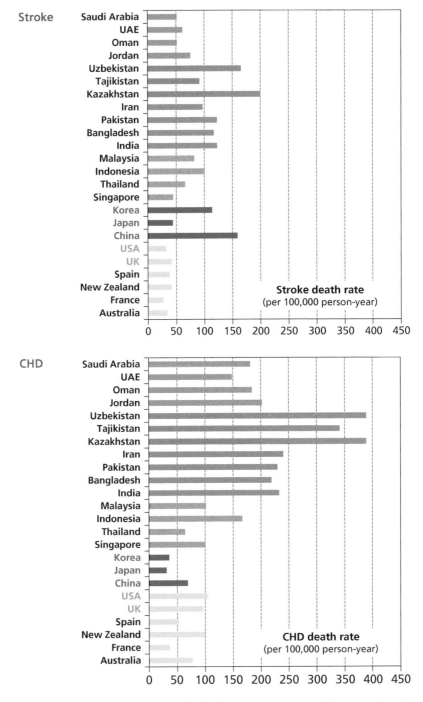

Figure 8.7 Age-standardized cardiovascular death rates per 100 000 in different regions of Asia in 2002 (data from the World Health Organization). CHD, coronary heart disease. *Source:* Ueshima et al. Circulation. 2008;118(25):2702–2709 [574].

Table 8.3 Cardiovascular disease in medicated patients with hypertension. HONEST study.

Cardiovascular events	No. of events	Incidence, events/1000 patient-years (95% CI)
Primary end point	280	6.46 (5.75–7.27)
Secondary end point	336	7.76 (6.98–8.64)
Stroke events[a]	127	2.92 (2.46–3.48)
Atherothrombotic cerebral infarction	43	0.99 (0.73–1.33)
Lacunar infarction	40	0.92 (0.67–1.25)
Cerebral haemorrhage	17	0.39 (0.24–0.63)
Unclassified cerebral infarction	13	0.30 (0.17–0.51)
Subarachnoid haemorrhage	8	0.18 (0.09–0.37)
Cardiogenic cerebral infarction	4	0.09 (0.03–0.24)
Unclassified stroke	3	0.07 (0.02–0.21)
Cardiac events	167	3.85 (3.30–4.48)
Coronary revascularisation procedure for angina pectoris[a]	77	1.77 (1.42–2.21)
Myocardial infarction[a]	45	1.03 (0.77–1.38)
Hospitalisation for heart failure	36	0.83 (0.60–1.15)
Hospitalisation for angina pectoris	13	0.30 (0.17–0.51)
All death	190	4.36 (3.78–5.02)
Cardiovascular death	46	1.05 (0.79–1.41)
Sudden death[a]	35	0.80 (0.58–1.12)
Aortic dissection	5	0.11 (0.05–0.28)
Arteriosclerosis obliterans	12	0.28 (0.16–0.48)

CI, confidence interval.
[a] Events comprising the primary end point. Cardiovascular death included fatal stroke, fatal myocardial infarction, and sudden death.
Source: Kario et al. Hypertension. 2014;64:989–996 [56].

in a Japanese population was almost comparable to that of a BMI of 30 kg/m^2 in a US population (Figure 8.10) [577, 578].

Obesity is known to increase salt sensitivity. Asians are genetically more likely to have salt sensitivity than Caucasians [579]. In addition, Asian individuals tend to have a higher dietary salt intake (Figure 8.11) [580]. Thus, the increase in salt sensitivity caused by mild obesity is enough to cause high BP in Asians who already have high salt sensitivity and high salt intake.

Body weight status is closely associated with cardiovascular prognosis. Obesity (BMI >28 kg/m^2) increases the risk of cardiovascular events, especially in adults aged <65 years, while lean (BMI <21 kg/m^2) is an also independent predictor of cardiovascular events in older patients aged ≥65 years [581]. In obese patients, atrial fibrillation is associated with poor cardiovascular prognosis, while AF is not a risk factor in nonobese patients [567].

Salt intake is gradually decreasing in Japan, but remains high (Figure 8.12). In a survey of patients with hypertension recruited from general practitioner-based clinics in Tochigi prefecture, the average salt intake (estimated by urinary

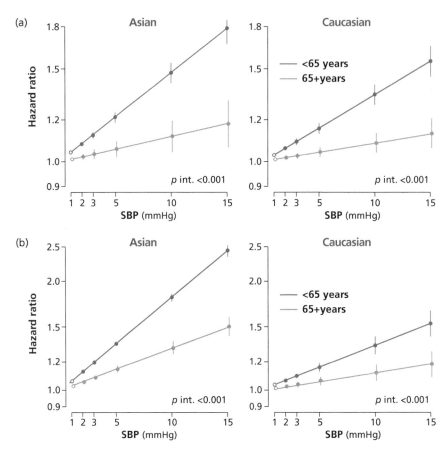

Figure 8.8 Asian populations are at greater cardiovascular risk related to hypertension. Risk of (a) fatal and nonfatal coronary heart disease, or (b) stroke. SBP, systolic blood pressure. *Source:* Perkovic et al. Hypertension. 2007;50:991–997 [575].

concentrations of sodium and creatinine) was 10.2 g/day, and the proportion of patients with SBP <130 mmHg was low (22.3%) (Figure 8.13). Salt restriction and maintaining a BMI <25 kg/m² are the two key prophylactic strategies against high BP, especially in Asian populations.

24-hour ambulatory BP profile in Asia

The 24-hour BP profile is determined partly by genetic factors, but it is also strongly affected by a variety of cultural factors (e.g. food, lifestyle, and traditions) and environmental factors (e.g. temperature, atmospheric pressure, humidity, and seasonal changes) [37, 156, 172]. BP variability may be greater in Asian populations than Western populations. Recent analysis of the International Ambulatory Blood Pressure Registry: Telemonitoring of Hypertension and Cardiovascular Risk Project (ARTEMIS) demonstrated that the prevalence of masked hypertension was higher in Asians than in Westerners [582]. In the same database, when office BP was comparable, Japanese patients with hypertension had a more exaggerated morning BP surge than similar Western patients

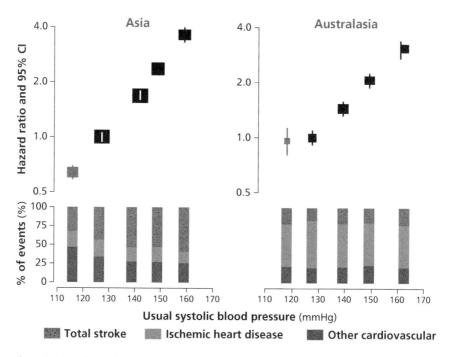

Figure 8.9 Usual systolic blood pressure and risks of cardiovascular death in Asia and Australasia (data from the Asia Pacific Cohort Studies Collaboration, which analyzed 425 325 study participants who were followed up for 3 million person-years). *Source:* Lawes et al. J Hypertens. 2003;21:707–716 [576].

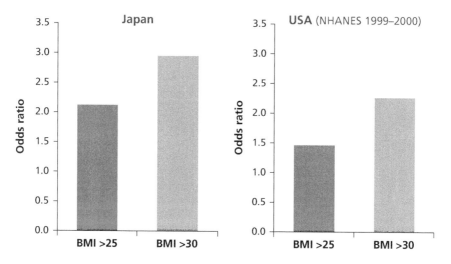

Figure 8.10 Ethnic differences in the impact of obesity on hypertension (Japan Morning Surge [JMS] study cohort, *n* = 12 000). Odds ratio values are for patients with prehypertension with normotension as the reference, adjusted for age and sex. NHANES, National Health and Nutrition Examination Survey. *Source:* Left: created based on data from Ishikawa et al. Hypertens Res. 2008;31:1323–1330 [577]; Right: created based on data from Greenlund et al. Arch Int Med. 2004;164;2113–2118 [578].

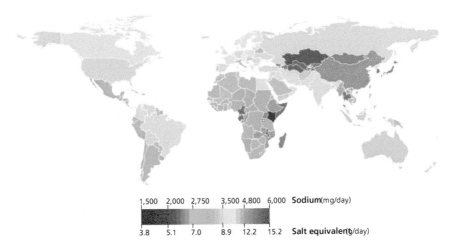

Figure 8.11 Worldwide salt intake in 2010 (age >20 years, men/women). *Source:* Reprinted from Powles et al. BMJ Open. 2013;3:e003733 [580], with permission from BMJ Publishing Group Ltd.

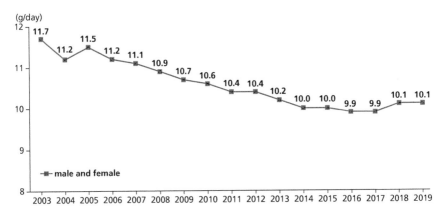

Figure 8.12 Salt intake in Japan. *Source:* Created based on data from 2019 National Health and Nutrition Survey. (Ministry of Health, Labour and Welfare; http://www.mhlw.go.jp/bunya/kenkou/kenkou_eiyou_chousa.html) accessed on November 1, 2021.

(Figure 8.14) [583]. In patients with drug-resistant hypertension, who were recruited using the same global entry criteria as used in the SYMPLICITY HTN-3 and HTN-J trials of catheter-based renal denervation, Japanese patients had higher morning BP levels and greater morning BP surges than the patients from other ethnic backgrounds, even when office BP was similar (Figure 8.15) [584]. In addition, data from a population cohort suggest that the nighttime BP fall might be smaller in Asians than in Westerners (Figure 8.16) [585]. In ABPM comparison studies, Asians are more likely to have isolated nocturnal hypertension than isolated daytime hypertension (Table 8.4) [36].

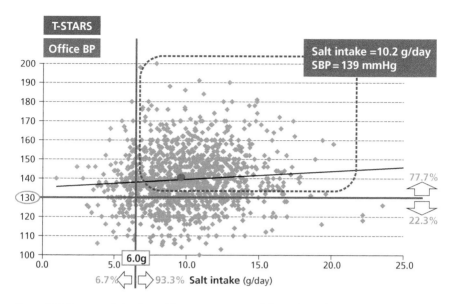

Figure 8.13 Data on salt intake and hypertension control from the Tochigi Salt Cardiovascular Risk Study (T-STARS; n = 4511 Japanese patients with hypertension). BP, blood pressure. *Source:* Kario. Essential Manual on Perfect 24-Hour Blood Pressure Management from Morning to Nocturnal Hypertension: Up-to-date for Anticipation Medicine. Wiley, 2018: 1–309 [24].

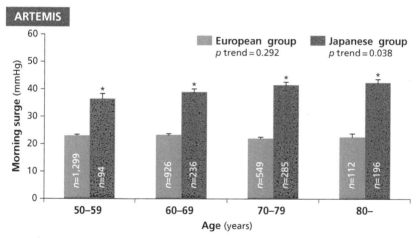

Values are expressed as means ± s.e.m. * - $p < 0.001$ vs. European group in the same category

Figure 8.14 Ethnic differences in the degree of morning blood pressure surge in the International Ambulatory Blood Pressure Registry: Telemonitoring of Hypertension and Cardiovascular Risk Project (ARTEMIS; 811 Japanese patients vs. 2887 Caucasians). s.e.m., standard error of the mean. *Source:* Hoshide et al. Hypertension. 2015;66:750–756 [583].

As well as differences between Asians and other ethnicities, patterns of diurnal BP and the prevalence of nocturnal hypertension might differ between countries in Asia. In our Asia collaboration study of ABPM, patients with hypertension from Thailand were more likely have riser and non-dipper patterns of nighttime BP than

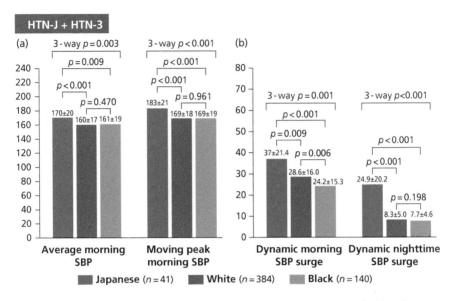

Figure 8.15 Ambulatory blood pressure monitoring (ABPM) parameters stratified by ethnicity. SBP, systolic blood pressure. (a) Average morning and moving peak morning SBP; (b) dynamic morning and nighttime SBP surges. *Source:* Kario et al. Circ J. 2017;81:1337–1345 [584].

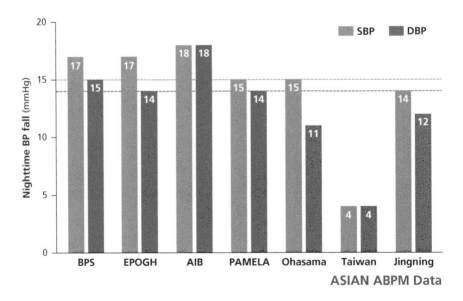

Figure 8.16 Nighttime blood pressure (BP) fall across populations from different regions. AIB, Allied Irish Bank study; BPS, Belgian population study; EPOGH, European Project on Genes of Hypertension; PAMELA, Pressioni, Arteriose Monitorate E Loro Associazioni, Monza, Italy; Ohasama, survey conducted in Ohasama, Iwate Prefecture, Japan; Taiwan, study conducted on the Taiwan and Kinmen (Quemoy) islands; Jingning, six villages of the Jingning County, China. DBP, diastolic BP; SBP, systolic BP. *Source:* Created based on data from Li et al. Blood Press Monit. 2005;10:125–134 [585].

Table 8.4 Prevalence of isolated nocturnal and daytime hypertension in various populations.

Ethnicity	Isolated nocturnal hypertension (%)	Isolated daytime hypertension (%)
Asians		
Chinese (n = 677)	10.9	4.9
Japanese (n = 1038)	10.5	6.0
Europeans		
East (n = 854)	7.9	13.9
West (n = 3268)	6.0	9.1
South Africans (n = 201)	10.2	6.6

Isolated nocturnal hypertension = nighttime blood pressure (BP) ≥120/70 mmHg and daytime BP <135/85 mmHg. Isolated daytime hypertension = daytime BP≥135/85 mmHg and nighttime BP<120/70 mmHg.
Source: Li and Wang Hypertension. 2013; 61: 278–283 [36].

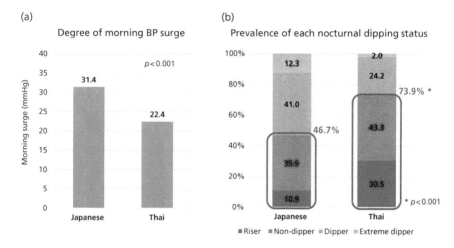

Figure 8.17 Differences in the degree of morning blood pressure (BP) surge and nocturnal dipping status between patients from Japan and Thailand with hypertension and suspected hypertension. (a) Degree of morning BP surge. (b) Prevalence of each nocturnal dipping status. *Source:* Created based on data from Tomitani et al. J Clin Hypertens (Greenwich). 2021; 23: 614–620 [561].

similar patients from Japan, while the morning BP surge was more exaggerated in Japanese compared with Thai patients (Figure 8.17) [561].

Asia BP@Home Study

A morning home BP-guided approach is the most effective strategy to achieve zero cardiovascular events in Asia [171, 184]. Asian data from two prospective observational studies (the Ohasama study [586] and the Japan Morning Surge Home Blood Pressure [J-HOP] study [189]) and two intervention studies (Hypertension Objective treatment based on Measurement by Electrical Devices of Blood Pressure [HOMED-BP] [188] and HONEST [56]) clearly demonstrated

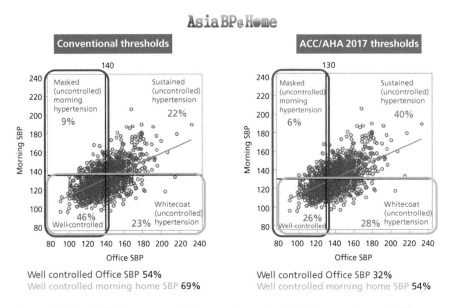

Well controlled Office SBP 54%
Well controlled morning home SBP **69%**

Well controlled Office SBP 32%
Well controlled morning home SBP **54%**

Figure 8.18 Systolic blood pressure (SBP) control status (AsiaBP@home study, $n = 1437$). ACC, American College of Cardiology; AHA, American Heart Association. *Source:* Kario et al. J Clin Hypertens (Greenwich). 2018;20(12):1686–1695 [573].

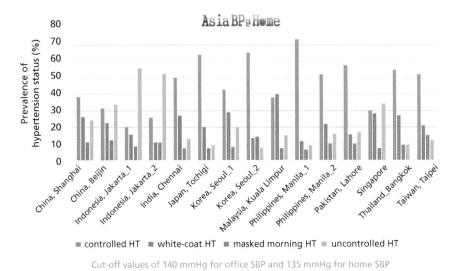

Figure 8.19 Country and regional differences in systolic blood pressure (SBP) control status based on different clinic and morning home blood pressure thresholds (15 Asian centers). HT, hypertension. *Source:* Kario et al. J Clin Hypertens (Greenwich). 2018;20(12):1686–1695 [573].

that morning home BP is the most important predictor of cardiovascular events, especially stroke, independent of office BP (Table 2.1).

Due to the local lifestyle in Asia, individuals are unlikely to measure evening home BP before dinner and instead take the evening home BP measurement just before going to bed, which is therefore the recommended approach in the region [181]. However, the measurement of evening home BP just before going to bed is strongly influenced by the individual's dinner (including alcohol consumption) and evening behavior (e.g. bathing in the evening is common in Asia) [263]. The importance of morning home BP as standard clinical practice needs to be stressed, because morning home BP has shown better reproducibility than evening home BP or office BP [587].

The Asia BP@Home study is the first home BP study to use the same protocol and the same HBPM device across all twelve participating Asian countries/ regions [521, 558, 572, 573]. BP was relatively well controlled in 68.2% of patients using a morning home systolic BP (SBP) cutoff <135 mmHg, and in 55.1% of patients using an office SBP cutoff of <140 mmHg. When cutoff values were changed to match those detailed in the 2017 American Heart Association/American College of Cardiology guidelines (SBP <130 mmHg) [178], 53.6% of patients were well controlled for morning home SBP (Figure 8.18) [572, 573]. In addition, as expected, marked regional, country-based, and ethnic differences in both office and morning home BP control status were identified (Figure 8.19). Masked uncontrolled morning hypertension was more common in patients with diabetes than in those without [521]. When countries were divided into East Asia, Southeast Asia, and South Asia regions, the multivariable-adjusted self-measured office and home resting heart rate was significantly higher in South Asia compared with East Asia and Southeast Asia (Figure 8.20) [558]. Given what is known about the impact of increased heart rate on heart disease, our findings suggest the possible benefit of regionally tailored clinical strategies for cardiovascular disease prevention.

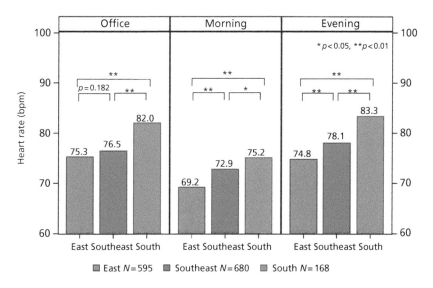

Figure 8.20 Regional differences in office and self-measured home heart rate in Asian patients with hypertension from the AsiaBP@Home study ($n = 1443$; adjusted for age, sex, body mass index, habitual alcohol consumption, current smoking habit, shift worker, hyperlipidemia, diabetes, chronic kidney disease, history of heart failure, beta-blocker use, and systolic blood pressure values. bpm: beats/minute. *Source:* Tomitani et al. J Clin Hypertens (Greenwich). 2021; 23: 606–613 [558].

References

1. Kario K. Nocturnal hypertension: new technology and evidence. *Hypertension*. 2018;71:997–1009. https://www.ahajournals.org/journal/hyp.
2. Kario K, Pickering TG, Umeda Y, Hoshide S, Hoshide Y, Morinari M, Murata M, Kuroda T, Schwartz JE and Shimada K. Morning surge in blood pressure as a predictor of silent and clinical cerebrovascular disease in elderly hypertensives: a prospective study. *Circulation*. 2003;107:1401–1406. https://www.ahajournals.org/journal/circ.
3. Kario K. Morning surge in blood pressure in hypertension: clinical relevance, prognosis significance and therapeutic approach. In: A. Berbari and G. Mancia, eds. *Special issues in hypertension*: Springer Inc.; 2012: 71–89.
4. Yano Y, Hoshide S, Tamaki N, Inokuchi T, Nagata M, Yokota N, Hidaka T, Kanemaru Y, Matsuda S, Kuwabara M, Shimada K and Kario K. Regional differences in hypertensive cardiovascular remodeling between fishing and farming communities in Japan. *Am J Hypertens*. 2011;24:437–443.
5. Sega R, Facchetti R, Bombelli M, Cesana G, Corrao G, Grassi G and Mancia G. Prognostic value of ambulatory and home blood pressures compared with office blood pressure in the general population: follow-up results from the Pressioni Arteriose Monitorate e Loro Associazioni (PAMELA) study. *Circulation*. 2005;111:1777–1783. https://www.ahajournals.org/journal/circ.
6. Boggia J, Li Y, Thijs L, Hansen TW, Kikuya M, Bjorklund-Bodegard K, Richart T, Ohkubo T, Kuznetsova T, Torp-Pedersen C, Lind L, Ibsen H, Imai Y, Wang J, Sandoya E, O'Brien E, Staessen JA and International Database on Ambulatory blood pressure monitoring in relation to Cardiovascular Outcomes (IDACO) investigators. Prognostic accuracy of day versus night ambulatory blood pressure: a cohort study. *Lancet*. 2007;370:1219–1229.
7. Kario K, Matsuo T, Kobayashi H, Imiya M, Matsuo M and Shimada K. Nocturnal fall of blood pressure and silent cerebrovascular damage in elderly hypertensive patients. Advanced silent cerebrovascular damage in extreme dippers. *Hypertension*. 1996;27:130–135. https://www.ahajournals.org/journal/hyp.
8. Kario K, Pickering TG, Matsuo T, Hoshide S, Schwartz JE and Shimada K. Stroke prognosis and abnormal nocturnal blood pressure falls in older hypertensives. *Hypertension*. 2001;38:852–857. https://www.ahajournals.org/journal/hyp.
9. Hoshide S, Kario K, Hoshide Y, Umeda Y, Hashimoto T, Kunii O, Ojima T and Shimada K. Associations between nondipping of nocturnal blood pressure decrease and cardiovascular target organ damage in strictly selected community-dwelling normotensives. *Am J Hypertens*. 2003;16:434–438.

10. Ohkubo T, Hozawa A, Yamaguchi J, Kikuya M, Ohmori K, Michimata M, Matsubara M, Hashimoto J, Hoshi H, Araki T, Tsuji I, Satoh H, Hisamichi S and Imai Y. Prognostic significance of the nocturnal decline in blood pressure in individuals with and without high 24-h blood pressure: the Ohasama study. *J Hypertens*. 2002;20:2183–2189. https://journals.lww.com/jhypertension/pages/default.aspx.

11. Kario K, Schwartz JE and Pickering TG. Changes of nocturnal blood pressure dipping status in hypertensives by nighttime dosing of alpha-adrenergic blocker, doxazosin: results from the HALT study. *Hypertension*. 2000;35:787–794. https://www.ahajournals.org/journal/hyp.

12. O'Brien E, Sheridan J and O'Malley K. Dippers and non-dippers. *Lancet*. 1988;2:397.

13. Shimada K, Kawamoto A, Matsubayashi K and Ozawa T. Silent cerebrovascular disease in the elderly. Correlation with ambulatory pressure. *Hypertension*. 1990;16:692–699. https://www.ahajournals.org/journal/hyp.

14. Kabutoya T, Hoshide S, Ishikawa J, Eguchi K, Shimada K and Kario K. The effect of pulse rate and blood pressure dipping status on the risk of stroke and cardiovascular disease in Japanese hypertensive patients. *Am J Hypertens*. 2010;23:749–755.

15. Kario K and Shimada K. Risers and extreme-dippers of nocturnal blood pressure in hypertension: antihypertensive strategy for nocturnal blood pressure. *Clin Exp Hypertens*. 2004;26:177–189.

16. Kario K, Hoshide S, Mizuno H, Kabutoya T, Nishizawa M, Yoshida T, Abe H, Katsuya T, Fujita Y, Okazaki O, Yano Y, Tomitani N, Kanegae H and JAMP Study Group. Nighttime blood pressure phenotype and cardiovascular prognosis: practitioner-based nationwide JAMP study. *Circulation*. 2020;142:1810–1820. https://www.ahajournals.org/journal/circ.

17. Fujiwara T, Hoshide S, Kanegae H and Kario K. Prognostic value of a riser pattern of nighttime blood pressure in very elderly adults of >/=80 years: a general practice-based prospective SEARCH study. *Am J Hypertens*. 2020;33:520–527.

18. Eguchi K, Pickering TG, Schwartz JE, Hoshide S, Ishikawa J, Ishikawa S, Shimada K and Kario K. Short sleep duration as an independent predictor of cardiovascular events in Japanese patients with hypertension. *Arch Intern Med*. 2008;168:2225–2231.

19. Ishikawa J, Shimizu M, Hoshide S, Eguchi K, Pickering TG, Shimada K and Kario K. Cardiovascular risks of dipping status and chronic kidney disease in elderly Japanese hypertensive patients. *J Clin Hypertens (Greenwich)*. 2008;10:787–794.

20. Komori T, Eguchi K, Saito T, Hoshide S and Kario K. Riser pattern is a novel predictor of adverse events in heart failure patients with preserved ejection fraction. *Circ J*. 2017;81:220–226.

21. Komori T, Eguchi K, Saito T, Hoshide S and Kario K. Riser pattern: another determinant of heart failure with preserved ejection fraction. *J Clin Hypertens (Greenwich)*. 2016;18:994–999.

22. Oba Y, Kabutoya T, Hoshide S, Eguchi K and Kario K. Association between nondipper pulse rate and measures of cardiac overload: The J-HOP Study. *J Clin Hypertens (Greenwich)*. 2017;19:402–409.

23. Ogoyama Y, Kabutoya T, Hoshide S and Kario K. The combination of non-dipper heart rate and high brain natriuretic peptide predicts cardiovascular events: the Japan morning surge-home blood pressure (J-HOP) Study. *Am J Hypertens*., 33: 430–438. 2020.

24. Kario K. *Essential Manual on Perfect 24-Hour Blood Pressure Management from Morning to Nocturnal Hypertension: Up-to-date for Anticipation Medicine*. Tokyo: Wiley; 2018; 1–309.

25. Yano Y, Hoshide S, Shimizu M, Eguchi K, Ishikawa J, Ishikawa S, Shimada K and Kario K. Association of home and ambulatory blood pressure changes with changes in cardiovascular biomarkers during antihypertensive treatment. *Am J Hypertens*. 2012; 25:306–312.

26. Nagai M, Hoshide S, Ishikawa J, Shimada K and Kario K. Ambulatory blood pressure as an independent determinant of brain atrophy and cognitive function in elderly hypertension. *J Hypertens*. 2008;26:1636–1641. https://journals.lww.com/jhypertension/pages/default.aspx.

27. Nagai M, Hoshide S, Ishikawa J, Shimada K and Kario K. Insular cortex atrophy as an independent determinant of disrupted diurnal rhythm of ambulatory blood pressure in elderly hypertension. *Am J Hypertens.* 2009;22:723–729.

28. Yano Y, Inokuchi T, Hoshide S, Kanemaru Y, Shimada K and Kario K. Association of poor physical function and cognitive dysfunction with high nocturnal blood pressure level in treated elderly hypertensive patients. *Am J Hypertens.* 2011;24:285–291.

29. Komori T, Eguchi K, Saito T, Nishimura Y, Hoshide S and Kario K. Riser blood pressure pattern is associated with mild cognitive impairment in heart failure patients. *Am J Hypertens.* 2016;29:194–201.

30. Komori T, Hoshide S, Tabei KI, Tomimoto H and Kario K. Quantitative evaluation of white matter hyperintensities in patients with heart failure using an innovative magnetic resonance image analysis method: association with disrupted circadian blood pressure variation. *J Clin Hypertens (Greenwich).* 2021;23:1089–1092.

31. Palatini P, Reboldi G, Beilin LJ, Eguchi K, Imai Y, Kario K, Ohkubo T, Pierdomenico SD, Saladini F, Schwartz JE, Wing L and Verdecchia P. Predictive value of night-time heart rate for cardiovascular events in hypertension. The ABP-International study. *Int J Cardiol.* 2013;168:1490–1495.

32. Komori T, Eguchi K, Tomizawa H, Ishikawa J, Hoshide S, Shimada K and Kario K. Factors associated with incident ischemic stroke in hospitalized heart failure patients: a pilot study. *Hypertens Res.* 2008;31:289–294.

33. Eguchi K, Pickering TG, Hoshide S, Ishikawa J, Ishikawa S, Schwartz JE, Shimada K and Kario K. Ambulatory blood pressure is a better marker than clinic blood pressure in predicting cardiovascular events in patients with/without type 2 diabetes. *Am J Hypertens.* 2008;21:443–450.

34. Hoshide S, Ishikawa J, Eguchi K, Ojima T, Shimada K and Kario K. Masked nocturnal hypertension and target organ damage in hypertensives with well-controlled self-measured home blood pressure. *Hypertens Res.* 2007;30:143–149.

35. Li Y, Staessen JA, Lu L, Li LH, Wang GL and Wang JG. Is isolated nocturnal hypertension a novel clinical entity? Findings from a Chinese population study. *Hypertension.* 2007;50:333–339. https://www.ahajournals.org/journal/hyp.

36. Li Y and Wang JG. Isolated nocturnal hypertension: a disease masked in the dark. *Hypertension.* 2013;61:278–283. https://www.ahajournals.org/journal/hyp.

37. Kario K. *Essential Manual of 24-Hour Blood Pressure Management from Morning to Nocturnal Hypertension.* London, UK: Wiley-Blackwell; 2015; 1–138.

38. Kario K. *Clinician's Manual on Early Morning Risk Management in Hypertension.* London, UK: Science Press; 2004.

39. Kimura G. Kidney and circadian blood pressure rhythm. *Hypertension.* 2008;51:827–828.

40. Kario K, Schwartz JE, Davidson KW and Pickering TG. Gender differences in associations of diurnal blood pressure variation, awake physical activity, and sleep quality with negative affect: the work site blood pressure study. *Hypertension.* 2001;38:997–1002. https://www.ahajournals.org/journal/hyp.

41. Kario K. Perfect 24-h management of hypertension: clinical relevance and perspectives. *J Hum Hypertens.* 2017;31:231–243.

42. Salles GF, Reboldi G, Fagard RH, Cardoso CR, Pierdomenico SD, Verdecchia P, Eguchi K, Kario K, Hoshide S, Polonia J, de la Sierra A, Hermida RC, Dolan E, O'Brien E, Roush GC and ABC- H Investigators. Prognostic effect of the nocturnal blood pressure fall in hypertensive patients: the ambulatory blood pressure collaboration in patients with hypertension (ABC-H) meta-analysis. *Hypertension.* 2016;67:693–700. https://www.ahajournals.org/journal/hyp.

43. Palatini P, Verdecchia P, Beilin LJ, Eguchi K, Imai Y, Kario K, Ohkubo T, Pierdomenico SD, Saladini F, Schwartz JE, Wing L, Signorotti S and Reboldi G. Association of extreme nocturnal dipping with cardiovascular events strongly depends on age. *Hypertension.* 2020;75:324–330. https://www.ahajournals.org/journal/hyp.

44. Viera AJ, Lin FC, Hinderliter AL, Shimbo D, Person SD, Pletcher MJ and Jacobs DR, Jr. Nighttime blood pressure dipping in young adults and coronary artery calcium 10-15

years later: the coronary artery risk development in young adults study. *Hypertension.* 2012;59:1157–1163. https://www.ahajournals.org/journal/hyp.

45. Watanabe N, Imai Y, Nagai K, Tsuji I, Satoh H, Sakuma M, Sakuma H, Kato J, Onodera–Kikuchi N, Yamada M, Abe F, Hisamichi S and Abe K. Nocturnal blood pressure and silent cerebrovascular lesions in elderly Japanese. *Stroke.* 1996;27:1319–1327. https://www.ahajournals.org/journal/str.

46. Siennicki-Lantz A, Reinprecht F, Axelsson J and Elmstahl S. Cerebral perfusion in the elderly with nocturnal blood pressure fall. *Eur J Neurol.* 2007;14:715–720.

47. Jerrard-Dunne P, Mahmud A and Feely J. Circadian blood pressure variation: relationship between dipper status and measures of arterial stiffness. *J Hypertens.* 2007;25:1233–1239. https://journals.lww.com/jhypertension/pages/default.aspx.

48. Kario K, Mitsuhashi T and Shimada K. Neurohumoral characteristics of older hypertensive patients with abnormal nocturnal blood pressure dipping. *Am J Hypertens.* 2002;15:531–537.

49. Muller JE, Tofler GH and Stone PH. Circadian variation and triggers of onset of acute cardiovascular disease. *Circulation.* 1989;79:733–743. https://www.ahajournals.org/journal/circ.

50. Kario K. Time for focus on morning hypertension: pitfall of current antihypertensive medication. *Am J Hypertens.* 2005;18:149–151.

51. Kario K, Ishikawa J, Pickering TG, Hoshide S, Eguchi K, Morinari M, Hoshide Y, Kuroda T and Shimada K. Morning hypertension: the strongest independent risk factor for stroke in elderly hypertensive patients. *Hypertens Res.* 2006;29:581–587.

52. Li Y, Thijs L, Hansen TW, Kikuya M, Boggia J, Richart T, Metoki H, Ohkubo T, Torp-Pedersen C, Kuznetsova T, Stolarz-Skrzypek K, Tikhonoff V, Malyutina S, Casiglia E, Nikitin Y, Sandoya E, Kawecka-Jaszcz K, Ibsen H, Imai Y, Wang J, Staessen JA and International Database on Ambulatory Blood Pressure Monitoring in Relation to Cardiovascular Outcomes Investigators. Prognostic value of the morning blood pressure surge in 5645 subjects from 8 populations. *Hypertension.* 2010;55:1040–1048. https://www.ahajournals.org/journal/hyp.

53. Kario K. Morning surge in blood pressure and cardiovascular risk: evidence and perspectives. *Hypertension.* 2010;56:765–773. https://www.ahajournals.org/journal/hyp.

54. Nishinaga M, Takata J, Okumiya K, Matsubayashi K, Ozawa T and Doi Y. High morning home blood pressure is associated with a loss of functional independence in the community-dwelling elderly aged 75 years or older. *Hypertens Res.* 2005;28:657–663.

55. Asayama K, Ohkubo T, Kikuya M, Obara T, Metoki H, Inoue R, Hara A, Hirose T, Hoshi H, Hashimoto J, Totsune K, Satoh H and Imai Y. Prediction of stroke by home "morning" versus "evening" blood pressure values: the Ohasama study. *Hypertension.* 2006;48:737–743. https://www.ahajournals.org/journal/hyp.

56. Kario K, Saito I, Kushiro T, Teramukai S, Ishikawa Y, Mori Y, Kobayashi F and Shimada K. Home blood pressure and cardiovascular outcomes in patients during antihypertensive therapy: primary results of HONEST, a large-scale prospective, real-world observational study. *Hypertension.* 2014;64:989–996. https://www.ahajournals.org/journal/hyp.

57. Kario K. Morning surge in blood pressure: a phenotype of systemic hemodynamic atherothrombotic syndrome. *Am J Hypertens.* 2015;28:7–9.

58. Kario K. Orthostatic hypertension-a new haemodynamic cardiovascular risk factor. *Nat Rev Nephrol.* 2013;9:726–738.

59. Bombelli M, Fodri D, Toso E, Macchiarulo M, Cairo M, Facchetti R, Dell'Oro R, Grassi G and Mancia G. Relationship among morning blood pressure surge, 24-hour blood pressure variability, and cardiovascular outcomes in a white population. *Hypertension.* 2014;64:943–950. https://www.ahajournals.org/journal/hyp.

60. Parati G, Vrijens B and Vincze G. Analysis and interpretation of 24-h blood pressure profiles: appropriate mathematical models may yield deeper understanding. *Am J Hypertens.* 2008;21:123–125; discussion 127-9.

61. Head GA, Chatzivlastou K, Lukoshkova EV, Jennings GL and Reid CM. A novel measure of the power of the morning blood pressure surge from ambulatory blood pressure recordings. *Am J Hypertens.* 2010;23:1074–1081.

62. Gosse P, Lasserre R, Minifie C, Lemetayer P and Clementy J. Blood pressure surge on rising. *J Hypertens.* 2004;22:1113–1118. https://journals.lww.com/jhypertension/pages/default.aspx.

63. Metoki H, Ohkubo T, Kikuya M, Asayama K, Obara T, Hashimoto J, Totsune K, Hoshi H, Satoh H and Imai Y. Prognostic significance for stroke of a morning pressor surge and a nocturnal blood pressure decline: the Ohasama study. *Hypertension.* 2006;47:149–154. https://www.ahajournals.org/journal/hyp.

64. Komori T, Hoshide S and Kario K. Differential effect of the morning blood pressure surge on prognoses between heart failure with reduced and preserved ejection fractions. *Circ J.* 2021;85:1535–1542.

65. Sheppard JP, Hodgkinson J, Riley R, Martin U, Bayliss S and McManus RJ. Prognostic significance of the morning blood pressure surge in clinical practice: a systematic review. *Am J Hypertens.* 2015;28:30–41. https://journals.lww.com/jhypertension/pages/default.aspx.

66. Verdecchia P, Angeli F, Mazzotta G, Garofoli M, Ramundo E, Gentile G, Ambrosio G and Reboldi G. Day–night dip and early-morning surge in blood pressure in hypertension: prognostic implications. *Hypertension.* 2012;60:34–42. https://www.ahajournals.org/journal/hyp.

67. Israel S, Israel A, Ben-Dov IZ and Bursztyn M. The morning blood pressure surge and all-cause mortality in patients referred for ambulatory blood pressure monitoring. *Am J Hypertens.* 2011;24:796–801.

68. Pierdomenico SD, Pierdomenico AM, Di Tommaso R, Coccina F, Di Carlo S, Porreca E and Cuccurullo F. Morning blood pressure surge, dipping, and risk of coronary events in elderly treated hypertensive patients. *Am J Hypertens.* 2016;29:39–45.

69. Pierdomenico SD, Pierdomenico AM, Coccina F, Lapenna D and Porreca E. Prognostic value of nondipping and morning surge in elderly treated hypertensive patients with controlled ambulatory blood pressure. *Am J Hypertens.* 2017;30:159–165.

70. Xie JC, Yan H, Zhao YX and Liu XY. Prognostic value of morning blood pressure surge in clinical events: a meta-analysis of longitudinal studies. *J Stroke Cerebrovasc Dis.* 2015;24:362–369.

71. Cheng HM, Wu CL, Sung SH, Lee JC, Kario K, Chiang CE, Huang CJ, Hsu PF, Chuang SY, Lakatta EG, Yin FCP, Chou P and Chen CH. Prognostic utility of morning blood pressure surge for 20-year all-cause and cardiovascular mortalities: results of a community-based study. *J Am Heart Assoc.* 2017;6(12):e007667, https://doi.org/10.1161/JAHA.117.007667.

72. Kuwajima I, Mitani K, Miyao M, Suzuki Y, Kuramoto K and Ozawa T. Cardiac implications of the morning surge in blood pressure in elderly hypertensive patients: relation to arising time. *Am J Hypertens.* 1995;8:29–33.

73. Marfella R, Gualdiero P, Siniscalchi M, Carusone C, Verza M, Marzano S, Esposito K and Giugliano D. Morning blood pressure peak, QT intervals, and sympathetic activity in hypertensive patients. *Hypertension.* 2003;41:237–243. https://www.ahajournals.org/journal/hyp.

74. Kaneda R, Kario K, Hoshide S, Umeda Y, Hoshide Y and Shimada K. Morning blood pressure hyper-reactivity is an independent predictor for hypertensive cardiac hypertrophy in a community-dwelling population. *Am J Hypertens.* 2005; 18:1528–1533.

75. Yano Y, Hoshide S, Inokuchi T, Kanemaru Y, Shimada K and Kario K. Association between morning blood pressure surge and cardiovascular remodeling in treated elderly hypertensive subjects. *Am J Hypertens.* 2009;22:1177–1182.

76. Soylu A, Yazici M, Duzenli MA, Tokac M, Ozdemir K and Gok H. Relation between abnormalities in circadian blood pressure rhythm and target organ damage in normotensives. *Circ J.* 2009;73:899–904.

77. Caliskan M, Caliskan Z, Gullu H, Keles N, Bulur S, Turan Y, Kostek O, Ciftci O, Guven A, Aung SM and Muderrisoglu H. Increased morning blood pressure surge and coronary

microvascular dysfunction in patient with early stage hypertension. *J Am Soc Hypertens.* 2014;8:652–659.

78. Zakopoulos NA, Tsivgoulis G, Barlas G, Papamichael C, Spengos K, Manios E, Ikonomidis I, Kotsis V, Spiliopoulou I, Vemmos K, Mavrikakis M and Moulopoulos SD. Time rate of blood pressure variation is associated with increased common carotid artery intima-media thickness. *Hypertension.* 2005;45:505–512. https://www.ahajournals.org/journal/hyp.

79. Marfella R, Siniscalchi M, Nappo F, Gualdiero P, Esposito K, Sasso FC, Cacciapuoti F, Di Filippo C, Rossi F, D'Amico M and Giugliano D. Regression of carotid atherosclerosis by control of morning blood pressure peak in newly diagnosed hypertensive patients. *Am J Hypertens.* 2005;18:308–318.

80. Marfella R, Siniscalchi M, Portoghese M, Di Filippo C, Ferraraccio F, Schiattarella C, Crescenzi B, Sangiuolo P, Ferraro G, Siciliano S, Cinone F, Mazzarella G, Martis S, Verza M, Coppola L, Rossi F, D'Amico M and Paolisso G. Morning blood pressure surge as a destabilizing factor of atherosclerotic plaque: role of ubiquitin-proteasome activity. *Hypertension.* 2007;49:784–791. https://www.ahajournals.org/journal/hyp.

81. Shimizu M, Ishikawa J, Yano Y, Hoshide S, Shimada K and Kario K. The relationship between the morning blood pressure surge and low-grade inflammation on silent cerebral infarct and clinical stroke events. *Atherosclerosis.* 2011;219:316–321.

82. Kario K. Treatment of early morning surges in blood pressure. In: D. Sicca and P. Toth, eds. *Clinical Challenges in Hypertension Management*, Oxford, UK: Atlas Medical Publishing; 2010: 27–38.

83. Chen CT, Li Y, Zhang J, Wang Y, Ling HW, Chen KM, Gao PJ and Zhu DL. Association between ambulatory systolic blood pressure during the day and asymptomatic intracranial arterial stenosis. *Hypertension.* 2014;63:61–67. https://www.ahajournals.org/journal/hyp.

84. Polonia J, Amado P, Barbosa L, Nazare J, Silva JA, Bertoquini S, Martins L and Carmona J. Morning rise, morning surge and daytime variability of blood pressure and cardiovascular target organ damage. A cross-sectional study in 743 subjects. *Rev Port Cardiol.* 2005;24:65–78.

85. Pucci G, Battista F, Anastasio F and Schillaci G. Morning pressor surge, blood pressure variability, and arterial stiffness in essential hypertension. *J Hypertens.* 2017;35:272–278. https://journals.lww.com/jhypertension/pages/default.aspx.

86. Pregowska-Chwala B, Prejbisz A, Kabat M, Pucilowska B, Paschalis-Purtak K, Florczak E, Klisiewicz A, Kusmierczyk-Droszcz B, Hanus K, Bursztyn M and Januszewicz A. Morning blood pressure surge and markers of cardiovascular alterations in untreated middle-aged hypertensive subjects. *J Am Soc Hypertens.* 2016;10:790–798.e2.

87. Alpaydin S, Turan Y, Caliskan M, Caliskan Z, Aksu F, Ozyildirim S, Buyukterzi Z, Kostek O and Muderrisoglu H. Morning blood pressure surge is associated with carotid intima-media thickness in prehypertensive patients. *Blood Press Monit.* 2017;22:131–136. https://journals.lww.com/bpmonitoring/pages/default.aspx.

88. Kario K, Shimada K, Schwartz JE, Matsuo T, Hoshide S and Pickering TG. Silent and clinically overt stroke in older Japanese subjects with white-coat and sustained hypertension. *J Am Coll Cardiol.* 2001;38:238–245.

89. Kario K, Pickering TG, Hoshide S, Eguchi K, Ishikawa J, Morinari M, Hoshide Y and Shimada K. Morning blood pressure surge and hypertensive cerebrovascular disease: role of the alpha adrenergic sympathetic nervous system. *Am J Hypertens.* 2004;17:668–675.

90. Fukuda M, Mizuno M, Yamanaka T, Motokawa M, Shirasawa Y, Nishio T, Miyagi S, Yoshida A and Kimura G. Patients with renal dysfunction require a longer duration until blood pressure dips during the night. *Hypertension.* 2008;52:1155–1160. https://www.ahajournals.org/journal/hyp.

91. Lurbe E, Redon J, Kesani A, Pascual JM, Tacons J, Alvarez V and Batlle D. Increase in nocturnal blood pressure and progression to microalbuminuria in type 1 diabetes. *N Engl J Med.* 2002;347:797–805.

92. Caramori ML, Pecis M and Azevedo MJ. Increase in nocturnal blood pressure and progression to microalbuminuria in diabetes. *N Engl J Med*. 2003;348:260–264; author reply 260-4.

93. Kawai T, Kamide K, Onishi M, Yamamoto-Hanasaki H, Baba Y, Hongyo K, Shimaoka I, Tatara Y, Takeya Y, Ohishi M and Rakugi H. Usefulness of the resistive index in renal Doppler ultrasonography as an indicator of vascular damage in patients with risks of atherosclerosis. *Nephrol Dial Transplant*. 2011;26:3256–3262.

94. Turak O, Afsar B, Siriopol D, Ozcan F, Cagli K, Yayla C, Oksuz F, Mendi MA, Kario K, Covic A and Kanbay M. Morning blood pressure surge as a predictor of development of chronic kidney disease. *J Clin Hypertens (Greenwich)*. 2016;18:444–448.

95. Ishikawa J, Kario K, Eguchi K, Morinari M, Hoshide S, Ishikawa S, Shimada K and J-More Group. Regular alcohol drinking is a determinant of masked morning hypertension detected by home blood pressure monitoring in medicated hypertensive patients with well-controlled clinic blood pressure: the Jichi Morning Hypertension Research (J-MORE) study. *Hypertens Res*. 2006;29:679–686.

96. Shimizu M, Ishikawa J, Eguchi K, Hoshide S, Shimada K and Kario K. Association of an abnormal blood glucose level and morning blood pressure surge in elderly subjects with hypertension. *Am J Hypertens*. 2009;22:611–616.

97. Ohira T, Tanigawa T, Tabata M, Imano H, Kitamura A, Kiyama M, Sato S, Okamura T, Cui R, Koike KA, Shimamoto T and Iso H. Effects of habitual alcohol intake on ambulatory blood pressure, heart rate, and its variability among Japanese men. *Hypertension*. 2009;53:13–19. https://www.ahajournals.org/journal/hyp.

98. Murakami S, Otsuka K, Kubo Y, Shinagawa M, Yamanaka T, Ohkawa S and Kitaura Y. Repeated ambulatory monitoring reveals a Monday morning surge in blood pressure in a community-dwelling population. *Am J Hypertens*. 2004;17:1179–1183.

99. Modesti PA, Morabito M, Bertolozzi I, Massetti L, Panci G, Lumachi C, Giglio A, Bilo G, Caldara G, Lonati L, Orlandini S, Maracchi G, Mancia G, Gensini GF and Parati G. Weather-related changes in 24-hour blood pressure profile: effects of age and implications for hypertension management. *Hypertension*. 2006;47:155–161. https://www.ahajournals.org/journal/hyp.

100. Murakami S, Otsuka K, Kono T, Soyama A, Umeda T, Yamamoto N, Morita H, Yamanaka G and Kitaura Y. Impact of outdoor temperature on prewaking morning surge and nocturnal decline in blood pressure in a Japanese population. *Hypertens Res*. 2011;34:70–73.

101. Kario K. Caution for winter morning surge in blood pressure: a possible link with cardiovascular risk in the elderly. *Hypertension*. 2006;47:139–140. https://www.ahajournals.org/journal/hyp.

102. Amin R, Somers VK, McConnell K, Willging P, Myer C, Sherman M, McPhail G, Morgenthal A, Fenchel M, Bean J, Kimball T and Daniels S. Activity-adjusted 24-hour ambulatory blood pressure and cardiac remodeling in children with sleep disordered breathing. *Hypertension*. 2008;51:84–91. https://www.ahajournals.org/journal/hyp.

103. Sheng CS, Cheng YB, Wei FF, Yang WY, Guo QH, Li FK, Huang QF, Thijs L, Staessen JA, Wang JG and Li Y. Diurnal blood pressure rhythmicity in relation to environmental and genetic cues in untreated referred patients. *Hypertension*. 2017;69:128–135. https://www.ahajournals.org/journal/hyp.

104. Kario K. Vascular damage in exaggerated morning surge in blood pressure. *Hypertension*. 2007;49:771–772. https://www.ahajournals.org/journal/hyp.

105. Otto ME, Svatikova A, Barretto RB, Santos S, Hoffmann M, Khandheria B and Somers V. Early morning attenuation of endothelial function in healthy humans. *Circulation*. 2004;109:2507–2510. https://www.ahajournals.org/journal/circ.

106. Linsell CR, Lightman SL, Mullen PE, Brown MJ and Causon RC. Circadian rhythms of epinephrine and norepinephrine in man. *J Clin Endocrinol Metab*. 1985;60:1210–1215.

107. Johnson AW, Hissen SL, Macefield VG, Brown R and Taylor CE. Magnitude of morning surge in blood pressure is associated with sympathetic but not cardiac baroreflex sensitivity. *Front Neurosci*. 2016;10:412.

108. Kawasaki T, Cugini P, Uezono K, Sasaki H, Itoh K, Nishiura M and Shinkawa K. Circadian variations of total renin, active renin, plasma renin activity and plasma aldosterone in clinically healthy young subjects. *Horm Metab Res*. 1990;22: 636–639.

109. Kario K, Yano Y, Matsuo T, Hoshide S, Eguchi K and Shimada K. Additional impact of morning haemostatic risk factors and morning blood pressure surge on stroke risk in older Japanese hypertensive patients. *Eur Heart J*. 2011;32:574–580.

110. Kario K, Yano Y, Matsuo T, Hoshide S, Asada Y and Shimada K. Morning blood pressure surge, morning platelet aggregation, and silent cerebral infarction in older Japanese hypertensive patients. *J Hypertens*. 2011;29:2433–2439. https://journals.lww.com/jhypertension/pages/default.aspx.

111. Mancia G, Fagard R, Narkiewicz K, Redon J, Zanchetti A, Bohm M, Christiaens T, Cifkova R, De Backer G, Dominiczak A, Galderisi M, Grobbee DE, Jaarsma T, Kirchhof P, Kjeldsen SE, Laurent S, Manolis AJ, Nilsson PM, Ruilope LM, Schmieder RE, Sirnes PA, Sleight P, Viigimaa M, Waeber B, Zannad F and Task Force Members. 2013 ESH/ESC Guidelines for the management of arterial hypertension: the Task Force for the management of arterial hypertension of the European Society of Hypertension (ESH) and of the European Society of Cardiology (ESC). *J Hypertens*. 2013;31:1281–1357. https://journals.lww.com/jhypertension/pages/default.aspx.

112. Kario K. Preceding linkage between a morning surge in blood pressure and small artery remodeling: an indicator of prehypertension? *J Hypertens*. 2007;25:1573–1575. https://journals.lww.com/jhypertension/pages/default.aspx.

113. Rizzoni D, Porteri E, Platto C, Rizzardi N, De Ciuceis C, Boari GE, Muiesan ML, Salvetti M, Zani F, Miclini M, Paiardi S, Castellano M and Rosei EA. Morning rise of blood pressure and subcutaneous small resistance artery structure. *J Hypertens*. 2007;25:1698–1703. https://journals.lww.com/jhypertension/pages/default.aspx.

114. Folkow B. Physiological aspects of primary hypertension. *Physiol Rev*. 1982; 62:347–504.

115. Schiffrin EL. Remodeling of resistance arteries in essential hypertension and effects of antihypertensive treatment. *Am J Hypertens*. 2004;17:1192–1200.

116. Panza JA, Epstein SE and Quyyumi AA. Circadian variation in vascular tone and its relation to alpha-sympathetic vasoconstrictor activity. *N Engl J Med*. 1991;325: 986–990.

117. Brandenberger G, Follenius M, Goichot B, Saini J, Spiegel K, Ehrhart J and Simon C. Twenty-four-hour profiles of plasma renin activity in relation to the sleep-wake cycle. *J Hypertens*. 1994;12:277–283. https://journals.lww.com/jhypertension/pages/default.aspx.

118. Naito Y, Tsujino T, Fujioka Y, Ohyanagi M and Iwasaki T. Augmented diurnal variations of the cardiac renin-angiotensin system in hypertensive rats. *Hypertension*. 2002;40:827–833. https://www.ahajournals.org/journal/hyp.

119. Tissot AC, Maurer P, Nussberger J, Sabat R, Pfister T, Ignatenko S, Volk HD, Stocker H, Muller P, Jennings GT, Wagner F and Bachmann MF. Effect of immunisation against angiotensin II with CYT006-AngQb on ambulatory blood pressure: a double-blind, randomised, placebo-controlled phase IIa study. *Lancet*. 2008;371:821–827.

120. Tochikubo O, Kawano Y, Miyajima E, Toshihiro N and Ishii M. Circadian variation of hemodynamics and baroreflex functions in patients with essential hypertension. *Hypertens Res*. 1997;20:157–166.

121. Eguchi K, Tomizawa H, Ishikawa J, Hoshide S, Pickering TG, Shimada K and Kario K. Factors associated with baroreflex sensitivity: association with morning blood pressure. *Hypertens Res*. 2007;30:723–728.

122. Kario K. Prognosis in relation to blood pressure variability: pro side of the argument. *Hypertension*. 2015;65:1163–1169; discussion 1169. https://www.ahajournals.org/journal/hyp.

123. Parati G, Ochoa JE, Lombardi C and Bilo G. Assessment and management of blood-pressure variability. *Nat Rev Cardiol*. 2013;10:143–155.

124. Kario K and Pickering TG. Blood pressure variability in elderly patients. *Lancet.* 2000;355:1645–1646.

125. Kikuya M, Ohkubo T, Metoki H, Asayama K, Hara A, Obara T, Inoue R, Hoshi H, Hashimoto J, Totsune K, Satoh H and Imai Y. Day-by-day variability of blood pressure and heart rate at home as a novel predictor of prognosis: the Ohasama study. *Hypertension.* 2008;52:1045–1050. https://www.ahajournals.org/journal/hyp.

126. Eguchi K, Ishikawa J, Hoshide S, Pickering TG, Schwartz JE, Shimada K and Kario K. Night time blood pressure variability is a strong predictor for cardiovascular events in patients with type 2 diabetes. *Am J Hypertens.* 2009;22:46–51.

127. Rothwell PM, Howard SC, Dolan E, O'Brien E, Dobson JE, Dahlof B, Sever PS and Poulter NR. Prognostic significance of visit-to-visit variability, maximum systolic blood pressure, and episodic hypertension. *Lancet.* 2010;375:895–905.

128. Matsui Y, O'Rourke MF, Hoshide S, Ishikawa J, Shimada K and Kario K. Combined effect of angiotensin II receptor blocker and either a calcium channel blocker or diuretic on day-by-day variability of home blood pressure: the Japan Combined Treatment With Olmesartan and a Calcium-Channel Blocker Versus Olmesartan and Diuretics Randomized Efficacy Study. *Hypertension.* 2012;59:1132–1138. https://www.ahajournals.org/journal/hyp.

129. Nagai M, Hoshide S, Ishikawa J, Shimada K and Kario K. Visit-to-visit blood pressure variations: new independent determinants for cognitive function in the elderly at high risk of cardiovascular disease. *J Hypertens.* 2012;30:1556–1563. https://journals.lww.com/jhypertension/pages/default.aspx.

130. Kawai T, Ohishi M, Ito N, Onishi M, Takeya Y, Yamamoto K, Kamide K and Rakugi H. Alteration of vascular function is an important factor in the correlation between visit-to-visit blood pressure variability and cardiovascular disease. *J Hypertens.* 2013;31:1387–1395; discussion 1395. https://journals.lww.com/jhypertension/pages/default.aspx.

131. Fukui M, Ushigome E, Tanaka M, Hamaguchi M, Tanaka T, Atsuta H, Ohnishi M, Oda Y, Hasegawa G and Nakamura N. Home blood pressure variability on one occasion is a novel factor associated with arterial stiffness in patients with type 2 diabetes. *Hypertens Res.* 2013;36:219–225.

132. Endo K, Kario K, Koga M, Nakagawara J, Shiokawa Y, Yamagami H, Furui E, Kimura K, Hasegawa Y, Okada Y, Okuda S, Namekawa M, Miyagi T, Osaki M, Minematsu K and Toyoda K. Impact of early blood pressure variability on stroke outcomes after thrombolysis: the SAMURAI rt-PA Registry. *Stroke.* 2013;44:816–818. https://www.ahajournals.org/journal/str.

133. Wei FF, Li Y, Zhang L, Xu TY, Ding FH, Wang JG and Staessen JA. Beat-to-beat, reading-to-reading, and day-to-day blood pressure variability in relation to organ damage in untreated Chinese. *Hypertension.* 2014;63:790–796. https://www.ahajournals.org/journal/hyp.

134. Nagai M, Hoshide S, Nishikawa M, Masahisa S and Kario K. Visit-to-visit blood pressure variability in the elderly: associations with cognitive impairment and carotid artery remodeling. *Atherosclerosis.* 2014;233:19–26.

135. Kagitani H, Hoshide S and Kario K. Optimal indicators of home BP variability in perimenopausal women and associations with albuminuria and reproducibility: The J-HOT home BP study. *Am J Hypertens.* 2015;28:586–594.

136. Rakugi H, Ogihara T, Saruta T, Kawai T, Saito I, Teramukai S, Shimada K, Katayama S, Higaki J, Odawara M, Tanahashi N, Kimura G and COLM Investigators. Preferable effects of olmesartan/calcium channel blocker to olmesartan/diuretic on blood pressure variability in very elderly hypertension: COLM study subanalysis. *J Hypertens.* 2015;33:2165–2172. https://journals.lww.com/jhypertension/pages/default.aspx.

137. Shibasaki S, Hoshide S, Eguchi K, Ishikawa J, Kario K and Japan Morning Surge-Home Blood Pressure Study Group. Increase trend in home blood pressure on a single occasion is associated with B-Type natriuretic peptide and the estimated glomerular filtration rate. *Am J Hypertens.* 2015;28:1098–1105. https://journals.lww.com/jhypertension/pages/default.aspx.

138. Kario K, Tomitani N, Matsumoto Y, Hamasaki H, Okawara Y, Kondo M, Nozue R, Yamagata H, Okura A and Hoshide S. Research and development of information and communication technology-based home blood pressure monitoring from morning to nocturnal hypertension. *Ann Glob Health.* 2016;82:254–273.

139. Imaizumi Y, Eguchi K, Taketomi A, Tsuchihashi T and Kario K. Exaggerated blood pressure variability in patients with pneumoconiosis: a pilot study. *Am J Hypertens.* 2014;27:1456–1463.

140. Kayano H, Koba S, Matsui T, Fukuoka H, Kaneko K, Shoji M, Toshida T, Watanabe N, Geshi E and Kobayashi Y. Impact of depression on masked hypertension and variability in home blood pressure in treated hypertensive patients. *Hypertens Res.* 2015;38:751–757.

141. Umemoto S, Ogihara T, Matsuzaki M, Rakugi H, Ohashi Y, Saruta T and Combination Therapy of Hypertension to Prevent Cardiovascular Events. Cope Trial Group effects of calcium channel blocker-based combinations on intra-individual blood pressure variability: post hoc analysis of the COPE trial. *Hypertens Res.* 2016;39:46–53.

142. Imaizumi Y, Eguchi K and Kario K. Coexistence of PM2.5 and low temperature is associated with morning hypertension in hypertensives. *Clin Exp Hypertens.* 2015;37:468–472.

143. Kario K, Eguchi K, Nakagawa Y, Motai K and Shimada K. Relationship between extreme dippers and orthostatic hypertension in elderly hypertensive patients. *Hypertension.* 1998;31:77–82. https://www.ahajournals.org/journal/hyp.

144. Kario K, Eguchi K, Hoshide S, Hoshide Y, Umeda Y, Mitsuhashi T and Shimada K. U-curve relationship between orthostatic blood pressure change and silent cerebrovascular disease in elderly hypertensives: orthostatic hypertension as a new cardiovascular risk factor. *J Am Coll Cardiol.* 2002;40:133–141.

145. Hoshide S, Matsui Y, Shibasaki S, Eguchi K, Ishikawa J, Ishikawa S, Kabutoya T, Schwartz JE, Pickering TG, Shimada K, Kario K and Japan Morning Surge-1 Study Group. Orthostatic hypertension detected by self-measured home blood pressure monitoring: a new cardiovascular risk factor for elderly hypertensives. *Hypertens Res.* 2008;31:1509–1516.

146. Kario K. New insight of morning blood pressure surge into the triggers of cardiovascular disease-synergistic resonance of blood pressure variability. *Am J Hypertens.* 2016;29:14–16.

147. Kario K. Orthostatic hypertension: a measure of blood pressure variation for predicting cardiovascular risk. *Circ J.* 2009;73:1002–1007.

148. Kario K and Wang JG. Could 130/80 mm Hg Be adopted as the diagnostic threshold and management goal of hypertension in consideration of the characteristics of asian populations? *Hypertension.* 2018;71:979–984. https://www.ahajournals.org/journal/hyp.

149. Jordan J, Ricci F, Hoffmann F, Hamrefors V and Fedorowski A. Orthostatic hypertension: critical appraisal of an overlooked condition. *Hypertension.* 2020;75:1151–1158.

150. Rahman M, Pradhan N, Chen Z, Kanthety R, Townsend RR, Tatsuoka C and Wright JT, Jr. Orthostatic hypertension and intensive blood pressure control; post-Hoc analyses of SPRINT. *Hypertension.* 2021;77:49–58. https://www.ahajournals.org/journal/hyp.

151. Sakakura K, Ishikawa J, Okuno M, Shimada K and Kario K. Exaggerated ambulatory blood pressure variability is associated with cognitive dysfunction in the very elderly and quality of life in the younger elderly. *Am J Hypertens.* 2007;20:720–727.

152. Cho N, Hoshide S, Nishizawa M, Fujiwara T and Kario K. Relationship between blood pressure variability and cognitive function in elderly patients with good blood pressure control. *Am J Hypertens.* 2018;31:293–298.

153. Nagai M, Hoshide S, Ishikawa J, Shimada K and Kario K. Visit-to-visit blood pressure variations: new independent determinants for carotid artery measures in the elderly at high risk of cardiovascular disease. *J Am Soc Hypertens.* 2011;5:184–192.

154. Nagai M, Hoshide S, Nishikawa M, Shimada K and Kario K. Sleep duration and insomnia in the elderly: associations with blood pressure variability and carotid artery remodeling. *Am J Hypertens.* 2013;26:981–989. https://journals.lww.com/jhypertension/pages/default.aspx.

155. Kario K. Systemic hemodynamic atherothrombotic syndrome: a blind spot in the current management of hypertension. *J Clin Hypertens (Greenwich).* 2015;17:328–331.

156. Kario K. Evidence and perspectives on the 24-hour management of hypertension: hemodynamic biomarker-initiated 'anticipation medicine' for zero cardiovascular event. *Prog Cardiovasc Dis.* 2016;59:262–281.

157. Kario K. Proposal of a new strategy for ambulatory blood pressure profile-based management of resistant hypertension in the era of renal denervation. *Hypertens Res.* 2013;36:478–484.

158. Kario K, Chirinos JA, Townsend RR, Weber MA, Scuteri A, Avolio A, Hoshide S, Kabutoya T, Tomiyama H, Node K, Ohishi M, Ito S, Kishi T, Rakugi H, Li Y, Chen CH, Park JB and Wang JG. Systemic hemodynamic atherothrombotic syndrome (SHATS) - coupling vascular disease and blood pressure variability: proposed concept from pulse of Asia. *Prog Cardiovasc Dis.* 2020;63:22–32.

159. Kario K. Systemic hemodynamic atherothrombotic syndrome (SHATS): diagnosis and severity assessment score. *J Clin Hypertens (Greenwich).* 2019;21:1011–1015.

160. Hoshide S, Kario K, Yano Y, Haimoto H, Yamagiwa K, Uchiba K, Nagasaka S, Matsui Y, Nakamura A, Fukutomi M, Eguchi K, Ishikawa J and J-HOP Study Group. Association of morning and evening blood pressure at home with asymptomatic organ damage in the J-HOP Study. *Am J Hypertens.* 2014;27:939–947.

161. Ito S, Nagasawa T, Abe M and Mori T. Strain vessel hypothesis: a viewpoint for linkage of albuminuria and cerebro-cardiovascular risk. *Hypertens Res.* 2009;32:115–121.

162. Briet M, Boutouyrie P, Laurent S and London GM. Arterial stiffness and pulse pressure in CKD and ESRD. *Kidney Int.* 2012;82:388–400.

163. Faraco G and Iadecola C. Hypertension: a harbinger of stroke and dementia. *Hypertension.* 2013;62:810–817. https://www.ahajournals.org/journal/hyp.

164. Amerena J., Julius S. (2005) Role of the nervous system in human hypertension. In: Hollenberg N.K. (eds) Atlas of Heart Diseases. Current Medicine Group, London.

165. Matsui Y, Eguchi K, Shibasaki S, Ishikawa J, Hoshide S, Shimada K, Kario K and Japan morning Surge-1 Study Group. Impact of arterial stiffness reduction on urinary albumin excretion during antihypertensive treatment: the Japan morning Surge-1 study. *J Hypertens.* 2010;28:1752–1760. https://journals.lww.com/jhypertension/pages/default.aspx.

166. Kario K. Thomas G. Pickering – a great mentor. *Blood Press Monit.* 2010;15:82–84.

167. Pickering TG, Eguchi K and Kario K. Masked hypertension: a review. *Hypertens Res.* 2007;30:479–488.

168. Kario K, Thijs L and Staessen JA. Blood pressure measurement and treatment decisions. *Circ Res.* 2019;124:990–1008.

169. Kario K and Pickering TG. White-coat hypertension or white-coat hypertension syndrome: which is accompanied by target organ damage? *Arch Intern Med.* 2000;160:3497–3498.

170. Eguchi K, Kario K and Shimada K. Greater impact of coexistence of hypertension and diabetes on silent cerebral infarcts. *Stroke.* 2003;34:2471–2474. https://www.ahajournals.org/journal/str.

171. Kario K. Global impact of 2017 American Heart Association/American College of cardiology hypertension guidelines: a perspective from Japan. *Circulation.* 2018;137:543–545. https://www.ahajournals.org/journal/circ.

172. Kario K, Tomitani N, Kanegae H, Yasui N, Nishizawa M, Fujiwara T, Shigezumi T, Nagai R and Harada H. Development of a new ICT-based multisensor blood pressure monitoring system for use in hemodynamic biomarker-initiated anticipation medicine for cardiovascular disease: the national IMPACT program project. *Prog Cardiovasc Dis.* 2017;60:435–449.

173. Watanabe T, Tomitani N and Kario K. Perspectives on an ambulatory blood pressure monitoring device with novel technology for pulse waveform analysis to detect arrhythmias. *J Clin Hypertens (Greenwich).* 2020;22:1525–1529.

174. Kabutoya T, Imai Y, Hoshide S and Kario K. Diagnostic accuracy of a new algorithm to detect atrial fibrillation in a home blood pressure monitor. *J Clin Hypertens (Greenwich).* 2017;19:1143–1147.

175. Kario K. Hemodynamic biomarker-initiated anticipation medicine in the future management of hypertension. *Am J Hypertens*. 2017;30:226–228.

176. Kario K, Schwartz JE and Pickering TG. Ambulatory physical activity as a determinant of diurnal blood pressure variation. *Hypertension*. 1999;34:685–691. https://www.ahajournals.org/journal/hyp.

177. Narita K, Hoshide S and Kario K. Improvement of actisensitivity after ventricular reverse remodeling in heart failure: new ICT-based multisensor ambulatory blood pressure monitoring. *Am J Hypertens*. 2020;33:161–164.

178. Whelton PK, Carey RM, Aronow WS, Casey DE, Jr., Collins KJ, Dennison Himmelfarb C, DePalma SM, Gidding S, Jamerson KA, Jones DW, MacLaughlin EJ, Muntner P, Ovbiagele B, Smith SC, Jr., Spencer CC, Stafford RS, Taler SJ, Thomas RJ, Williams KA, Sr., Williamson JD and Wright JT, Jr. 2017 ACC/AHA/AAPA/ABC/ACPM/AGS/APhA/ASH/ASPC/NMA/PCNA guideline for the prevention, detection, evaluation, and management of high blood pressure in adults: executive summary: a report of the American College of Cardiology/American Heart Association Task Force on Clinical Practice Guidelines. *Hypertension*. 2018;71:1269–1324. https://www.ahajournals.org/journal/hyp.

179. Sprint Research Group, Wright JT, Jr., Williamson JD, Whelton PK, Snyder JK, Sink KM, Rocco MV, Reboussin DM, Rahman M, Oparil S, Lewis CE, Kimmel PL, Johnson KC, Goff DC, Jr., Fine LJ, Cutler JA, Cushman WC, Cheung AK and Ambrosius WT. A randomized trial of intensive versus standard blood-pressure control. *N Engl J Med*. 2015;373:2103–2116.

180. Kario K. PREFACE: "the lower the better" association between white-coat effect-excluded blood pressure and cardiovascular events in high-risk hypertension: insights from SPRINT *Curr Hypertens Rev*. 2016;12:2–10.

181. Shimamoto K, Ando K, Fujita T, Hasebe N, Higaki J, Horiuchi M, Imai Y, Imaizumi T, Ishimitsu T, Ito M, Ito S, Itoh H, Iwao H, Kai H, Kario K, Kashihara N, Kawano Y, Kim-Mitsuyama S, Kimura G, Kohara K, Komuro I, Kumagai H, Matsuura H, Miura K, Morishita R, Naruse M, Node K, Ohya Y, Rakugi H, Saito I, Saitoh S, Shimada K, Shimosawa T, Suzuki H, Tamura K, Tanahashi N, Tsuchihashi T, Uchiyama M, Ueda S, Umemura S and Japanese Society of Hypertension Committee for Guidelines for the Management of Hypertension. The Japanese society of hypertension guidelines for the management of hypertension (JSH 2014). *Hypertens Res*. 2014;37:253–390.

182. Krause T, Lovibond K, Caulfield M, McCormack T, Williams B and Guideline Development Group. Management of hypertension: summary of NICE guidance. *BMJ*. 2011;343:d4891.

183. Park S, Buranakitjaroen P, Chen CH, Chia YC, Divinagracia R, Hoshide S, Shin J, Siddique S, Sison J, Soenarta AA, Sogunuru GP, Tay JC, Turana Y, Wang JG, Zhang Y, Kario K and HOPE Asia Network. Expert panel consensus recommendations for home blood pressure monitoring in Asia: the Hope Asia Network. *J Hum Hypertens*. 2018;32:249–258.

184. Kario K, Park S, Buranakitjaroen P, Chia YC, Chen CH, Divinagracia R, Hoshide S, Shin J, Siddique S, Sison J, Soenarta AA, Sogunuru GP, Tay JC, Turana Y, Wong L, Zhang Y and Wang JG. Guidance on home blood pressure monitoring: a statement of the HOPE Asia Network. *J Clin Hypertens (Greenwich)*. 2018;20:456–461.

185. Kario K, Park S, Chia YC, Sukonthasarn A, Turana Y, Shin J, Chen CH, Buranakitjaroen P, Divinagracia R, Nailes J, Hoshide S, Siddique S, Sison J, Soenarta AA, Sogunuru GP, Tay JC, Teo BW, Zhang YQ, Van Minh H, Tomitani N, Kabutoya T, Verma N, Wang TD and Wang JG. 2020 Consensus summary on the management of hypertension in Asia from the HOPE Asia Network. *J Clin Hypertens (Greenwich)*. 2020;22:351–362.

186. Bobrie G, Chatellier G, Genes N, Clerson P, Vaur L, Vaisse B, Menard J and Mallion JM. Cardiovascular prognosis of "masked hypertension" detected by blood pressure self-measurement in elderly treated hypertensive patients. *JAMA*. 2004;291:1342–1349.

187. Fagard RH, Van Den Broeke C and De Cort P. Prognostic significance of blood pressure measured in the office, at home and during ambulatory monitoring in older patients in general practice. *J Hum Hypertens*. 2005;19:801–807.

188. Asayama K, Ohkubo T, Metoki H, Obara T, Inoue R, Kikuya M, Thijs L, Staessen JA, Imai Y and Hypertension Objective Treatment Based on Measurement by Electrical Devices of Blood Pressure. Cardiovascular outcomes in the first trial of antihypertensive therapy guided by self-measured home blood pressure. *Hypertens Res.* 2012;35:1102–1110.

189. Hoshide S, Yano Y, Haimoto H, Yamagiwa K, Uchiba K, Nagasaka S, Matsui Y, Nakamura A, Fukutomi M, Eguchi K, Ishikawa J, Kario K and J-HOP Study Group. Morning and evening home blood pressure and risks of incident stroke and coronary artery disease in the Japanese general practice population: the Japan morning surge-home blood pressure study. *Hypertension.* 2016;68:54–61. https://www.ahajournals.org/journal/hyp.

190. Kario K, Kanegae H, Tomitani N, Okawara Y, Fujiwara T, Yano Y and Hoshide S. Nighttime blood pressure measured by home blood pressure monitoring as an independent predictor of cardiovascular events in general practice. *Hypertension.* 2019;73:1240–1248. https://www.ahajournals.org/journal/hyp.

191. Fujiwara T, Yano Y, Hoshide S, Kanegae H and Kario K. Association of cardiovascular outcomes with masked hypertension defined by home blood pressure monitoring in a Japanese general practice population. *JAMA Cardiol.* 2018;3:583–590.

192. Kario K, Shimbo D, Hoshide S, Wang JG, Asayama K, Ohkubo T, Imai Y, McManus RJ, Kollias A, Niiranen TJ, Parati G, Williams B, Weber MA, Vongpatanasin W, Muntner P and Stergiou GS. Emergence of home blood pressure-guided management of hypertension based on global evidence. *Hypertension.* 2019:229–236. https://www.ahajournals.org/journal/hyp.

193. Chobanian AV, Bakris GL, Black HR, Cushman WC, Green LA, Izzo JL, Jr., Jones DW, Materson BJ, Oparil S, Wright JT, Jr., Roccella EJ, and National Heart L, Blood Institute Joint National Committee on Prevention DE, Treatment of High Blood P and National High Blood Pressure Education Program Coordinating Committee. The seventh report of the joint national committee on prevention, detection, evaluation, and treatment of high blood pressure: the JNC 7 report. *JAMA.* 2003;289:2560–2572.

194. Ohkubo T, Imai Y, Tsuji I, Nagai K, Kato J, Kikuchi N, Nishiyama A, Aihara A, Sekino M, Kikuya M, Ito S, Satoh H and Hisamichi S. Home blood pressure measurement has a stronger predictive power for mortality than does screening blood pressure measurement: a population-based observation in Ohasama, Japan. *J Hypertens.* 1998;16:971–975. https://journals.lww.com/jhypertension/pages/default.aspx.

195. Kawauchi D, Hoshide S and Kario K. Morning home blood pressure and cardiovascular events in a Japanese general practice population over 80 years old: the J-HOP study. *Am J Hypertens.* 2018;31:1190–1196.

196. Shimizu H, Hoshide S, Kanegae H and Kario K. Cardiovascular outcome and home blood pressure in relation to silent myocardial ischemia in a clinical population: the J-HOP study. *J Clin Hypertens (Greenwich).* 2020;22:2214–2220.

197. Kario K, Saito I, Kushiro T, Teramukai S, Tomono Y, Okuda Y and Shimada K. Morning home blood pressure is a strong predictor of coronary artery disease: the HONEST study. *J Am Coll Cardiol.* 2016;67:1519–1527.

198. Kushiro T, Kario K, Saito I, Teramukai S, Sato Y, Okuda Y and Shimada K. Increased cardiovascular risk of treated white coat and masked hypertension in patients with diabetes and chronic kidney disease: the HONEST Study. *Hypertens Res.* 2017;40:87–95.

199. Kamoi K, Miyakoshi M, Soda S, Kaneko S and Nakagawa O. Usefulness of home blood pressure measurement in the morning in type 2 diabetic patients. *Diabetes Care.* 2002;25:2218–2223.

200. Saito I, Kario K, Kushiro T, Teramukai S, Yaginuma M, Zenimura N, Mori Y, Okuda Y and Shimada K. Home blood pressure and cardiovascular outcomes in very elderly patients receiving antihypertensive drug therapy: a subgroup analysis of Home blood pressure measurement with Olmesartan Naive patients to Establish Standard Target blood pressure (HONEST) study. *Clin Exp Hypertens.* 2018;40:407–413.

201. Kario K, Iwashita M, Okuda Y, Sugiyama M, Saito I, Kushiro T, Teramukai S and Shimada K. Morning home blood pressure and cardiovascular events in Japanese hypertensive patients. *Hypertension*. 2018;72:854–861. https://www.ahajournals.org/journal/hyp.

202. Saito I, Kario K, Kushiro T, Teramukai S, Yaginuma M, Mori Y, Okuda Y and Shimada K. Home blood pressure and cardiovascular risk in treated hypertensive patients: the prognostic value of the first and second measurements and the difference between them in the HONEST study. *Hypertens Res*. 2016;39:857–862.

203. Kario K, Hasebe N, Okumura K, Yamashita T, Akao M, Atarashi H, Ikeda T, Koretsune Y, Shimizu W, Tsutsui H, Toyoda K, Hirayama A, Yasaka M, Yamaguchi T, Teramukai S, Kimura T, Kaburagi J, Takita A and Inoue H. High prevalence of masked uncontrolled morning hypertension in elderly non-valvular atrial fibrillation patients: home blood pressure substudy of the ANAFIE Registry. *J Clin Hypertens (Greenwich)*. 2021;23:73–82.

204. Matsui Y, Eguchi K, Shibasaki S, Shimizu M, Ishikawa J, Shimada K and Kario K. Association between the morning-evening difference in home blood pressure and cardiac damage in untreated hypertensive patients. *J Hypertens*. 2009;27:712–720. https://journals.lww.com/jhypertension/pages/default.aspx.

205. Matsui Y, Eguchi K, Shibasaki S, Ishikawa J, Shimada K and Kario K. Morning hypertension assessed by home monitoring is a strong predictor of concentric left ventricular hypertrophy in patients with untreated hypertension. *J Clin Hypertens (Greenwich)*. 2010;12:776–783.

206. Shibuya Y, Ikeda T and Gomi T. Morning rise of blood pressure assessed by home blood pressure monitoring is associated with left ventricular hypertrophy in hypertensive patients receiving long-term antihypertensive medication. *Hypertens Res*. 2007;30:903–911.

207. Johansson JK, Niiranen TJ, Puukka PJ and Jula AM. Prognostic value of the variability in home-measured blood pressure and heart rate: the Finn-Home Study. *Hypertension*. 2012;59:212–218. https://www.ahajournals.org/journal/hyp.

208. Eguchi K, Matsui Y, Shibasaki S, Hoshide S, Kabutoya T, Ishikawa J, Ishikawa S, Shimada K, Kario K and Japan Morning Surge-1 Study Group. Controlling evening BP as well as morning BP is important in hypertensive patients with prediabetes/diabetes: the JMS-1 study. *Am J Hypertens*. 2010;23:522–527.

209. Matsui Y, Ishikawa J, Eguchi K, Shibasaki S, Shimada K and Kario K. Maximum value of home blood pressure: a novel indicator of target organ damage in hypertension. *Hypertension*. 2011;57:1087–1093. https://www.ahajournals.org/journal/hyp.

210. Hoshide S, Yano Y, Mizuno H, Kanegae H and Kario K. Day-by-day variability of home blood pressure and incident cardiovascular disease in clinical practice: the J-HOP study (Japan Morning Surge-Home Blood Pressure). *Hypertension*. 2018;71:177–184. https://www.ahajournals.org/journal/hyp.

211. Ishiyama Y, Hoshide S, Kanegae H and Kario K. Increased arterial stiffness amplifies the association between home blood pressure variability and cardiac overload: the J-HOP study. *Hypertension*. 2020;75:1600–1606. https://www.ahajournals.org/journal/hyp.

212. Toriumi S, Hoshide S, Nagai M and Kario K. Day-to-day blood pressure variability as a phenotype in a high-risk patient. *Geriatr Gerontol Int*. 2014;14:1005–1006.

213. Hoshide S, Parati G, Matsui Y, Shibazaki S, Eguchi K and Kario K. Orthostatic hypertension: home blood pressure monitoring for detection and assessment of treatment with doxazosin. *Hypertens Res*. 2012;35:100–106.

214. Narita K, Hoshide S, Fujiwara T, Kanegae H and Kario K. Seasonal variation of home blood pressure and its association with target organ damage: the J-HOP study (Japan Morning Surge-Home Blood Pressure). *Am J Hypertens*. 2020;33:620–628.

215. Kario K. Home blood pressure monitoring: current status and new developments. *Am J Hypertens*. 2021;34:783–794.

216. Umishio W, Ikaga T, Kario K, Fujino Y, Hoshi T, Ando S, Suzuki M, Yoshimura T, Yoshino H, Murakami S and on behalf of the SWH Survey Group. Cross-sectional analysis of the relationship between home blood pressure and indoor temperature in

winter: a nationwide Smart Wellness Housing Survey in Japan. *Hypertension.* 2019;74:756–766. https://www.ahajournals.org/journal/hyp.

217. Umishio W, Ikaga T, Kario K, Fujino Y, Hoshi T, Ando S, Suzuki M, Yoshimura T, Yoshino H, Murakami S and Smart Wellness Housing Survey Group. Intervention study of the effect of insulation retrofitting on home blood pressure in winter: a nationwide Smart Wellness Housing survey. *J Hypertens.* 2020;38:2510–2518. https://journals.lww.com/jhypertension/pages/default.aspx.

218. Tomitani N, Hoshide S and Kario K. Self-measured worksite blood pressure and its association with organ damage in working adults: Japan Morning Surge Home Blood Pressure (J-HOP) worksite study. *J Clin Hypertens (Greenwich).* 2021;23:53–60.

219. Kuwabara M, Harada K, Hishiki Y and Kario K. Validation of two watch-type wearable blood pressure monitors according to the ANSI/AAMI/ISO81060-2:2013 guidelines: Omron HEM-6410T-ZM and HEM-6410T-ZL. *J Clin Hypertens (Greenwich).* 2019;21:853–858.

220. Kario K, Shimbo D, Tomitani N, Kanegae H, Schwartz JE and Williams B. The first study comparing a wearable watch-type blood pressure monitor with a conventional ambulatory blood pressure monitor on in-office and out-of-office settings. *J Clin Hypertens (Greenwich).* 2020;22:135–141.

221. Kario K. Management of hypertension in the digital era: small wearable monitoring devices for remote blood pressure monitoring. *Hypertension.* 2020;76:640–650. https://www.ahajournals.org/journal/hyp.

222. Tomitani N, Kanegae H, Suzuki Y, Kuwabara M and Kario K. Stress-induced blood pressure elevation self-measured by a wearable watch-type device. *Am J Hypertens.* 2021;34:377–382.

223. Kario K, Hoshide S, Shimizu M, Yano Y, Eguchi K, Ishikawa J, Ishikawa S and Shimada K. Effect of dosing time of angiotensin II receptor blockade titrated by self-measured blood pressure recordings on cardiorenal protection in hypertensives: the Japan Morning Surge-Target Organ Protection (J-TOP) study. *J Hypertens.* 2010;28:1574–1583.

224. Ishikawa J, Hoshide S, Eguchi K, Ishikawa S, Shimada K, Kario K and Japan Morning Surge-Home Blood Pressure Study Investigators Group. Nighttime home blood pressure and the risk of hypertensive target organ damage. *Hypertension.* 2012;60:921–928.

225. Ishikawa J, Shimizu M, Sugiyama Edison E, Yano Y, Hoshide S, Eguchi K, Kario K and J-TOP Study Investigators Group. Assessment of the reductions in night-time blood pressure and dipping induced by antihypertensive medication using a home blood pressure monitor. *J Hypertens.* 2014;32:82–89. https://journals.lww.com/jhypertension/pages/default.aspx.

226. Kario K, Hoshide S, Haimoto H, Yamagiwa K, Uchiba K, Nagasaka S, Yano Y, Eguchi K, Matsui Y, Shimizu M, Ishikawa J, Ishikawa S and J-HOP Study Group. Sleep blood pressure self-measured at home as a novel determinant of organ damage: Japan morning surge home blood pressure (J-HOP) study. *J Clin Hypertens (Greenwich).* 2015;17:340–348.

227. Kario K, Tomitani N, Kanegae H, Ishii H, Uchiyama K, Yamagiwa K, Shiraiwa T, Katsuya T, Yoshida T, Kanda K, Hasegawa S and Hoshide S. Comparative effects of an angiotensin II receptor blocker (ARB)/diuretic vs. ARB/calcium-channel blocker combination on uncontrolled nocturnal hypertension evaluated by information and communication technology-based nocturnal home blood pressure monitoring- the NOCTURNE study. *Circ J.* 2017;81:948–957.

228. Fujiwara T, Tomitani N, Kanegae H and Kario K. Comparative effects of valsartan plus either cilnidipine or hydrochlorothiazide on home morning blood pressure surge evaluated by information and communication technology-based nocturnal home blood pressure monitoring. *J Clin Hypertens (Greenwich).* 2018;20:159–167.

229. Shirasaki O, Yamashita S, Kawara S, Tagami K, Ishikawa J, Shimada K and Kario K. A new technique for detecting sleep apnea-related "midnight" surge of blood pressure. *Hypertens Res.* 2006;29:695–702.

230. Shirasaki O, Kuwabara M, Saito M, Tagami K, Washiya S and Kario K. Development and clinical application of a new technique for detecting 'sleep blood pressure surges' in sleep apnea patients based on a variable desaturation threshold. *Hypertens Res.* 2011;34:922–928.

231. Kario K, Kuwabara M, Hoshide S, Nagai M and Shimpo M. Effects of nighttime single-dose administration of vasodilating vs sympatholytic antihypertensive agents on sleep blood pressure in hypertensive patients with sleep apnea syndrome. *J Clin Hypertens (Greenwich).* 2014;16:459–466.

232. Kuwabara M, Hamasaki H, Tomitani N, Shiga T and Kario K. Novel triggered nocturnal blood pressure monitoring for sleep apnea syndrome: distribution and reproducibility of hypoxia-triggered nocturnal blood pressure measurements. *J Clin Hypertens (Greenwich).* 2017;19:30–37.

233. Kario K and Hamasaki H. Nocturnal blood pressure surge behind morning surge in obstructive sleep apnea syndrome: another phenotype of systemic hemodynamic atherothrombotic syndrome. *J Clin Hypertens (Greenwich).* 2015;17:682–685.

234. Yoshida T, Kuwabara M, Hoshide S and Kario K. Recurrence of stroke caused by nocturnal hypoxia-induced blood pressure surge in a young adult male with severe obstructive sleep apnea syndrome. *J Am Soc Hypertens.* 2016;10:201–204.

235. Kario K. Sleep and circadian cardiovascular medicine. In: R. Vasan and D. Sawyer, eds. *Encyclopedia of Caridovascular Research and Medicine,* Amsterdam: Elsevier; 2018: 424–437.

236. Kuwabara M, Harada K, Hishiki Y and Kario K. Validation of a wrist-type home nocturnal blood pressure monitor in the sitting and supine position according to the ANSI/AAMI/ISO81060-2:2013 guidelines: Omron HEM-9600T. *J Clin Hypertens (Greenwich).* 2019;21:463–469.

237. Kuwabara M, Harada K, Hishiki Y, Ohkubo T, Kario K and Imai Y. Validation of a wrist-type home nocturnal blood pressure monitor in the sitting and supine position according to the ANSI/AAMI/ISO81060-2:2013 guidelines: Omron HEM-9601T. *J Clin Hypertens (Greenwich).* 2020;22:970–978.

238. Kario K, Tomitani N, Iwashita C, Shiga T and Kanegae H. Simultaneous self-monitoring comparison of a supine algorithm-equipped wrist nocturnal home blood pressure monitoring device with an upper arm device. *J Clin Hypertens (Greenwich).* 2021;23:793–801.

239. Tomitani N, Kanegae H and Kario K. Comparison of nighttime measurement schedules using a wrist-type nocturnal home blood pressure monitoring device. *J Clin Hypertens (Greenwich).* 2021;23:1144-1149.

240. Coleman A, Freeman P, Steel S and Shennan A. Validation of the Omron 705IT (HEM-759-E) oscillometric blood pressure monitoring device according to the British Hypertension Society protocol. *Blood Press Monit.* 2006;11:27–32. https://journals.lww.com/bpmonitoring/pages/default.aspx.

241. Takahashi H, Yoshika M and Yokoi T. Validation of two automatic devices: Omron HEM-7252G-HP and Omron HEM-7251G for self-measurement of blood pressure according to the European Society of Hypertension International Protocol revision 2010. *Blood Press Monit.* 2015;20:286–290. https://journals.lww.com/bpmonitoring/pages/default.aspx.

242. Viera AJ and Hinderliter AL. Validation of the HEM-780REL with easy wrap cuff for self-measurement of blood pressure according to the European Society of Hypertension International Protocol. *Blood Press Monit.* 2007;12:335–338. https://journals.lww.com/bpmonitoring/pages/default.aspx.

243. Kuwabara M, Tomitani N, Shiga T and Kario K. Polysomnography-derived sleep parameters as a determinant of nocturnal blood pressure profile in patients with obstructive sleep apnea. *J Clin Hypertens (Greenwich).* 2018;20:1039–1048.

244. Asayama K, Fujiwara T, Hoshide S, Ohkubo T, Kario K, Stergiou GS, Parati G, White WB, Weber MA, Imai Y and International Expert Group of Nocturnal Home Blood Pressure. Nocturnal blood pressure measured by home devices: evidence and

perspective for clinical application. *J Hypertens*. 2019;37:905–916. https://journals.lww. com/jhypertension/pages/default.aspx.

245. Fujiwara T, Hoshide S, Kanegae H and Kario K. Cardiovascular event risks associated with masked nocturnal hypertension defined by home blood pressure monitoring in the J-HOP nocturnal blood pressure study. *Hypertension*. 2020;76:259–266. https:// www.ahajournals.org/journal/hyp.

246. Mokwatsi GG, Hoshide S, Kanegae H, Fujiwara T, Negishi K, Schutte AE and Kario K. Direct comparison of home versus ambulatory defined nocturnal hypertension for predicting cardiovascular events: the Japan morning surge-home blood pressure (J-HOP) study. *Hypertension*. 2020;76:554–561. https://www.ahajournals.org/journal/hyp.

247. Kario K, Hettrick DA, Prejbisz A and Januszewicz A. Obstructive sleep apnea-induced neurogenic nocturnal hypertension: a potential role of renal denervation? *Hypertension*. 2021;77:1047–1060. https://www.ahajournals.org/journal/hyp.

248. Kario K. Obstructive sleep apnea syndrome and hypertension: ambulatory blood pressure. *Hypertens Res*. 2009;32:428–432.

249. Sasaki N, Nagai M, Mizuno H, Kuwabara M, Hoshide S and Kario K. Associations between characteristics of obstructive sleep apnea and nocturnal blood pressure surge. *Hypertension*. 2018;72:1133–1140. https://www.ahajournals.org/journal/hyp.

250. Kario K. Obstructive sleep apnea syndrome and hypertension: mechanism of the linkage and 24-h blood pressure control. *Hypertens Res*. 2009;32:537–541.

251. Khan SU, Duran CA, Rahman H, Lekkala M, Saleem MA and Kaluski E. A meta-analysis of continuous positive airway pressure therapy in prevention of cardiovascular events in patients with obstructive sleep apnoea. *Eur Heart J*. 2018;39:2291–2297.

252. McEvoy RD, Antic NA, Heeley E, Luo Y, Ou Q, Zhang X, Mediano O, Chen R, Drager LF, Liu Z, Chen G, Du B, McArdle N, Mukherjee S, Tripathi M, Billot L, Li Q, Lorenzi-Filho G, Barbe F, Redline S, Wang J, Arima H, Neal B, White DP, Grunstein RR, Zhong N, Anderson CS, and Save Investigators and Coordinators. CPAP for prevention of cardiovascular events in obstructive sleep apnea. *N Engl J Med*. 2016;375:919–931.

253. Umemura S, Arima H, Arima S, Asayama K, Dohi Y, Hirooka Y, Horio T, Hoshide S, Ikeda S, Ishimitsu T, Ito M, Ito S, Iwashima Y, Kai H, Kamide K, Kanno Y, Kashihara N, Kawano Y, Kikuchi T, Kitamura K, Kitazono T, Kohara K, Kudo M, Kumagai H, Matsumura K, Matsuura H, Miura K, Mukoyama M, Nakamura S, Ohkubo T, Ohya Y, Okura T, Rakugi H, Saitoh S, Shibata H, Shimosawa T, Suzuki H, Takahashi S, Tamura K, Tomiyama H, Tsuchihashi T, Ueda S, Uehara Y, Urata H and Hirawa N. The Japanese society of hypertension guidelines for the management of hypertension (JSH 2019). *Hypertens Res*. 2019;42:1235–1481.

254. Williams B, Mancia G, Spiering W, Agabiti Rosei E, Azizi M, Burnier M, Clement DL, Coca A, de Simone G, Dominiczak A, Kahan T, Mahfoud F, Redon J, Ruilope L, Zanchetti A, Kerins M, Kjeldsen SE, Kreutz R, Laurent S, Lip GYH, McManus R, Narkiewicz K, Ruschitzka F, Schmieder RE, Shlyakhto E, Tsioufis C, Aboyans V, Desormais I and ESC Scientific Document Group. 2018 ESC/ESH Guidelines for the management of arterial hypertension. *Eur Heart J*. 2018;39:3021–3104.

255. Kanegae H, Oikawa T, Suzuki K, Okawara Y and Kario K. Developing and validating a new precise risk-prediction model for new-onset hypertension: the Jichi Genki hypertension prediction model (JG model). *J Clin Hypertens (Greenwich)*. 2018;20:880–890.

256. Julius S, Nesbitt SD, Egan BM, Weber MA, Michelson EL, Kaciroti N, Black HR, Grimm RH, Jr., Messerli FH, Oparil S, Schork MA and Trial of Preventing Hypertension Study, Investigators. Feasibility of treating prehypertension with an angiotensin-receptor blocker. *N Engl J Med*. 2006;354:1685–97.

257. Kanegae H, Oikawa T and Kario K. Should pre-hypertension be treated? *Curr Hypertens Rep*. 2017;19:91.

258 Kanegae H, Oikawa T, Okawara Y, Hoshide S and Kario K. Which blood pressure measurement, systolic or diastolic, better predicts future hypertension in normotensive young adults? *J Clin Hypertens (Greenwich)*. 2017;19:603–610.

259. Tanaka A, Tomiyama H, Maruhashi T, Matsuzawa Y, Miyoshi T, Kabutoya T, Kario K, Sugiyama S, Munakata M, Ito H, Ueda S, Vlachopoulos C, Higashi Y, Inoue T, Node K and Physiological Diagnosis Criteria for Vascular Failure Committee. Physiological diagnostic criteria for vascular failure. *Hypertension.* 2018;72:1060–1071. https://www.ahajournals.org/journal/hyp.

260. Kario K, Kanegae H, Oikawa T and Suzuki K. Hypertension is predicted by both large and small artery disease. *Hypertension.* 2019;73:75–83. https://www.ahajournals.org/journal/hyp.

261. Kario K, Kabutoya T, Fujiwara T, Negishi K, Nishizawa M, Yamamoto M, Yamagiwa K, Kawashima A, Yoshida T, Nakazato J, Matsui Y, Sekizuka H, Abe H, Abe Y, Fujita Y, Sato K, Narita K, Tsuchiya N, Kubota Y, Hashizume T and Hoshide S. Rationale, design, and baseline characteristics of the Cardiovascular Prognostic COUPLING Study in Japan (the COUPLING Registry). *J Clin Hypertens (Greenwich).* 2020;22:465–474.

262. Kabutoya T, Hoshide S, Fujiwara T, Negishi K, Nishizawa M, Yamamoto M, Yamagiwa K, Kawashima A, Yoshida T, Nakazato J, Matsui Y, Sekizuka H, Abe H, Abe Y, Fujita Y, Sato K, Narita K, Tsuchiya N, Kubota Y, Hashizume T and Kario K. Age-related difference of the association of cardiovascular risk factors with the cardio-ankle vascular index in the Cardiovascular Prognostic Coupling Study in Japan (the Coupling Registry). *J Clin Hypertens (Greenwich).* 2020;22:1208–1215.

263. Fujiwara T, Hoshide S, Nishizawa M, Matsuo T and Kario K. Difference in evening home blood pressure between before dinner and at bedtime in Japanese elderly hypertensive patients. *J Clin Hypertens (Greenwich).* 2017;19:731–739.

264. Pickering TG, Miller NH, Ogedegbe G, Krakoff LR, Artinian NT, Goff D and American Heart A, American Society of H and Preventive Cardiovascular Nurses Association. Call to action on use and reimbursement for home blood pressure monitoring: executive summary: a joint scientific statement from the American Heart Association, American Society Of Hypertension, and Preventive Cardiovascular Nurses Association. *Hypertension.* 2008;52:1–9. https://www.ahajournals.org/journal/hyp.

265. Fujiwara T and Kario K. Comparison of waiting room and examination room blood pressure with home blood pressure level in a rural clinical practice. *J Clin Hypertens (Greenwich).* 2017;19:1051–1053.

266. Fujiwara T, Nishizawa M, Hoshide S, Kanegae H and Kario K. Comparison of different schedules of nocturnal home blood pressure measurement using an information/communication technology-based device in hypertensive patients. *J Clin Hypertens (Greenwich).* 2018;20:1633–1641.

267. Kario K. Proposal of RAS-diuretic vs. RAS-calcium antagonist strategies in high-risk hypertension: insight from the 24-hour ambulatory blood pressure profile and central pressure. *J Am Soc Hypertens.* 2010;4:215–218.

268. Kario K. Hypertension: benefits of strict blood-pressure lowering in hypertension. *Nat Rev Cardiol.* 2016;13:125–126.

269. Ruilope LM, Dukat A, Bohm M, Lacourciere Y, Gong J and Lefkowitz MP. Blood-pressure reduction with LCZ696, a novel dual-acting inhibitor of the angiotensin II receptor and neprilysin: a randomised, double-blind, placebo-controlled, active comparator study. *Lancet.* 2010;375:1255–1266.

270. Kario K, Sun N, Chiang FT, Supasyndh O, Baek SH, Inubushi-Molessa A, Zhang Y, Gotou H, Lefkowitz M and Zhang J. Efficacy and safety of LCZ696, a first-in-class angiotensin receptor neprilysin inhibitor, in Asian patients with hypertension: a randomized, double-blind, placebo-controlled study. *Hypertension.* 2014;63:698–705. https://www.ahajournals.org/journal/hyp.

271. Bavishi C, Messerli FH, Kadosh B, Ruilope LM and Kario K. Role of neprilysin inhibitor combinations in hypertension: insights from hypertension and heart failure trials. *Eur Heart J.* 2015;36:1967–1973.

272. Williams B, Cockcroft JR, Kario K, Zappe DH, Brunel PC, Wang Q and Guo W. Effects of sacubitril/valsartan versus olmesartan on central hemodynamics in the elderly with

systolic hypertension: the PARAMETER study. *Hypertension.* 2017;69:411–420. https://www.ahajournals.org/journal/hyp.

273. Wang TD, Tan RS, Lee HY, Ihm SH, Rhee MY, Tomlinson B, Pal P, Yang F, Hirschhorn E, Prescott MF, Hinder M and Langenickel TH. Effects of sacubitril/valsartan (LCZ696) on natriuresis, diuresis, blood pressures, and NT-proBNP in salt-sensitive hypertension. *Hypertension.* 2017;69:32–41. https://www.ahajournals.org/journal/hyp.

274. Kario K. The sacubitril/valsartan, a first-in-class, angiotensin receptor neprilysin inhibitor (ARNI): potential uses in hypertension, heart failure, and beyond. *Curr Cardiol Rep.* 2018;20:5.

275. Kario K, Weber M and Ferrannini E. Nocturnal hypertension in diabetes: potential target of sodium/glucose cotransporter 2 (SGLT2) inhibition. *J Clin Hypertens (Greenwich).* 2018;20:424–428.

276. McMurray JJ, Packer M, Desai AS, Gong J, Lefkowitz MP, Rizkala AR, Rouleau JL, Shi VC, Solomon SD, Swedberg K, Zile MR and PARADIGM-HF Investigators and Committees. Angiotensin-neprilysin inhibition versus enalapril in heart failure. *N Engl J Med.* 2014;371:993–1004.

277. Neal B, Perkovic V, Mahaffey KW, de Zeeuw D, Fulcher G, Erondu N, Shaw W, Law G, Desai M, Matthews DR and Group CPC. Canagliflozin and cardiovascular and renal events in type 2 diabetes. *N Engl J Med.* 2017;377:644–657.

278. Zinman B, Wanner C, Lachin JM, Fitchett D, Bluhmki E, Hantel S, Mattheus M, Devins T, Johansen OE, Woerle HJ, Broedl UC, Inzucchi SE and Empa-Reg Outcome Investigators. Empagliflozin, cardiovascular outcomes, and mortality in type 2 diabetes. *N Engl J Med.* 2015;373:2117–2128.

279. Wanner C, Inzucchi SE, Lachin JM, Fitchett D, von Eynatten M, Mattheus M, Johansen OE, Woerle HJ, Broedl UC, Zinman B and Empa-Reg Outcome Investigators. Empagliflozin and progression of kidney disease in type 2 diabetes. *N Engl J Med.* 2016;375:323–334.

280. Kario K and Williams B. Nocturnal hypertension and heart failure: mechanisms, evidence, and new treatments. *Hypertension.* 2021;78:564–577. https://doi.org/10.1161/HYPERTENSIONAHA.121.17440.

281. Kario K, Bhatt DL, Brar S, Cohen SA, Fahy M and Bakris GL. Effect of catheter-based renal denervation on morning and nocturnal blood pressure: insights from SYMPLICITY HTN-3 and SYMPLICITY HTN-Japan. *Hypertension.* 2015;66:1130–1137. https://www.ahajournals.org/journal/hyp.

282. Kario K, Bhatt DL, Kandzari DE, Brar S, Flack JM, Gilbert C, Oparil S, Robbins M, Townsend RR and Bakris G. Impact of renal denervation on patients with obstructive sleep apnea and resistant hypertension- insights from the SYMPLICITY HTN-3 trial. *Circ J.* 2016;80:1404–1412.

283. Townsend RR, Mahfoud F, Kandzari DE, Kario K, Pocock S, Weber MA, Ewen S, Tsioufis K, Tousoulis D, Sharp ASP, Watkinson AF, Schmieder RE, Schmid A, Choi JW, East C, Walton A, Hopper I, Cohen DL, Wilensky R, Lee DP, Ma A, Devireddy CM, Lea JP, Lurz PC, Fengler K, Davies J, Chapman N, Cohen SA, DeBruin V, Fahy M, Jones DE, Rothman M, Bohm M and Spyral HTN-Off Med trial investigators. Catheter-based renal denervation in patients with uncontrolled hypertension in the absence of antihypertensive medications (SPYRAL HTN-OFF MED): a randomised, sham-controlled, proof-of-concept trial. *Lancet.* 2017;390:2160–2170.

284. Kario K. Are melatonin and its receptor agonist specific antihypertensive modulators of resistant hypertension caused by disrupted circadian rhythm? *J Am Soc Hypertens.* 2011;5:354–8.

285. Ettehad D, Emdin CA, Kiran A, Anderson SG, Callender T, Emberson J, Chalmers J, Rodgers A and Rahimi K. Blood pressure lowering for prevention of cardiovascular disease and death: a systematic review and meta-analysis. *Lancet.* 2016;387:957–967.

286. Kario K. Differential approaches are much needed for "real world" management of hypertension in the era of "hypertension paradox". *Curr Hypertens Rev.* 2018;14:2–5.

287. Kario K, Abe T and Kanegae H. Impact of pre-existing hypertension and control status before atrial fibrillation onset on cardiovascular prognosis in patients with non-valvular atrial fibrillation: a real-world database analysis in Japan. *J Clin Hypertens (Greenwich).* 2020;22:431–437.

288. Nakano M, Eguchi K, Sato T, Onoguchi A, Hoshide S and Kario K. Effect of intensive salt-restriction education on clinic, home, and ambulatory blood pressure levels in treated hypertensive patients during a 3-month education period. *J Clin Hypertens (Greenwich).* 2016;18:385–392.

289. He FJ and MacGregor GA. Beneficial effects of potassium on human health. *Physiol Plant.* 2008;133:725–735.

290. Whelton PK and He J. Health effects of sodium and potassium in humans. *Curr Opin Lipidol.* 2014;25:75–79.

291. D'Elia L, Barba G, Cappuccio FP and Strazzullo P. Potassium intake, stroke, and cardiovascular disease a meta-analysis of prospective studies. *J Am Coll Cardiol.* 2011;57:1210–1219.

292. Zhang Z, Cogswell ME, Gillespie C, Fang J, Loustalot F, Dai S, Carriquiry AL, Kuklina EV, Hong Y, Merritt R and Yang Q. Association between usual sodium and potassium intake and blood pressure and hypertension among U.S. adults: NHANES 2005–2010. *PLoS One.* 2013;8:e75289.

293. Stone MS, Martyn L and Weaver CM. Potassium intake, bioavailability, hypertension, and glucose control. *Nutrients.* 2016;8(7):444. https://doi.org/10.3390/nu8070444.

294. Weaver CM. Potassium and health. *Adv Nutr.* 2013;4:368S–377S.

295. Writing Group Members, Mozaffarian D, Benjamin EJ, Go AS, Arnett DK, Blaha MJ, Cushman M, Das SR, de Ferranti S, Despres JP, Fullerton HJ, Howard VJ, Huffman MD, Isasi CR, Jimenez MC, Judd SE, Kissela BM, Lichtman JH, Lisabeth LD, Liu S, Mackey RH, Magid DJ, McGuire DK, Mohler ER, 3rd, Moy CS, Muntner P, Mussolino ME, Nasir K, Neumar RW, Nichol G, Palaniappan L, Pandey DK, Reeves MJ, Rodriguez CJ, Rosamond W, Sorlie PD, Stein J, Towfighi A, Turan TN, Virani SS, Woo D, Yeh RW, Turner MB and American Heart Association Statistics Committee and Stroke Statistics Subcommittee. Heart disease and stroke statistics-2016 update: a report from the American Heart Association. *Circulation.* 2016;133:e38–360. https://www.ahajournals.org/journal/circ.

296. Filippini T, Violi F, D'Amico R and Vinceti M. The effect of potassium supplementation on blood pressure in hypertensive subjects: a systematic review and meta-analysis. *Int J Cardiol.* 2017;230:127–135.

297. Dickinson HO, Nicolson DJ, Campbell F, Beyer FR and Mason J. Potassium supplementation for the management of primary hypertension in adults. *Cochrane Database Syst Rev.* 2006:CD004641.

298. Hunter RW and Bailey MA. Hyperkalemia: pathophysiology, risk factors and consequences. *Nephrol Dial Transplant.* 2019;34:iii2–iii11.

299. Zhang X, Li Y, Del Gobbo LC, Rosanoff A, Wang J, Zhang W and Song Y. Effects of magnesium supplementation on blood pressure: a meta-analysis of randomized double-blind placebo-controlled trials. *Hypertension.* 2016;68:324–333. https://www.ahajournals.org/journal/hyp.

300. Cormick G, Ciapponi A, Cafferata ML and Belizan JM. Calcium supplementation for prevention of primary hypertension. *Cochrane Database Syst. Rev.* 2015:CD010037.

301. Dickinson HO, Nicolson DJ, Cook JV, Campbell F, Beyer FR, Ford GA and Mason J. Calcium supplementation for the management of primary hypertension in adults. *Cochrane Database Syst. Rev.* 2006:CD004639.

302. Eicher JD, Maresh CM, Tsongalis GJ, Thompson PD and Pescatello LS. The additive blood pressure lowering effects of exercise intensity on post-exercise hypotension. *Am Heart J.* 2010;160:513–520.

303. Borjesson M, Onerup A, Lundqvist S and Dahlof B. Physical activity and exercise lower blood pressure in individuals with hypertension: narrative review of 27 RCTs. *Br J Sports Med*. 2016;50:356–361.

304. St-Onge MP, Grandner MA, Brown D, Conroy MB, Jean-Louis G, Coons M, Bhatt DL, and American Heart Association Obesity BCD, Nutrition Committees of the Council on L, Cardiometabolic H, Council on Cardiovascular Disease in the Young, Council on Clinical Cardiology and Stroke Council. Sleep duration and quality: impact on lifestyle behaviors and cardiometabolic health: a scientific statement from the American Heart Association. *Circulation*. 2016;134:e367–e386.

305. Grandner MA, Alfonso-Miller P, Fernandez-Mendoza J, Shetty S, Shenoy S and Combs D. Sleep: important considerations for the prevention of cardiovascular disease. *Curr Opin Cardiol*. 2016;31:551–565.

306. Friedman O, Shukla Y and Logan AG. Relationship between self-reported sleep duration and changes in circadian blood pressure. *Am J Hypertens*. 2009;22:1205–1211.

307. Kwok CS, Kontopantelis E, Kuligowski G, Gray M, Muhyaldeen A, Gale CP, Peat GM, Cleator J, Chew-Graham C, Loke YK and Mamas MA. Self-reported sleep duration and quality and cardiovascular disease and mortality: a dose-response meta-analysis. *J Am Heart Assoc*. 2018;7:e008552.

308. Cappuccio FP, Cooper D, D'Elia L, Strazzullo P and Miller MA. Sleep duration predicts cardiovascular outcomes: a systematic review and meta-analysis of prospective studies. *Eur Heart J*. 2011;32:1484–1492.

309. Itani O, Jike M, Watanabe N and Kaneita Y. Short sleep duration and health outcomes: a systematic review, meta-analysis, and meta-regression. *Sleep Med*. 2017;32: 246–256.

310. Jike M, Itani O, Watanabe N, Buysse DJ and Kaneita Y. Long sleep duration and health outcomes: a systematic review, meta-analysis and meta-regression. *Sleep Med Rev*. 2018;39:25–36.

311. Krittanawong C, Tunhasiriwet A, Wang Z, Zhang H, Farrell AM, Chirapongsathorn S, Sun T, Kitai T and Argulian E. Association between short and long sleep durations and cardiovascular outcomes: a systematic review and meta-analysis. *Eur Heart J Acute Cardiovasc Care*. 2019;8:762–770.

312. Kario K, Nomura A, Harada N, Tanigawa T, So R, Nakagawa K, Suzuki S, Okura A, Hida E and Satake K. A multicenter clinical trial to assess the efficacy of the digital therapeutics for essential hypertension: rationale and design of the HERB-DH1 trial. *J Clin Hypertens (Greenwich)*. 2020;22:1713–1722.

313. Kario K, Nomura A, Harada N, Okura A, Nakagawa K, Tanigawa T, Hida E. Efficacy of a digital therapeutics system in the management of essential hypertension: the HERB-DH1 pivotal trial. *Eur Heart J*. 2021; 42: 4111–4122.

314. Elliott HL. Benefits of twenty-four-hour blood pressure control. *J Hypertens Suppl*. 1996;14:S15–S19.

315. Hoshide S, Yano Y, Kanegae H and Kario K. Effect of lowering home blood pressure on subclinical cardiovascular disease in masked uncontrolled hypertension. *J Am Coll Cardiol*. 2018;71:2858–2859.

316. Triggle DJ. Calcium channel antagonists: clinical uses--past, present and future. *Biochem Pharmacol*. 2007;74:1–9.

317. Eguchi K, Kario K, Hoshide Y, Hoshide S, Ishikawa J, Morinari M, Ishikawa S and Shimada K. Comparison of valsartan and amlodipine on ambulatory and morning blood pressure in hypertensive patients. *Am J Hypertens*. 2004;17:112–117.

318. Kario K, Kimura K and Node K. Nearly half of uncontrolled hypertensive patients could be controlled by high-dose titration of amlodipine in the clinical setting: the ACHIEVE study. *Curr Hypertens Rev*. 2011;7:102–110.

319. Kario K and Shimada K. Differential effects of amlodipine on ambulatory blood pressure in elderly hypertensive patients with different nocturnal reductions in blood pressure. *Am J Hypertens*. 1997;10:261–268.

320. Wang JG, Kario K, Lau T, Wei YQ, Park CG, Kim CH, Huang J, Zhang W, Li Y, Yan P, Hu D and Asian Pacific Heart Association. Use of dihydropyridine calcium channel blockers in the management of hypertension in Eastern Asians: a scientific statement from the Asian Pacific Heart Association. *Hypertens Res.* 2011;34:423–430.

321. Mizuno H, Hoshide S, Tomitani N and Kario K. Comparison of ambulatory blood pressure-lowering effects of higher doses of different calcium antagonists in uncontrolled hypertension: the Calcium Antagonist Controlled-Release High-Dose Therapy in Uncontrolled Refractory Hypertensive Patients (CARILLON) Study. *Blood Press.* 2017;26:284–293.

322. Kario K, Ando S, Kido H, Nariyama J, Takiuchi S, Yagi T, Shimizu T, Eguchi K, Ohno M, Kinoshita O and Yamada T. The effects of the L/N-type calcium channel blocker (cilnidipine) on sympathetic hyperactive morning hypertension: results from ACHIEVE-ONE. *J Clin Hypertens (Greenwich).* 2013;15:133–142.

323. Kario K, Nariyama J, Kido H, Ando S, Takiuchi S, Eguchi K, Niijima Y, Ando T and Noda M. Effect of a novel calcium channel blocker on abnormal nocturnal blood pressure in hypertensive patients. *J Clin Hypertens (Greenwich).* 2013;15:465–472.

324. Eguchi K, Tomizawa H, Ishikawa J, Hoshide S, Fukuda T, Numao T, Shimada K and Kario K. Effects of new calcium channel blocker, azelnidipine, and amlodipine on baroreflex sensitivity and ambulatory blood pressure. *J Cardiovasc Pharmacol.* 2007;49:394–400.

325. Kario K, Uehara Y, Shirayama M, Takahashi M, Shiosakai K, Hiramatsu K, Komiya M and Shimada K. Study of sustained blood pressure-lowering effect of azelnidipine guided by self-measured morning and evening home blood pressure: subgroup analysis of the At-HOME study. *Drugs R D.* 2013;13:75–85.

326. Kuramoto K, Ichikawa S, Hirai A, Kanada S, Nakachi T and Ogihara T. Azelnidipine and amlodipine: a comparison of their pharmacokinetics and effects on ambulatory blood pressure. *Hypertens Res.* 2003;26:201–208.

327. Kario K, Sato Y, Shirayama M, Takahashi M, Shiosakai K, Hiramatsu K, Komiya M and Shimada K. Inhibitory effects of azelnidipine tablets on morning hypertension. *Drugs R D.* 2013;13:63–73.

328. Nonaka H, Emoto N, Ikeda K, Fukuya H, Rohman MS, Raharjo SB, Yagita K, Okamura H and Yokoyama M. Angiotensin II induces circadian gene expression of clock genes in cultured vascular smooth muscle cells. *Circulation.* 2001;104:1746–1748. https://www.ahajournals.org/journal/circ.

329. Kuroda T, Kario K, Hoshide S, Hashimoto T, Nomura Y, Saito Y, Mito H and Shimada K. Effects of bedtime vs. morning administration of the long-acting lipophilic angiotensin-converting enzyme inhibitor trandolapril on morning blood pressure in hypertensive patients. *Hypertens Res.* 2004;27:15–20.

330. Ogihara T, Nakao K, Fukui T, Fukiyama K, Ueshima K, Oba K, Sato T, Saruta T and Candesartan Antihypertensive Survival Evaluation in Japan Trial Group. Effects of candesartan compared with amlodipine in hypertensive patients with high cardiovascular risks: candesartan antihypertensive survival evaluation in Japan trial. *Hypertension.* 2008;51:393–398. https://www.ahajournals.org/journal/hyp.

331. Kasanuki H, Hagiwara N, Hosoda S, Sumiyoshi T, Honda T, Haze K, Nagashima M, Yamaguchi J, Origasa H, Urashima M, Ogawa H and Investigators H.-C. Angiotensin II receptor blocker-based vs. non-angiotensin II receptor blocker-based therapy in patients with angiographically documented coronary artery disease and hypertension: the Heart Institute of Japan Candesartan Randomized Trial for Evaluation in Coronary Artery Disease (HIJ-CREATE). *Eur Heart J.* 2009;30:1203–1212.

332. Suzuki H, Kanno Y and Efficacy of Candesartan on Outcome in Saitama Trial Group. Effects of candesartan on cardiovascular outcomes in Japanese hypertensive patients. *Hypertens Res.* 2005;28:307–314.

333. Neutel J and Smith DH. Evaluation of angiotensin II receptor blockers for 24-hour blood pressure control: meta-analysis of a clinical database. *J Clin Hypertens (Greenwich).* 2003;5:58–63.

334. Inada Y, Ojima M, Kanagawa R, Misumi Y, Nishikawa K and Naka T. Pharmacologic properties of candesartan cilexetil--possible mechanisms of long-acting antihypertensive action. *J Hum Hypertens.* 1999;13 Suppl. 1:S75–S80.

335. Eguchi K, Kario K and Shimada K. Comparison of candesartan with lisinopril on ambulatory blood pressure and morning surge in patients with systemic hypertension. *Am J Cardiol.* 2003;92:621–624.

336. Fukuda M, Yamanaka T, Mizuno M, Motokawa M, Shirasawa Y, Miyagi S, Nishio T, Yoshida A and Kimura G. Angiotensin II type 1 receptor blocker, olmesartan, restores nocturnal blood pressure decline by enhancing daytime natriuresis. *J Hypertens.* 2008;26:583–588. https://journals.lww.com/jhypertension/pages/default.aspx.

337. Kario K, Saito I, Kushiro T, Teramukai S, Ishikawa Y, Hiramatsu K, Kobayashi F and Shimada K. Effect of the angiotensin II receptor antagonist olmesartan on morning home blood pressure in hypertension: HONEST study at 16 weeks. *J Hum Hypertens.* 2013;27:721–728.

338. Kario K, Saito I, Kushiro T, Teramukai S, Yaginuma M, Mori Y, Okuda Y, Kobayashi F and Shimada K. Persistent olmesartan-based blood pressure-lowering effects on morning hypertension in Asians: the HONEST study. *Hypertens Res.* 2016;39:334–341.

339. Kario K, Saito I, Kushiro T, Teramukai S, Ishikawa Y, Kobayashi F and Shimada K. Effects of olmesartan-based treatment on masked, white-coat, poorly controlled, and well-controlled hypertension: HONEST study. *J Clin Hypertens (Greenwich).* 2014;16:442–450.

340. Kario K, Saito I, Kushiro T, Teramukai S, Mori Y, Hiramatsu K, Kobayashi F and Shimada K. Enhanced blood pressure-lowering effect of olmesartan in hypertensive patients with chronic kidney disease-associated sympathetic hyperactivity: HONEST study. *J Clin Hypertens (Greenwich).* 2013;15:555–561.

341. Rakugi H, Kario K, Enya K, Igeta M and Ikeda Y. Effect of azilsartan versus candesartan on nocturnal blood pressure variation in Japanese patients with essential hypertension. *Blood Press.* 2013;22 Suppl. 1:22–28.

342. Rakugi H, Kario K, Enya K, Sugiura K and Ikeda Y. Effect of azilsartan versus candesartan on morning blood pressure surges in Japanese patients with essential hypertension. *Blood Press Monit.* 2014;19:164–169. https://journals.lww.com/bpmonitoring/pages/default.aspx.

343. Kario K and Hoshide S. Age-related difference in the sleep pressure-lowering effect between an angiotensin II receptor blocker and a calcium channel blocker in Asian hypertensives: the ACS1 Study. *Hypertension.* 2015;65:729–735. https://www.ahajournals.org/journal/hyp.

344. Kario K and Hoshide S. Age- and sex-related differences in efficacy with an angiotensin II receptor blocker and a calcium channel blocker in Asian hypertensive patients. *J Clin Hypertens (Greenwich).* 2016;18:672–678.

345. Uzu T and Kimura G. Diuretics shift circadian rhythm of blood pressure from nondipper to dipper in essential hypertension. *Circulation.* 1999;100:1635–1638. https://www.ahajournals.org/journal/circ.

346. Ishikawa J, Eguchi K, Hoshide S, Shimada K and Kario K. Relationship between the change in left ventricular hypertrophy and asleep blood pressure after sodium restriction and/or diuretic treatment. *Blood Press Monit.* 2011;16:172–179. https://journals.lww.com/bpmonitoring/pages/default.aspx.

347. Pickering TG, Levenstein M and Walmsley P. Nighttime dosing of doxazosin has peak effect on morning ambulatory blood pressure. Results of the HALT Study. Hypertension and Lipid Trial Study Group. *Am J Hypertens.* 1994;7:844–847.

348. Kario K, Matsui Y, Shibasaki S, Eguchi K, Ishikawa J, Hoshide S, Ishikawa S, Kabutoya T, Schwartz JE, Pickering TG, Shimada K and Japan Morning Surge-1 Study Group. An alpha-adrenergic blocker titrated by self-measured blood pressure recordings lowered blood pressure and microalbuminuria in patients with morning hypertension: the Japan Morning Surge-1 Study. *J Hypertens.* 2008;26:1257–1265. https://journals.lww.com/jhypertension/pages/default.aspx.

349. Shibasaki S, Eguchi K, Matsui Y, Ishikawa J, Hoshide S, Ishikawa S, Kabutoya T, Pickering TG, Shimada K, Kario K and Japan Morning Surge-1 Study Group. Adrenergic

blockade improved insulin resistance in patients with morning hypertension: the Japan Morning Surge-1 Study. *J Hypertens.* 2009;27:1252–1257. https://journals.lww.com/jhypertension/pages/default.aspx.

350. Kario K, Ito S, Itoh H, Rakugi H, Okuda Y, Yoshimura M and Yamakawa S. Effect of the nonsteroidal mineralocorticoid receptor blocker, esaxerenone, on nocturnal hypertension: a post hoc analysis of the ESAX-HTN study. *Am J Hypertens.* 2021;34:540-551.

351. Arai K, Homma T, Morikawa Y, Ubukata N, Tsuruoka H, Aoki K, Ishikawa H, Mizuno M and Sada T. Pharmacological profile of CS-3150, a novel, highly potent and selective non-steroidal mineralocorticoid receptor antagonist. *Eur J Pharmacol.* 2015;761:226–234.

352. Ito S, Satoh M, Tamaki Y, Gotou H, Charney A, Okino N, Akahori M and Zhang J. Safety and efficacy of LCZ696, a first-in-class angiotensin receptor neprilysin inhibitor, in Japanese patients with hypertension and renal dysfunction. *Hypertens Res.* 2015;38:269–275.

353. Kario K, Tamaki Y, Okino N, Gotou H, Zhu M and Zhang J. LCZ696, a First-in-class angiotensin receptor-neprilysin inhibitor: the first clinical experience in patients with severe hypertension. *J Clin Hypertens (Greenwich).* 2016;18:308–314.

354. Supasyndh O, Sun N, Kario K, Hafeez K and Zhang J. Long-term (52-week) safety and efficacy of Sacubitril/valsartan in Asian patients with hypertension. *Hypertens Res.* 2017;40:472–476.

355. Supasyndh O, Wang J, Hafeez K, Zhang Y, Zhang J and Rakugi H. Efficacy and safety of Sacubitril/Valsartan (LCZ696) compared with olmesartan in elderly Asian patients (>/=65 Years) with systolic hypertension. *Am J Hypertens.* 2017;30:1163–1169.

356. Wang JG, Yukisada K, Sibulo A, Jr., Hafeez K, Jia Y and Zhang J. Efficacy and safety of sacubitril/valsartan (LCZ696) add-on to amlodipine in Asian patients with systolic hypertension uncontrolled with amlodipine monotherapy. *J Hypertens.* 2017;35:877–885. https://journals.lww.com/jhypertension/pages/default.aspx.

357. Solomon SD, Zile M, Pieske B, Voors A, Shah A, Kraigher-Krainer E, Shi V, Bransford T, Takeuchi M, Gong J, Lefkowitz M, Packer M, McMurray JJ and Prospective comparison of ARNI with A. R. B. on Management Of heart failUre with preserved ejectioN fracTion Investigators. The angiotensin receptor neprilysin inhibitor LCZ696 in heart failure with preserved ejection fraction: a phase 2 double-blind randomised controlled trial. *Lancet.* 2012;380:1387–1395.

358. Moorhouse RC, Webb DJ, Kluth DC and Dhaun N. Endothelin antagonism and its role in the treatment of hypertension. *Curr Hypertens Rep.* 2013;15:489–496.

359. da Silva AA, Kuo JJ, Tallam LS and Hall JE. Role of endothelin-1 in blood pressure regulation in a rat model of visceral obesity and hypertension. *Hypertension.* 2004;43:383–387.

360. Yuan W, Cheng G, Li B, Li Y, Lu S, Liu D, Xiao J, Zhao Z. Endothelin-receptor antagonist can reduce blood pressure in patients with hypertension: a meta-analysis. *Blood Press.* 2017; 26: 139–149.

361. Weber MA, Black H, Bakris G, Krum H, Linas S, Weiss R, Linseman JV, Wiens BL, Warren MS and Lindholm LH. A selective endothelin-receptor antagonist to reduce blood pressure in patients with treatment-resistant hypertension: a randomised, double-blind, placebo-controlled trial. *Lancet.* 2009;374:1423–1431.

362. Verweij P, Danaietash P, Flamion B, Menard J and Bellet M. Randomized dose-response study of the new dual endothelin receptor antagonist aprocitentan in hypertension. *Hypertension.* 2020;75:956–965. https://www.ahajournals.org/journal/hyp.

363. Williams B, Poulter NR, Brown MJ, Davis M, McInnes GT, Potter JF, Sever PS, Thom SM and BHS guidelines working party for the British Hypertension Society. British Hypertension Society guidelines for hypertension management 2004 (BHS-IV): summary. *BMJ.* 2004;328:634–640.

364. Unger T, Borghi C, Charchar F, Khan NA, Poulter NR, Prabhakaran D, Ramirez A, Schlaich M, Stergiou GS, Tomaszewski M, Wainford RD, Williams B and Schutte AE. 2020 International Society of Hypertension global hypertension practice guidelines.

J Hypertens. 2020;38:982–1004. https://journals.lww.com/jhypertension/pages/default.aspx.

365. Wald DS, Law M, Morris JK, Bestwick JP and Wald NJ. Combination therapy versus monotherapy in reducing blood pressure: meta-analysis on 11,000 participants from 42 trials. *Am J Med.* 2009;122:290–300.

366. Egan BM, Bandyopadhyay D, Shaftman SR, Wagner CS, Zhao Y and Yu-Isenberg KS. Initial monotherapy and combination therapy and hypertension control the first year. *Hypertension.* 2012;59:1124–1131. https://www.ahajournals.org/journal/hyp.

367. Osterberg L and Blaschke T. Adherence to medication. *N Engl J Med.* 2005;353:487–497.

368. Gupta AK, Arshad S and Poulter NR. Compliance, safety, and effectiveness of fixed-dose combinations of antihypertensive agents: a meta-analysis. *Hypertension.* 2010;55:399–407. https://www.ahajournals.org/journal/hyp.

369. Matsui Y, Eguchi K, O'Rourke MF, Ishikawa J, Miyashita H, Shimada K and Kario K. Differential effects between a calcium channel blocker and a diuretic when used in combination with angiotensin II receptor blocker on central aortic pressure in hypertensive patients. *Hypertension.* 2009;54:716–723. https://www.ahajournals.org/journal/hyp.

370. Matsui Y, Eguchi K, Ishikawa J, Shimada K and Kario K. Urinary albumin excretion during angiotensin II receptor blockade: comparison of combination treatment with a diuretic or a calcium-channel blocker. *Am J Hypertens.* 2011;24:466–473.

371. Eguchi K, Hoshide S, Kabutoya T, Shimada K and Kario K. Is very low dose hydrochlorothiazide combined with candesartan effective in uncontrolled hypertensive patients? *Blood Press Monit.* 2010;15:308–311. https://journals.lww.com/bpmonitoring/pages/default.aspx.

372. Yano Y, Hoshide S, Tamaki N, Nagata M, Sasaki K, Kanemaru Y, Shimada K and Kario K. Efficacy of eplerenone added to renin-angiotensin blockade in elderly hypertensive patients: the Jichi-Eplerenone Treatment (JET) study. *J Renin Angiotensin Aldosterone Syst.* 2011;12:340–347.

373. Fukutomi M, Hoshide S, Eguchi K, Watanabe T, Shimada K and Kario K. Differential effects of strict blood pressure lowering by losartan/hydrochlorothiazide combination therapy and high-dose amlodipine monotherapy on microalbuminuria: the ALPHABET study. *J Am Soc Hypertens.* 2012;6:73–82.

374. Mizuno H, Hoshide S, Fukutomi M and Kario K. Differing effects of aliskiren/amlodipine combination and high-dose amlodipine monotherapy on ambulatory blood pressure and target organ protection. *J Clin Hypertens (Greenwich).* 2016;18:70–78.

375. Fukutomi M, Hoshide S, Mizuno H and Kario K. Differential effects of aliskiren/amlodipine combination and high-dose amlodipine monotherapy on endothelial function in elderly hypertensive patients. *Am J Hypertens.* 2014;27:14–20.

376. Kario K, Hoshide S, Uchiyama K, Yoshida T, Okazaki O, Noshiro T, Aoki H, Mizuno H and Matsumoto Y. Dose timing of an angiotensin II receptor blocker/calcium channel blocker combination in hypertensive patients with paroxysmal atrial fibrillation. *J Clin Hypertens (Greenwich).* 2016;18:1036–1044.

377. Fujiwara T, Hoshide S, Yano Y, Kanegae H and Kario K. Comparison of morning vs bedtime administration of the combination of valsartan/amlodipine on nocturnal brachial and central blood pressure in patients with hypertension. *J Clin Hypertens (Greenwich).* 2017;19:1319–1326.

378. Kario K, Matsuda S, Nagahama S, Kurose Y, Sugii H, Teshima T and Suzuki N. Single-pill combination of cilnidipine, an L-/N-type calcium channel blocker, and valsartan effectively reduces home pulse pressure in patients with uncontrolled hypertension and sympathetic hyperactivity: The HOPE-Combi survey. *J Clin Hypertens (Greenwich).* 2020;22:457–464.

379. Pedrosa RP, Drager LF, Gonzaga CC, Sousa MG, de Paula LK, Amaro AC, Amodeo C, Bortolotto LA, Krieger EM, Bradley TD and Lorenzi-Filho G. Obstructive sleep apnea:

the most common secondary cause of hypertension associated with resistant hypertension. *Hypertension*. 2011;58:811–817. https://www.ahajournals.org/journal/hyp.

380. Pimenta E, Gaddam KK, Oparil S, Aban I, Husain S, Dell'Italia LJ and Calhoun DA. Effects of dietary sodium reduction on blood pressure in subjects with resistant hypertension: results from a randomized trial. *Hypertension*. 2009;54:475–481. https://www.ahajournals.org/journal/hyp.

381. Uzu T, Ishikawa K, Fujii T, Nakamura S, Inenaga T and Kimura G. Sodium restriction shifts circadian rhythm of blood pressure from nondipper to dipper in essential hypertension. *Circulation*. 1997;96:1859–1862. https://www.ahajournals.org/journal/circ.

382. Nishizaka MK, Zaman MA and Calhoun DA. Efficacy of low-dose spironolactone in subjects with resistant hypertension. *Am J Hypertens*. 2003;16:925–930.

383. Williams B, MacDonald TM, Morant S, Webb DJ, Sever P, McInnes G, Ford I, Cruickshank JK, Caulfield MJ, Salsbury J, Mackenzie I, Padmanabhan S, Brown MJ and British Hypertension Society's Pathway Studies Group. Spironolactone versus placebo, bisoprolol, and doxazosin to determine the optimal treatment for drug-resistant hypertension (PATHWAY-2): a randomised, double-blind, crossover trial. *Lancet*. 2015;386:2059–2068.

384. Ferrannini E. Sodium-glucose co-transporters and their inhibition: clinical physiology. *Cell Metab*. 2017;26:27–38.

385. Kario K, Ferdinand KC and O'Keefe JH. Control of 24-hour blood pressure with SGLT2 inhibitors to prevent cardiovascular disease. *Prog Cardiovasc Dis*. 2020;63:249–262.

386. Weber MA, Mansfield TA, Cain VA, Iqbal N, Parikh S and Ptaszynska A. Blood pressure and glycaemic effects of dapagliflozin versus placebo in patients with type 2 diabetes on combination antihypertensive therapy: a randomised, double-blind, placebo-controlled, phase 3 study. *Lancet Diabetes Endocrinol*. 2016;4:211–220.

387. Kario K, Ferdinand KC and Vongpatanasin W. Are SGLT2 inhibitors new hypertension drugs? *Circulation*. 2021;143:1750-1753. https://www.ahajournals.org/journal/circ.

388. Ferdinand KC, Izzo JL, Lee J, Meng L, George J, Salsali A and Seman L. Antihyperglycemic and blood pressure effects of empagliflozin in black patients with type 2 diabetes mellitus and hypertension. *Circulation*. 2019;139:2098–2109. https://www.ahajournals.org/journal/circ.

389. Papadopoulou E, Loutradis C, Tzatzagou G, Kotsa K, Zografou I, Minopoulou I, Theodorakopoulou MP, Tsapas A, Karagiannis A and Sarafidis P. Dapagliflozin decreases ambulatory central blood pressure and pulse wave velocity in patients with type 2 diabetes: a randomized, double-blind, placebo-controlled clinical trial. *J Hypertens*. 2021;39:749–758. https://journals.lww.com/jhypertension/pages/default.aspx.

390. Kario K, Hoshide S, Okawara Y, Tomitani N, Yamauchi K, Ohbayashi H, Itabashi N, Matsumoto Y and Kanegae H. Effect of canagliflozin on nocturnal home blood pressure in Japanese patients with type 2 diabetes mellitus: The SHIFT-J study. *J Clin Hypertens (Greenwich)*. 2018;20:1527–1535.

391. Kario K, Okada K, Murata M, Suzuki D, Yamagiwa K, Abe Y, Usui I, Tsuchiya N, Iwashita C, Harada N, Okawara Y, Ishibashi S and Hoshide S. Effects of luseogliflozin on arterial properties in patients with type 2 diabetes mellitus: the multicenter, exploratory LUSCAR study. *J Clin Hypertens (Greenwich)*. 2020;22:1585–1593.

392. Kario K, Okada K, Kato M, Nishizawa M, Yoshida T, Asano T, Uchiyama K, Niijima Y, Katsuya T, Urata H, Osuga JI, Fujiwara T, Yamazaki S, Tomitani N and Kanegae H. 24-hour blood pressure-lowering effect of an SGLT-2 inhibitor in patients with diabetes and uncontrolled nocturnal hypertension: results from the randomized, placebo-controlled SACRA study. *Circulation*. 2018;139:2089–2097. https://www.ahajournals.org/journal/circ.

393. Okada K, Hoshide S, Kato M, Kanegae H, Ishibashi S and Kario K. Safety and efficacy of empagliflozin in elderly Japanese patients with type 2 diabetes mellitus: a post hoc analysis of data from the SACRA study. *J Clin Hypertens (Greenwich)*. 2021;23:860-869.

394. Piepoli MF, Hoes AW, Agewall S, Albus C, Brotons C, Catapano AL, Cooney MT, Corra U, Cosyns B, Deaton C, Graham I, Hall MS, Hobbs FDR, Lochen ML, Lollgen H,

Marques-Vidal P, Perk J, Prescott E, Redon J, Richter DJ, Sattar N, Smulders Y, Tiberi M, van der Worp HB, van Dis I, Verschuren WMM, Binno S and ESC Scientific Document Group. 2016 European Guidelines on cardiovascular disease prevention in clinical practice: The Sixth Joint Task Force of the European Society of Cardiology and Other Societies on Cardiovascular Disease Prevention in Clinical Practice (constituted by representatives of 10 societies and by invited experts) Developed with the special contribution of the European Association for Cardiovascular Prevention & Rehabilitation (EACPR). *Eur Heart J.* 2016;37:2315–2381.

395. Bredemeier M, Lopes LM, Eisenreich MA, Hickmann S, Bongiorno GK, d'Avila R, Morsch ALB, da Silva Stein F and Campos GGD. Xanthine oxidase inhibitors for prevention of cardiovascular events: a systematic review and meta-analysis of randomized controlled trials. *BMC Cardiovasc Disord.* 2018;18:24.

396. Kario K, Nishizawa M, Kiuchi M, Kiyosue A, Tomita F, Ohtani H, Abe Y, Kuga H, Miyazaki S, Kasai T, Hongou M, Yasu T, Kuramochi J, Fukumoto Y, Hoshide S and Hisatome I. Comparative effects of topiroxostat and febuxostat on arterial properties in hypertensive patients with hyperuricemia. *J Clin Hypertens (Greenwich).* 2021;23:334–344.

397. Zhang DY, Cheng YB, Guo QH, Shan XL, Wei FF, Lu F, Sheng CS, Huang QF, Yang CH, Li Y and Wang JG. Treatment of masked hypertension with a Chinese herbal formula: a randomized, placebo-controlled trial. *Circulation.* 2020;142:1821–1830. https://www.ahajournals.org/journal/circ.

398. Thoenes M, Neuberger HR, Volpe M, Khan BV, Kirch W and Bohm M. Antihypertensive drug therapy and blood pressure control in men and women: an international perspective. *J Hum Hypertens.* 2010;24:336–344.

399. Persell SD. Prevalence of resistant hypertension in the United States, 2003–2008. *Hypertension.* 2011;57:1076–1080. https://www.ahajournals.org/journal/hyp.

400. Sim JJ, Bhandari SK, Shi J, Liu IL, Calhoun DA, McGlynn EA, Kalantar-Zadeh K and Jacobsen SJ. Characteristics of resistant hypertension in a large, ethnically diverse hypertension population of an integrated health system. *Mayo Clin Proc.* 2013;88:1099–1107.

401. Burnier M and Egan BM. Adherence in hypertension. *Circ Res.* 2019;124:1124–1140.

402. Vrijens B, Vincze G, Kristanto P, Urquhart J and Burnier M. Adherence to prescribed antihypertensive drug treatments: longitudinal study of electronically compiled dosing histories. *BMJ.* 2008;336:1114–1117.

403. Hill MN, Miller NH, Degeest S, American Society of Hypertension Writing Group, Materson BJ, Black HR, Izzo JL, Jr., Oparil S and Weber MA. Adherence and persistence with taking medication to control high blood pressure. *J Am Soc Hypertens.* 2011;5:56–63.

404. Brinker S, Pandey A, Ayers C, Price A, Raheja P, Arbique D, Das SR, Halm EA, Kaplan NM and Vongpatanasin W. Therapeutic drug monitoring facilitates blood pressure control in resistant hypertension. *J Am Coll Cardiol.* 2014;63:834–835.

405. Ceral J, Habrdova V, Vorisek V, Bima M, Pelouch R and Solar M. Difficult-to-control arterial hypertension or uncooperative patients? The assessment of serum antihypertensive drug levels to differentiate non-responsiveness from non-adherence to recommended therapy. *Hypertens Res.* 2011;34:87–90.

406. Strauch B, Petrak O, Zelinka T, Rosa J, Somloova Z, Indra T, Chytil L, Maresova V, Kurcova I, Holaj R, Wichterle D and Widimsky J, Jr. Precise assessment of noncompliance with the antihypertensive therapy in patients with resistant hypertension using toxicological serum analysis. *J Hypertens.* 2013;31:2455–2461. https://journals.lww.com/jhypertension/pages/default.aspx.

407. Tomaszewski M, White C, Patel P, Masca N, Damani R, Hepworth J, Samani NJ, Gupta P, Madira W, Stanley A and Williams B. High rates of non-adherence to antihypertensive treatment revealed by high-performance liquid chromatography-tandem mass spectrometry (HP LC-MS/MS) urine analysis. *Heart.* 2014;100:855–861.

408. Osborn JW and Foss JD. Renal nerves and long-term control of arterial pressure. *Compr Physiol.* 2017;7:263–320.
409. Polhemus DJ, Trivedi RK, Gao J, Li Z, Scarborough AL, Goodchild TT, Varner KJ, Xia H, Smart FW, Kapusta DR and Lefer DJ. Renal sympathetic denervation protects the failing heart via inhibition of neprilysin activity in the kidney. *J Am Coll Cardiol.* 2017;70:2139–2153.
410. Kario K, Hettrick DA and Esler MD. Device-based treatment in hypertension: at the forefront of renal denervation. *Cardiovasc Dis.* 2021; 1: 112-127.
411. Smithwick RH. Hypertensive cardiovascular disease; effect of thoracolumbar splanchnicectomy on mortality and survival rates. *J Am Med Assoc.* 1951;147:1611–1615.
412. Krum H, Schlaich M, Whitbourn R, Sobotka PA, Sadowski J, Bartus K, Kapelak B, Walton A, Sievert H, Thambar S, Abraham WT and Esler M. Catheter-based renal sympathetic denervation for resistant hypertension: a multicentre safety and proof-of-principle cohort study. *Lancet.* 2009;373:1275–1281.
413. Symplicity HTNI, Esler MD, Krum H, Sobotka PA, Schlaich MP, Schmieder RE and Bohm M. Renal sympathetic denervation in patients with treatment-resistant hypertension (The Symplicity HTN-2 Trial): a randomised controlled trial. *Lancet.* 2010;376:1903–1909.
414. Bhatt DL, Kandzari DE, O'Neill WW, D'Agostino R, Flack JM, Katzen BT, Leon MB, Liu M, Mauri L, Negoita M, Cohen SA, Oparil S, Rocha-Singh K, Townsend RR, Bakris GL and for the SYMPLICITY HTN-3 Investigators. A controlled trial of renal denervation for resistant hypertension. *N Engl J Med.* 2014;370:1393–401.
415. Kario K, Ogawa H, Okumura K, Okura T, Saito S, Ueno T, Haskin R, Negoita M, Shimada K and Symplicity HTN- Japan Investigators. SYMPLICITY HTN-Japan - First Randomized Controlled Trial of Catheter-Based Renal Denervation in Asian Patients -. *Circ J.* 2015;79:1222–1229.
416. Kario K, Yamamoto E, Tomita H, Okura T, Saito S, Ueno T, Yasuhara D, Shimada K and Symplicity HTN- Japan Investigators. Sufficient and persistent blood pressure reduction in the final long-term results from SYMPLICITY HTN-Japan- safety and efficacy of renal denervation at 3 years. *Circ J.* 2019;83:622–629.
417. Azizi M, Sapoval M, Gosse P, Monge M, Bobrie G, Delsart P, Midulla M, Mounier-Véhier C, Courand PY, Lantelme P, Denolle T, Dourmap-Collas C, Trillaud H, Pereira H, Plouin PF, Chatellier G; Renal Denervation for Hypertension (DENERHTN) investigators. Optimum and stepped care standardised antihypertensive treatment with or without renal denervation for resistant hypertension (DENERHTN): a multicentre, open-label, randomised controlled trial. *Lancet.* 2015;385:1957–1965.
418. Azizi M, Pereira H, Hamdidouche I, Gosse P, Monge M, Bobrie G, Delsart P, Mounier-Vehier C, Courand PY, Lantelme P, Denolle T, Dourmap-Collas C, Girerd X, Michel Halimi J, Zannad F, Ormezzano O, Vaisse B, Herpin D, Ribstein J, Chamontin B, Mourad JJ, Ferrari E, Plouin PF, Jullien V, Sapoval M, Chatellier G and Investigators D. Adherence to antihypertensive treatment and the blood pressure-lowering effects of renal denervation in the renal denervation for hypertension (DENERHTN) trial. *Circulation.* 2016;134:847–857. https://www.ahajournals.org/journal/circ.
419. Kandzari DE, Bhatt DL, Brar S, Devireddy CM, Esler M, Fahy M, Flack JM, Katzen BT, Lea J, Lee DP, Leon MB, Ma A, Massaro J, Mauri L, Oparil S, O'Neill WW, Patel MR, Rocha-Singh K, Sobotka PA, Svetkey L, Townsend RR and Bakris GL. Predictors of blood pressure response in the SYMPLICITY HTN-3 trial. *Eur Heart J.* 2015;36:219–227.
420. Kandzari DE, Bhatt DL, Sobotka PA, O'Neill WW, Esler M, Flack JM, Katzen BT, Leon MB, Massaro JM, Negoita M, Oparil S, Rocha-Singh K, Straley C, Townsend RR and Bakris G. Catheter-based renal denervation for resistant hypertension: rationale and design of the SYMPLICITY HTN-3 trial. *Clin Cardiol.* 2012;35:528–535.
421. Kandzari DE, Kario K, Mahfoud F, Cohen SA, Pilcher G, Pocock S, Townsend R, Weber MA and Bohm M. The SPYRAL HTN Global Clinical Trial Program: Rationale and design

for studies of renal denervation in the absence (SPYRAL HTN OFF-MED) and presence (SPYRAL HTN ON-MED) of antihypertensive medications. *Am Heart J.* 2016;171:82–91.

422. Mahfoud F, Tunev S, Ewen S, Cremers B, Ruwart J, Schulz-Jander D, Linz D, Davies J, Kandzari DE, Whitbourn R, Bohm M and Melder RJ. Impact of lesion placement on efficacy and safety of catheter-based radiofrequency renal denervation. *J Am Coll Cardiol.* 2015;66:1766–1775.

423. Henegar JR, Zhang Y, Hata C, Narciso I, Hall ME and Hall JE. Catheter-based radiofrequency renal denervation: location effects on renal norepinephrine. *Am J Hypertens.* 2015;28:909–914.

424. Pekarskiy SE, Baev AE, Mordovin VF, Semke GV, Ripp TM, Falkovskaya AU, Lichikaki VA, Sitkova ES, Zubanova IV and Popov SV. Denervation of the distal renal arterial branches vs. conventional main renal artery treatment: a randomized controlled trial for treatment of resistant hypertension. *J Hypertens.* 2017;35:369–375. https://journals.lww.com/jhypertension/pages/default.aspx.

425. Fengler K, Ewen S, Hollriegel R, Rommel KP, Kulenthiran S, Lauder L, Cremers B, Schuler G, Linke A, Bohm M, Mahfoud F and Lurz P. Blood pressure response to main renal artery and combined main renal artery plus branch renal denervation in patients with resistant hypertension. *J Am Heart Assoc.* 2017;6(8):e006196.

426. Kandzari DE, Böhm M, Mahfoud F, Townsend RR, Weber MA, Pocock S, Tsioufis K, Tousoulis D, Choi JW, East C, Brar S, Cohen SA, Fahy M, Pilcher G, Kario K and Spyral HTN-On Med Trial Investigators. Effect of renal denervation on blood pressure in the presence of antihypertensive drugs: 6-month efficacy and safety results from the SPYRAL HTN-ON MED proof-of-concept randomised trial. *Lancet.* 2018;391:2346–2355.

427. Böhm M, Kario K, Kandzari DE, Mahfoud F, Weber MA, Schmieder RE, Tsioufis K, Pocock S, Konstantinidis D, Choi JW, East C, Lee DP, Ma A, Ewen S, Cohen DL, Wilensky R, Devireddy CM, Lea J, Schmid A, Weil J, Agdirlioglu T, Reedus D, Jefferson BK, Reyes D, D'Souza R, Sharp ASP, Sharif F, Fahy M, DeBruin V, Cohen SA, Brar S, Townsend RR and SPYRAL HTN-OFF MED Pivotal Investigators. Efficacy of catheter-based renal denervation in the absence of antihypertensive medications (SPYRAL HTN-OFF MED Pivotal): a multicentre, randomised, sham-controlled trial. *Lancet.* 2020;395:1444–1451.

428. Sakakura K, Roth A, Ladich E, Shen K, Coleman L, Joner M and Virmani R. Controlled circumferential renal sympathetic denervation with preservation of the renal arterial wall using intraluminal ultrasound: a next-generation approach for treating sympathetic overactivity. *EuroIntervention.* 2015;10:1230–1238.

429. Mauri L, Kario K, Basile J, Daemen J, Davies J, Kirtane AJ, Mahfoud F, Schmieder RE, Weber M, Nanto S and Azizi M. A multinational clinical approach to assessing the effectiveness of catheter-based ultrasound renal denervation: The RADIANCE-HTN and REQUIRE clinical study designs. *Am Heart J.* 2018;195:115–129.

430. Mabin T, Sapoval M, Cabane V, Stemmett J and Iyer M. First experience with endovascular ultrasound renal denervation for the treatment of resistant hypertension. *EuroIntervention.* 2012;8:57–61.

431. Mahfoud F, Renkin J, Sievert H, Bertog S, Ewen S, Bohm M, Lengele JP, Wojakowski W, Schmieder R, van der Giet M, Parise H, Haratani N, Pathak A and Persu A. Alcohol-mediated renal denervation using the peregrine system infusion catheter for treatment of hypertension. *JACC Cardiovasc Interv.* 2020;13:471–484.

432. Qian PC, Barry MA, Lu J, Al-Raisi S, Mina A, Ryan J, Bandodkar S, Alvarez S, James V, Ronquillo J, Varikatt W, Clayton Z, Chong J, Kovoor P, Pouliopoulos J, McEwan A, Thiagalingam A and Thomas SP. Transcatheter microwave ablation can deliver deep and circumferential perivascular nerve injury without significant arterial injury to provide effective renal denervation. *J Hypertens.* 2019;37:2083–2092. https://journals.lww.com/jhypertension/pages/default.aspx.

433. Waksman R, Barbash IM, Chan R, Randolph P, Makuria AT and Virmani R. Beta radiation for renal nerve denervation: initial feasibility and safety. *EuroIntervention.* 2013;9:738–744.

434. Chen H, Ji M, Zhang Y, Xu Y, Qiao L, Shen L and Ge J. References efficiency and safety of renal denervation via cryoablation (Cryo-RDN) in Chinese patients with uncontrolled hypertension: study protocol for a randomized controlled trial. *Trials.* 2019;20:653.

435. Forssell C, Bjarnegard N and Nystrom FH. A pilot study of perioperative external circumferential cryoablation of human renal arteries for sympathetic denervation. *Vasc Specialist Int.* 2020;36:151–157.

436. Baik J, Song WH, Yim D, Lee S, Yang S, Lee HY, Choi EK, Jeong CW and Park SM. Laparoscopic renal denervation system for treating resistant hypertension: overcoming limitations of catheter-based approaches. *IEEE Trans Biomed Eng.* 2020;67:3425–3437.

437. Liu Y, Zhu B, Zhu L, Zhao L, Ding D, Liu Z, Fan Z, Zhao Q, Zhang Y, Wang J and Gao C. Clinical outcomes of laparoscopic-based renal denervation plus adrenalectomy vs adrenalectomy alone for treating resistant hypertension caused by unilateral aldosterone-producing adenoma. *J Clin Hypertens (Greenwich).* 2020;22:1606–1615.

438. Azizi M, Schmieder RE, Mahfoud F, Weber MA, Daemen J, Davies J, Basile J, Kirtane AJ, Wang Y, Lobo MD, Saxena M, Feyz L, Rader F, Lurz P, Sayer J, Sapoval M, Levy T, Sanghvi K, Abraham J, Sharp ASP, Fisher NDL, Bloch MJ, Reeve-Stoffer H, Coleman L, Mullin C, Mauri L and RADIANCE-HTN Investigators. Endovascular ultrasound renal denervation to treat hypertension (RADIANCE-HTN SOLO): a multicentre, international, single-blind, randomised, sham-controlled trial. *Lancet.* 2018;391:2335–2345.

439. Kario K, Weber MA, Mahfoud F, Kandzari DE, Schmieder RE, Kirtane AJ, Bohm M, Hettrick DA, Townsend RR and Tsioufis KP. Changes in 24–hour patterns of blood pressure in hypertension following renal denervation therapy. *Hypertension.* 2019:244–249. https://www.ahajournals.org/journal/hyp.

440. Azizi M, Schmieder RE, Mahfoud F, Weber MA, Daemen J, Lobo MD, Sharp ASP, Bloch MJ, Basile J, Wang Y, Saxena M, Lurz P, Rader F, Sayer J, Fisher NDL, Fouassier D, Barman NC, Reeve-Stoffer H, McClure C, Kirtane AJ and Investigators R-H. Six-month results of treatment-blinded medication titration for hypertension control following randomization to endovascular ultrasound renal denervation or a sham procedure in the RADIANCE-HTN SOLO trial. *Circulation.* 2019;139:2542–2553.

441. He FJ, Marciniak M, Visagie E, Markandu ND, Anand V, Dalton RN and MacGregor GA. Effect of modest salt reduction on blood pressure, urinary albumin, and pulse wave velocity in white, black, and Asian mild hypertensives. *Hypertension.* 2009;54: 482–488.

442. Park JB, Kario K and Wang JG. Systolic hypertension: an increasing clinical challenge in Asia. *Hypertens Res.* 2015;38:227–236.

443. Kario K, Chen CH, Park S, Park CG, Hoshide S, Cheng HM, Huang QF and Wang JG. Consensus document on improving hypertension management in Asian patients, taking into account Asian characteristics. *Hypertension.* 2018;71:375–382. https://www.ahajournals.org/journal/hyp.

444. Kim BK, Bohm M, Mahfoud F, Mancia G, Park S, Hong MK, Kim HS, Park SJ, Park CG, Seung KB, Gwon HC, Choi DJ, Ahn TH, Kim CJ, Kwon HM, Esler M and Jang YS. Renal denervation for treatment of uncontrolled hypertension in an Asian population: results from the Global SYMPLICITY Registry in South Korea (GSR Korea). *J Hum Hypertens.* 2016;30:315–321.

445. Lee CK, Wang TD, Lee YH, Fahy M, Lee CH, Sung SH, Kao HL, Wu YW and Lin TH. Efficacy and safety of renal denervation for patients with uncontrolled hypertension in Taiwan: 3-year results from the Global SYMPLICITY Registry-Taiwan (GSR-Taiwan). *Acta Cardiol Sin.* 2019;35:618–626.

446. Mahfoud F. Three-year safety and efficacy in the Global Simplicity Registry: impact of anti-hypertensive medication burden on blood pressure reduction. 2020;2021:Presented at EuroPCR. 2020. Available from: https://www.pcronline.com/Cases-resources-images/Resources/Course-videos-slides/2020/Abstracts-on-Renal-denervation-PCR-e-Course-2020.

447. Mahfoud F, Mancia G, Schmieder R, Narkiewicz K, Ruilope L, Schlaich M, Whitbourn R, Zirlik A, Zeller T, Stawowy P, Cohen SA, Fahy M and Bohm M. Renal denervation in high-risk patients with hypertension. *J Am Coll Cardiol.* 2020;75:2879–2888.

448. Sanders MF, Reitsma JB, Morpey M, Gremmels H, Bots ML, Pisano A, Bolignano D, Zoccali C and Blankestijn PJ. Renal safety of catheter-based renal denervation: systematic review and meta-analysis. *Nephrol Dial Transplant.* 2017;32:1440–1447.

449. Sardar P, Bhatt DL, Kirtane AJ, Kennedy KF, Chatterjee S, Giri J, Soukas PA, White WB, Parikh SA and Aronow HD. Sham-controlled randomized trials of catheter-based renal denervation in patients with hypertension. *J Am Coll Cardiol.* 2019;73:1633–1642.

450. Stavropoulos K, Patoulias D, Imprialos K, Doumas M, Katsimardou A, Dimitriadis K, Tsioufis C and Papademetriou V. Efficacy and safety of renal denervation for the management of arterial hypertension: a systematic review and meta-analysis of randomized, sham-controlled, catheter-based trials. *J Clin Hypertens (Greenwich).* 2020;22: 572–584.

451. Townsend RR, Walton A, Hettrick DA, Hickey GL, Weil J, Sharp ASP, Blankestijn PJ, Bohm M and Mancia G. Review and meta-analysis of renal artery damage following percutaneous renal denervation with radiofrequency renal artery ablation. *EuroIntervention.* 2020;16:89–96.

452. Mahfoud F, Bohm M, Schmieder R, Narkiewicz K, Ewen S, Ruilope L, Schlaich M, Williams B, Fahy M and Mancia G. Effects of renal denervation on kidney function and long-term outcomes: 3-year follow-up from the Global SYMPLICITY Registry. *Eur Heart J.* 2019;40:3474–3482.

453. Kario K, Bohm M, Mahfoud F, Townsend RR, Weber MA, Patel M, Tyson CC, Weil J, Agdirlioglu T, Cohen SA, Fahy M and Kandzari DE. Twenty-four-hour ambulatory blood pressure reduction patterns after renal denervation in the SPYRAL HTN-OFF MED trial. *Circulation.* 2018;138:1602–1604.

454. Kario K, Weber MA, Bohm M, Townsend RR, Mahfoud F, Schmieder RE, Tsioufis K, Cohen SA, Fahy M and Kandzari DE. Effect of renal denervation in attenuating the stress of morning surge in blood pressure: post-hoc analysis from the SPYRAL HTN-ON MED trial. *Clin Res Cardiol.* 2021;110: 725-731.

455. Mompeo B, Maranillo E, Garcia-Touchard A, Larkin T and Sanudo J. The gross anatomy of the renal sympathetic nerves revisited. *Clin Anat.* 2016;29:660–664.

456. Garcia-Touchard A, Maranillo E, Mompeo B and Sanudo JR. Microdissection of the human renal nervous system: implications for performing renal denervation procedures. *Hypertension.* 2020;76:1240–1246. https://www.ahajournals.org/journal/hyp.

457. Kandzari DE, Mahfoud F, Bhatt DL, Bohm M, Weber MA, Townsend RR, Hettrick DA, Schmieder RE, Tsioufis K and Kario K. Confounding factors in renal denervation trials: revisiting old and identifying new challenges in trial design of device therapies for hypertension. *Hypertension.* 2020;76:1410–1417. https://www.ahajournals.org/journal/hyp.

458. Bohm M, Mahfoud F, Townsend RR, Kandzari DE, Pocock S, Ukena C, Weber MA, Hoshide S, Patel M, Tyson CC, Weil J, Agdirlioglu T, Fahy M and Kario K. Ambulatory heart rate reduction after catheter-based renal denervation in hypertensive patients not receiving anti-hypertensive medications: data from SPYRAL HTN-OFF MED, a randomized, sham-controlled, proof-of-concept trial. *Eur Heart J.* 2019;40:743–751.

459. Kario K, Ikemoto T, Kuwabara M, Ishiyama H, Saito K and Hoshide S. Catheter-based renal denervation reduces hypoxia-triggered nocturnal blood pressure peak in obstructive sleep apnea syndrome. *J Clin Hypertens (Greenwich).* 2016;18:707–709.

460. Warchol-Celinska E, Prejbisz A, Kadziela J, Florczak E, Januszewicz M, Michalowska I, Dobrowolski P, Kabat M, Sliwinski P, Klisiewicz A, Topor-Madry R, Narkiewicz K, Somers VK, Sobotka PA, Witkowski A and Januszewicz A. Renal denervation in resistant hypertension and obstructive sleep apnea: randomized proof-of-concept phase II trial. *Hypertension.* 2018;72:381–390. https://www.ahajournals.org/journal/hyp.

461. Okon T, Rohnert K, Stiermaier T, Rommel KP, Muller U, Fengler K, Schuler G, Desch S and Lurz P. Invasive aortic pulse wave velocity as a marker for arterial stiffness predicts outcome of renal sympathetic denervation. *EuroIntervention.* 2016;12:e684–e692.

462. Mahfoud F, Bakris G, Bhatt DL, Esler M, Ewen S, Fahy M, Kandzari D, Kario K, Mancia G, Weber M and Bohm M. Reduced blood pressure-lowering effect of catheter-based renal denervation in patients with isolated systolic hypertension: data from SYMPLICITY HTN-3 and the Global SYMPLICITY Registry. *Eur Heart J.* 2017;38:93–100.

463. Ewen S, Ukena C, Linz D, Kindermann I, Cremers B, Laufs U, Wagenpfeil S, Schmieder RE, Bohm M and Mahfoud F. Reduced effect of percutaneous renal denervation on blood pressure in patients with isolated systolic hypertension. *Hypertension.* 2015;65:193–199. https://www.ahajournals.org/journal/hyp.

464. Fengler K, Rommel KP, Hoellriegel R, Blazek S, Besler C, Desch S, Schuler G, Linke A and Lurz P. Pulse wave velocity predicts response to renal denervation in isolated systolic hypertension. *J Am Heart Assoc.* 2017;6(5):e005879.

465. Schmieder RE, Hogerl K, Jung S, Bramlage P, Veelken R and Ott C. Patient preference for therapies in hypertension: a cross-sectional survey of German patients. *Clin Res Cardiol.* 2019;108:1331–1342.

466. Schmieder RE, Kandzari DE, Wang TD, Lee YH, Lazarus G and Pathak A. Differences in patient and physician perspectives on pharmaceutical therapy and renal denervation for the management of hypertension. *J Hypertens.* 2021;39:162–168. https://journals.lww.com/jhypertension/pages/default.aspx.

467. Zhou HH, Koshakji RP, Silberstein DJ, Wilkinson GR and Wood AJ. Racial differences in drug response. Altered sensitivity to and clearance of propranolol in men of Chinese descent as compared with American whites. *N Engl J Med.* 1989;320:565–570.

468. Kario K, Kim BK, Aoki J, Wong AY, Lee YH, Wongpraparut N, Nguyen QN, Ahmad WAW, Lim ST, Ong TK and Wang TD. Renal denervation in Asia: consensus statement of the asia renal denervation consortium. *Hypertension.* 2020;75:590–602. https://www.ahajournals.org/journal/hyp.

469. Omboni S. Connected health in hypertension management. *Front Cardiovasc Med.* 2019;6:76.

470. Omboni S, McManus RJ, Bosworth HB, Chappell LC, Green BB, Kario K, Logan AG, Magid DJ, McKinstry B, Margolis KL, Parati G and Wakefield BJ. Evidence and recommendations on the use of telemedicine for the management of arterial hypertension: an international expert position paper. *Hypertension* 2020;76:1368–1383. https://www.ahajournals.org/journal/hyp.

471. Kario K, Tomitani N, Kanegae H, Yasui N, Nagai R and Harada H. The further development of out-of-office BP monitoring: Japan's ImPACT Program Project's achievements, impact, and direction. *J Clin Hypertens (Greenwich).* 2019;21:344–349.

472. Sabbahi A, Arena R, Elokda A and Phillips SA. Exercise and hypertension: uncovering the mechanisms of vascular control. *Prog Cardiovasc Dis.* 2016;59:226–234.

473. Oktay AA, Lavie CJ, Kokkinos PF, Parto P, Pandey A and Ventura HO. The interaction of cardiorespiratory fitness with obesity and the obesity paradox in cardiovascular disease. *Prog Cardiovasc Dis.* 2017;60:30–44.

474. Lee DC, Brellenthin AG, Thompson PD, Sui X, Lee IM and Lavie CJ. Running as a key lifestyle medicine for longevity. *Prog Cardiovasc Dis.* 2017;60:45–55.

475. Wang JG, Kario K, Park JB and Chen CH. Morning blood pressure monitoring in the management of hypertension. *J Hypertens.* 2017;35:1554–1563.

476. Reilly JP and White CJ. Renal denervation for resistant hypertension. *Prog Cardiovasc Dis.* 2016;59:295–302.

477. Kanegae H, Suzuki K, Fukatani K, Ito T, Harada N and Kario K. Highly precise risk prediction model for new-onset hypertension using artificial intelligence techniques. *J Clin Hypertens (Greenwich).* 2020;22:445–450.

478. Koshimizu H, Kojima R, Kario K and Okuno Y. Prediction of blood pressure variability using deep neural networks. *Int J Med Informatics*. 2020;136:104067.

479. Kario K, Schwartz JE, Gerin W, Robayo N, Maceo E and Pickering TG. Psychological and physical stress-induced cardiovascular reactivity and diurnal blood pressure variation in women with different work shifts. *Hypertens Res*. 2002;25:543–551.

480. Kokubo A, Kuwabara M, Nakajima H, Tomitani N, Yamashita S, Shiga T and Kario K. Automatic detection algorithm for establishing standard to identify "surge blood pressure". *Med Biol Eng Comput*. 2020;58:1393–1404.

481. Webb AJS, Lawson A, Wartolowska K, Mazzucco S and Rothwell PM. Progression of beat-to-beat blood pressure variability despite best medical management. *Hypertension*. 2021;77:193–201. https://www.ahajournals.org/journal/hyp.

482. Webb AJS, Mazzucco S, Li L and Rothwell PM. Prognostic significance of blood pressure variability on beat-to-beat monitoring after transient ischemic attack and stroke. *Stroke*. 2018;49:62–67. https://www.ahajournals.org/journal/str.

483. Kario K, Nishizawa M, Hoshide S, Shimpo M, Ishibashi Y, Kunii O and Shibuya K. Development of a disaster cardiovascular prevention network. *Lancet*. 2011;378:1125–1127.

484. Nishizawa M, Hoshide S, Shimpo M and Kario K. Disaster hypertension: experience from the great East Japan earthquake of 2011. *Curr Hypertens Rep*. 2012;14: 375–381.

485. JCS, JSH and JCC Joint Working Group. Guidelines for Disaster Medicine for Patients With Cardiovascular Diseases (JCS 2014/JSH 2014/JCC 2014) – Digest Version. *Circ J*. 2016;80:261–284.

486. Kario K, Matsuo T, Shimada K and Pickering TG. Factors associated with the occurrence and magnitude of earthquake-induced increases in blood pressure. *Am J Med*. 2001;111:379–84.

487. Kario K. Disaster hypertension - its characteristics, mechanism, and management. *Circ J*. 2012;76:553–562.

488. Kario K. Management of high casual blood pressure in a disaster situation: the 1995 Hanshin–Awaji earthquake. *Am J Hypertens*. 1998;11:1138–1139.

489. Kario K, Matsuo T, Ishida T and Shimada K. "White coat" hypertension and the Hanshin–Awaji earthquake. *Lancet* 1995;345:1365.

490. Kario K, Matsuo T, Kobayashi H, Yamamoto K and Shimada K. Earthquake-induced potentiation of acute risk factors in hypertensive elderly patients: possible triggering of cardiovascular events after a major earthquake. *J Am Coll Cardiol*. 1997;29:926–933.

491. Kario K, McEwen BS and Pickering TG. Disasters and the heart: a review of the effects of earthquake-induced stress on cardiovascular disease. *Hypertens Res*. 2003;26:355–367.

492. Nishizawa M, Hoshide S, Okawara Y, Shimpo M, Matsuo T and Kario K. Aftershock triggers augmented pressor effects in survivors: follow-up of the Great East Japan Earthquake. *Am J Hypertens*. 2015;28:1405–1408.

493. Nishizawa M, Hoshide S, Okawara Y, Matsuo T and Kario K. Strict blood pressure control achieved using an ICT-based home blood pressure monitoring system in a catastrophically damaged area after a disaster. *J Clin Hypertens (Greenwich)*. 2017;19:26–29.

494. Nishizawa M, Fujiwara T, Hoshide S, Sato K, Okawara Y, Tomitani N, Matsuo T and Kario K. Winter morning surge in blood pressure after the Great East Japan Earthquake. *J Clin Hypertens (Greenwich)*. 2019;21:208–216.

495. Hoshide S, Nishizawa M, Okawara Y, Harada N, Kunii O, Shimpo M and Kario K. Salt intake and risk of disaster hypertension among evacuees in a shelter after the Great East Japan earthquake. *Hypertension*. 2019;74:564–571. https://www.ahajournals.org/journal/hyp.

496. Santia. ISD. Characteristics of COVID-19 patients dying in Italy. Report based on data available on March 20th, 2020. 2020:https://www.epicentro.iss.it/coronavirus/bollettino/Report-COVID-2019_20_marzo_eng.pdf Accessed 23 Mar 2021.

497. Ferrario CM, Jessup J, Chappell MC, Averill DB, Brosnihan KB, Tallant EA, Diz DI and Gallagher PE. Effect of angiotensin-converting enzyme inhibition and angiotensin II receptor blockers on cardiac angiotensin-converting enzyme 2. *Circulation.* 2005;111:2605–2610. https://www.ahajournals.org/journal/circ.

498. Ishiyama Y, Gallagher PE, Averill DB, Tallant EA, Brosnihan KB and Ferrario CM. Upregulation of angiotensin-converting enzyme 2 after myocardial infarction by blockade of angiotensin II receptors. *Hypertension.* 2004;43:970–976. https://www.ahajournals.org/journal/hyp.

499. Li J, Wang X, Chen J, Zhang H and Deng A. Association of renin-angiotensin system inhibitors with severity or risk of death in patients with hypertension hospitalized for coronavirus disease 2019 (COVID-19) infection in Wuhan, China. *JAMA Cardiol.* 2020;5:825–830.

500. Kario K, Morisawa Y, Sukonthasarn A, Turana Y, Chia YC, Park S, Wang TD, Chen CH, Tay JC, Li Y, Wang JG and Hypertension Cardiovascular Outcome Prevention EiAN. COVID-19 and hypertension-evidence and practical management: Guidance from the HOPE Asia Network. *J Clin Hypertens (Greenwich).* 2020;22:1109–1119.

501. Yang G, Tan Z, Zhou L, Yang M, Peng L, Liu J, Cai J, Yang R, Han J, Huang Y and He S. Effects of angiotensin II receptor blockers and ACE (angiotensin-converting enzyme) inhibitors on virus infection, inflammatory status, and clinical outcomes in patients with COVID-19 and hypertension: a single-center retrospective study. *Hypertension.* 2020;76:51–58. https://www.ahajournals.org/journal/hyp.

502. Zhang P, Zhu L, Cai J, Lei F, Qin JJ, Xie J, Liu YM, Zhao YC, Huang X, Lin L, Xia M, Chen MM, Cheng X, Zhang X, Guo D, Peng Y, Ji YX, Chen J, She ZG, Wang Y, Xu Q, Tan R, Wang H, Lin J, Luo P, Fu S, Cai H, Ye P, Xiao B, Mao W, Liu L, Yan Y, Liu M, Chen M, Zhang XJ, Wang X, Touyz RM, Xia J, Zhang BH, Huang X, Yuan Y, Loomba R, Liu PP and Li H. Association of inpatient use of angiotensin-converting enzyme inhibitors and angiotensin II receptor blockers with mortality among patients with hypertension hospitalized With COVID-19. *Circ Res.* 2020;126:1671–1681.

503. Kario K and HOPE Asia Network. The HOPE Asia Network for "zero" cardiovascular events in Asia. *J Clin Hypertens (Greenwich).* 2018;20:212–214.

504. Kario K, Chia YC, Sukonthasarn A, Turana Y, Shin J, Chen CH, Buranakitjaroen P, Nailes J, Hoshide S, Siddique S, Sison J, Soenarta AA, Sogunuru GP, Tay JC, Teo BW, Zhang YQ, Park S, Minh HV, Tomitani N, Kabutoya T, Verma N, Wang TD and Wang JG. Diversity of and initiatives for hypertension management in Asia-why we need the HOPE Asia Network. *J Clin Hypertens (Greenwich).* 2020;22:331–343.

505. Kario K and Wang J. Towards "zero" cardiovascular events in Asia: the HOPE Asia network. *JACC Asia.* 2021; 1: 121–124.

506. Weber MA and Lackland DT. Hypertension: cardiovascular benefits of lowering blood pressure. *Nat Rev Nephrol.* 2016;12:202–204.

507. Campbell NR, Khalsa T, World Hypertension League E, Lackland DT, Niebylski ML, Nilsson PM, Redburn KA, Orias M, Zhang XH, International Society of Hypertension E, Burrell L, Horiuchi M, Poulter NR, Prabhakaran D, Ramirez AJ, Schiffrin EL, Touyz RM, Wang JG, Weber MA, World Stroke Organization; International Diabetes Federation; International Council of Cardiovascular Prevention and Rehabilitation; International Society of Nephrology. High Blood Pressure 2016: Why Prevention and Control Are Urgent and Important. The World Hypertension League, International Society of Hypertension, World Stroke Organization, International Diabetes Foundation, International Council of Cardiovascular Prevention and Rehabilitation, International Society of Nephrology. *J Clin Hypertens (Greenwich).* 2016;18:714–717.

508. Weber MA and Lackland DT. Contributions to hypertension public policy and clinical practice: a review of recent reports. *J Clin Hypertens (Greenwich).* 2016;18:1063–1070.

509. Yano Y, Briasoulis A, Bakris GL, Hoshide S, Wang JG, Shimada K and Kario K. Effects of antihypertensive treatment in Asian populations: a meta-analysis of prospective randomized controlled studies (CARdiovascular protectioN group in Asia: CARNA). *J Am Soc Hypertens.* 2014;8:103–116.

510. Hoshide S, Wang JG, Park S, Chen CH, Cheng HM, Huang QF, Park CG and Kario K. Treatment considerations of clinical physician on hypertension management in Asia. *Curr Hypertens Rev.* 2016;12:164–168.

511. Chia YC, Buranakitjaroen P, Chen CH, Divinagracia R, Hoshide S, Park S, Shin J, Siddique S, Sison J, Soenarta AA, Sogunuru GP, Tay JC, Turana Y, Wang JG, Wong L, Zhang Y, Kario K and HOPE Asia Network. Current status of home blood pressure monitoring in Asia: statement from the HOPE Asia Network. *J Clin Hypertens (Greenwich).* 2017;19:1192–1201.

512. Kario K, Shin J, Chen CH, Buranakitjaroen P, Chia YC, Divinagracia R, Nailes J, Hoshide S, Siddique S, Sison J, Soenarta AA, Sogunuru GP, Tay JC, Teo BW, Turana Y, Zhang Y, Park S, Van Minh H and Wang JG. Expert panel consensus recommendations for ambulatory blood pressure monitoring in Asia: the HOPE Asia Network. *J Clin Hypertens (Greenwich).* 2019;21:1250–1283.

513. Kario K, Hoshide S, Chia YC, Buranakitjaroen P, Siddique S, Shin J, Turana Y, Park S, Tsoi K, Chen CH, Cheng HM, Fujiwara T, Li Y, Huynh VM, Nagai M, Nailes J, Sison J, Soenarta AA, Sogunuru GP, Sukonthasarn A, Tay JC, Teo BW, Verma N, Wang TD, Zhang Y and Wang JG. Guidance on ambulatory blood pressure monitoring: a statement from the HOPE Asia Network. *J Clin Hypertens (Greenwich).* 2021;23:411–421.

514. Kario K. The HOPE Asia Network activity for "zero" cardiovascular events in Asia: overview 2020. *J Clin Hypertens (Greenwich).* 2020;22:321–330.

515. Chia YC, Kario K, Turana Y, Nailes J, Tay JC, Siddique S, Park S, Shin J, Buranakitjaroen P, Chen CH, Divinagracia R, Hoshide S, Minh HV, Sison J, Soenarta AA, Sogunuru GP, Sukonthasarn A, Teo BW, Verma N, Zhang Y, Wang TD and Wang JG. Target blood pressure and control status in Asia. *J Clin Hypertens (Greenwich).* 2020;22:344–350.

516. Wang JG, Chia YC, Chen CH, Park S, Hoshide S, Tomitani N, Kabutoya T, Shin J, Turana Y, Soenarta AA, Tay JC, Buranakitjaroen P, Nailes J, Van Minh H, Siddique S, Sison J, Sogunuru GP, Sukonthasarn A, Teo BW, Verma N, Zhang YQ, Wang TD and Kario K. What is new in the 2018 Chinese hypertension guideline and the implication for the management of hypertension in Asia? *J Clin Hypertens (Greenwich).* 2020;22:363–368.

517. Hoshide S, Kario K, Tomitani N, Kabutoya T, Chia YC, Park S, Shin J, Turana Y, Tay JC, Buranakitjaroen P, Chen CH, Nailes J, Minh HV, Siddique S, Sison J, Soenarta AA, Sogunuru GP, Sukonthasarn A, Teo BW, Verma N, Zhang Y, Wang TD and Wang JG. Highlights of the 2019 Japanese Society of Hypertension Guidelines and perspectives on the management of Asian hypertensive patients. *J Clin Hypertens (Greenwich).* 2020;22:369-377.

518. Wang JG, Bu PL, Chen LY, Chen X, Chen YY, Cheng WL, Chu SL, Cui ZQ, Dai QY, Feng YQ, Jiang XJ, Jiang YN, Li WH, Li Y, Li Y, Lin JX, Liu J, Mu JJ, Peng YX, Song L, Sun NL, Wang Y, Xi Y, Xie LD, Xue H, Yu J, Yu W, Zhang YQ and Zhu ZM. 2019 Chinese Hypertension League guidelines on home blood pressure monitoring. *J Clin Hypertens (Greenwich).* 2020;22:378–383.

519. Shin J, Kario K, Chia YC, Turana Y, Chen CH, Buranakitjaroen P, Divinagracia R, Nailes J, Hoshide S, Siddique S, Sison J, Soenarta AA, Sogunuru GP, Tay JC, Teo BW, Zhang YQ, Park S, Van Minh H, Kabutoya T, Verma N, Wang TD and Wang JG. Current status of ambulatory blood pressure monitoring in Asian countries: a report from the HOPE Asia Network. *J Clin Hypertens (Greenwich).* 2020;22:384–390.

520. Cheng HM, Chuang SY, Wang TD, Kario K, Buranakitjaroen P, Chia YC, Divinagracia R, Hoshide S, Minh HV, Nailes J, Park S, Shin J, Siddique S, Sison J, Soenarta AA, Sogunuru GP, Sukonthasarn A, Tay JC, Teo BW, Turana Y, Verma N, Zhang Y, Wang JG and Chen CH. Central blood pressure for the management of hypertension: Is it a practical clinical tool in current practice? *J Clin Hypertens (Greenwich).* 2020;22:391–406.

521. Chia YC, Kario K, Tomitani N, Park S, Shin J, Turana Y, Tay JC, Buranakitjaroen P, Chen CH, Hoshide S, Nailes J, Minh HV, Siddique S, Sison J, Soenarta AA, Sogunuru GP, Sukonthasarn A, Teo BW, Verma N, Zhang Y, Wang TD and Wang JG. Comparison of day-to-day blood pressure variability in hypertensive patients with type 2 diabetes mellitus to those without diabetes: Asia BP@Home Study. *J Clin Hypertens (Greenwich).* 2020;22:407–414.

522. Turana Y, Tengkawan J, Chia YC, Teo BW, Shin J, Sogunuru GP, Soenarta AA, Minh HV, Buranakitjaroen P, Chen CH, Nailes J, Hoshide S, Park S, Siddique S, Sison J, Sukonthasarn A, Tay JC, Wang TD, Verma N, Zhang YQ, Wang JG and Kario K. High blood pressure in dementia: how low can we go? *J Clin Hypertens (Greenwich)*. 2020;22:415–422.

523. Soenarta AA, Buranakitjaroen P, Chia YC, Chen CH, Nailes J, Hoshide S, Minh HV, Park S, Shin J, Siddique S, Sison J, Sogunuru GP, Sukonthasarn A, Tay JC, Teo BW, Turana Y, Verma N, Wang TD, Zhang YQ, Wang JG and Kario K. An overview of hypertension and cardiac involvement in Asia: focus on heart failure. *J Clin Hypertens (Greenwich)*. 2020; 22:423-430.

524. Park S, Kario K, Chia YC, Turana Y, Chen CH, Buranakitjaroen P, Nailes J, Hoshide S, Siddique S, Sison J, Soenarta AA, Sogunuru GP, Tay JC, Teo BW, Zhang YQ, Shin J, Van Minh H, Tomitani N, Kabutoya T, Sukonthasarn A, Verma N, Wang TD, Wang JG and Network HA. The influence of the ambient temperature on blood pressure and how it will affect the epidemiology of hypertension in Asia. *J Clin Hypertens (Greenwich)*. 2020;22:438–444.

525. Hoshide S, Kabutoya T, Ueno H and Kario K. Class effect of xanthine oxidase inhibitors on flow-mediated dilatation in hypertensive patients: a randomized controlled trial. *J Clin Hypertens (Greenwich)*. 2020;22:451–456.

526. Guo QH, Zhang YQ and Wang JG. Asian management of hypertension: current status, home blood pressure, and specific concerns in China. *J Clin Hypertens (Greenwich)*. 2020;22:475–478.

527. Sogunuru GP and Mishra S. Asian management of hypertension: current status, home blood pressure, and specific concerns in India. *J Clin Hypertens (Greenwich)*. 2020;22:479–482.

528. Turana Y, Tengkawan J and Soenarta AA. Asian management of hypertension: current status, home blood pressure, and specific concerns in Indonesia. *J Clin Hypertens (Greenwich)*. 2020;22:483–485.

529. Kabutoya T, Hoshide S and Kario K. Asian management of hypertension: current status, home blood pressure, and specific concerns in Japan. *J Clin Hypertens (Greenwich)*. 2020;22:486–492.

530. Park S and Shin J. Asian management of hypertension: current status, home blood pressure, and specific concerns in Korea. *J Clin Hypertens (Greenwich)*. 2020;22:493–496.

531. Chia YC and Kario K. Asian management of hypertension: current status, home blood pressure, and specific concerns in Malaysia. *J Clin Hypertens (Greenwich)*. 2020;22:497–500.

532. Siddique S. Asian management of hypertension: current status, home blood pressure, and specific concerns in Pakistan. *J Clin Hypertens (Greenwich)*. 2020;22:501–503.

533. Sison J, Divinagracia R and Nailes J. Asian management of hypertension: current status, home blood pressure, and specific concerns in Philippines (a country report). *J Clin Hypertens (Greenwich)*. 2020;22:504–507.

534. Tay JC and Teo BW. Asian management of hypertension: current status, home blood pressure, and specific concerns in Singapore. *J Clin Hypertens (Greenwich)*. 2020;22:508–510.

535. Cheng HM, Lin HJ, Wang TD and Chen CH. Asian management of hypertension: current status, home blood pressure, and specific concerns in Taiwan. *J Clin Hypertens (Greenwich)*. 2020;22:511–514.

536. Buranakitjaroen P, Wanthong S and Sukonthasarn A. Asian management of hypertension: current status, home blood pressure, and specific concerns in Thailand. *J Clin Hypertens (Greenwich)*. 2020;22:515–518.

537. Van Huynh M, Nguyen Lan V, Van Huy T, Cao Thuc S, Tran Kim S, To M, Duong Thanh B and Hoang Anh T. Asian management of hypertension: current status, home blood pressure, and specific concerns in Vietnam. *J Clin Hypertens (Greenwich)*. 2020;22:519–521.

538. Kario K. HOPE Asia Network Activity 2021-collaboration and perspectives of Asia academic activity. *J Clin Hypertens (Greenwich)*. 2021;23:408–410.

539. Chia YC, Turana Y, Sukonthasarn A, Zhang Y, Shin J, Cheng HM, Tay JC, Tsoi K, Siddique S, Verma N, Buranakitjaroen P, Sogunuru GP, Nailes J, Van Minh H, Park S, Teo BW, Chen CH, Wang TD, Soenarta AA, Hoshide S, Wang JG and Kario K. Comparison of guidelines for the management of hypertension: similarities and differences between international and Asian countries; perspectives from HOPE-Asia Network. *J Clin Hypertens (Greenwich)*. 2021;23:422–434.

540. Wang JG, Li Y, Chia YC, Cheng HM, Minh HV, Siddique S, Sogunuru GP, Tay JC, Teo BW, Tsoi K, Turana Y, Wang TD, Zhang YQ and Kario K. Telemedicine in the management of hypertension: evolving technological platforms for blood pressure telemonitoring. *J Clin Hypertens (Greenwich)*. 2021;23:435–439.

541. Siddique S, Hameed Khan A, Shahab H, Zhang YQ, Chin Tay J, Buranakitjaroen P, Turana Y, Verma N, Chen CH, Cheng HM, Wang TD, Van Minh H, Chia YC and Kario K. Office blood pressure measurement: a comprehensive review. *J Clin Hypertens (Greenwich)*. 2021;23:440–449.

542. Huang JF, Li Y, Shin J, Chia YC, Sukonthasarn A, Turana Y, Chen CH, Cheng HM, Ann Soenarta A, Tay JC, Wang TD, Kario K and Wang JG. Characteristics and control of the 24-hour ambulatory blood pressure in patients with metabolic syndrome. *J Clin Hypertens (Greenwich)*. 2021;23:450–456.

543. Fujiwara T, Hoshide S, Tomitani N, Cheng HM, Soenarta AA, Turana Y, Chen CH, Minh HV, Sogunuru GP, Tay JC, Wang TD, Chia YC, Verma N, Li Y, Wang JG and Kario K. Clinical significance of nocturnal home blood pressure monitoring and nocturnal hypertension in Asia. *J Clin Hypertens (Greenwich)*. 2021;23:457–466.

544. Tsai TY, Cheng HM, Chuang SY, Chia YC, Soenarta AA, Minh HV, Siddique S, Turana Y, Tay JC, Kario K and Chen CH. Isolated systolic hypertension in Asia. *J Clin Hypertens (Greenwich)*. 2021;23:467–474.

545. Teo BW, Chan GC, Leo CCH, Tay JC, Chia YC, Siddique S, Turana Y, Chen CH, Cheng HM, Hoshide S, Minh HV, Sogunuru GP, Wang TD and Kario K. Hypertension and chronic kidney disease in Asian populations. *J Clin Hypertens (Greenwich)*. 2021;23:475–480.

546. Wang TD, Lee CK, Chia YC, Tsoi K, Buranakitjaroen P, Chen CH, Cheng HM, Tay JC, Teo BW, Turana Y, Sogunuru GP, Wang JG and Kario K. Hypertension and erectile dysfunction: the role of endovascular therapy in Asia. *J Clin Hypertens (Greenwich)*. 2021;23:481–488.

547. Hoshide S, Kario K, Chia YC, Siddique S, Buranakitjaroen P, Tsoi K, Tay JC, Turana Y, Chen CH, Cheng HM, Huynh VM, Park S, Soenarta AA, Sogunuru GP, Wang TD and Wang JG. Characteristics of hypertension in obstructive sleep apnea: an Asian experience. *J Clin Hypertens (Greenwich)*. 2021;23:489–495.

548. Matsubayashi H, Nagai M, Dote K, Turana Y, Siddique S, Chia YC, Chen CH, Cheng HM, Van Minh H, Verma N, Chin Tay J, Wee Teo B and Kario K. Long sleep duration and cardiovascular disease: associations with arterial stiffness and blood pressure variability. *J Clin Hypertens (Greenwich)*. 2021;23:496–503.

549. Turana Y, Tengkawan J, Chia YC, Shin J, Chen CH, Park S, Tsoi K, Buranakitjaroen P, Soenarta AA, Siddique S, Cheng HM, Tay JC, Teo BW, Wang TD and Kario K. Mental health problems and hypertension in the elderly: review from the HOPE Asia Network. *J Clin Hypertens (Greenwich)*. 2021;23:504–512.

550. Turana Y, Tengkawan J, Chia YC, Nathaniel M, Wang JG, Sukonthasarn A, Chen CH, Minh HV, Buranakitjaroen P, Shin J, Siddique S, Nailes JM, Park S, Teo BW, Sison J, Ann Soenarta A, Hoshide S, Tay JC, Prasad Sogunuru G, Zhang Y, Verma N, Wang TD and Kario K. Hypertension and stroke in Asia: a comprehensive review from HOPE Asia. *J Clin Hypertens (Greenwich)*. 2021;23:513–521.

551. Chan GC, Teo BW, Tay JC, Chen CH, Cheng HM, Wang TD, Turana Y, Kario K, Chia YC, Tsoi K, Sogunuru GP and Nailes J. Hypertension in a multi-ethnic Asian population of Singapore. *J Clin Hypertens (Greenwich)*. 2021;23:522–528.

552. Minh HV, Tien HA, Sinh CT, Thang DC, Chen CH, Tay JC, Siddique S, Wang TD, Sogunuru GP, Chia YC and Kario K. Assessment of preferred methods to measure insulin resistance in Asian patients with hypertension. *J Clin Hypertens (Greenwich)*. 2021;23:529–537.

553. Chang HC, Cheng HM, Chen CH, Wang TD, Soenarta AA, Turana Y, Teo BW, Tay JC, Tsoi K, Wang JG and Kario K. Dietary intervention for the management of hypertension in Asia. *J Clin Hypertens (Greenwich)*. 2021;23:538–544.

554. Sukonthasarn A, Chia YC, Wang JG, Nailes J, Buranakitjaroen P, Van Minh H, Verma N, Hoshide S, Shin J, Turana Y, Tay JC, Teo BW, Siddique S, Sison J, Zhang YQ, Wang TD, Chen CH and Kario K. The feasibility of polypill for cardiovascular disease prevention in Asian Population. *J Clin Hypertens (Greenwich)*. 2021;23:545–555.

555. Lin DS, Wang TD, Buranakitjaroen P, Chen CH, Cheng HM, Chia YC, Sukonthasarn A, Tay JC, Teo BW, Turana Y, Wang JG and Kario K. Angiotensin receptor neprilysin inhibitor as a novel antihypertensive drug: evidence from Asia and around the globe. *J Clin Hypertens (Greenwich)*. 2021;23:556–567.

556. Tsoi K, Yiu K, Lee H, Cheng HM, Wang TD, Tay JC, Teo BW, Turana Y, Soenarta AA, Sogunuru GP, Siddique S, Chia YC, Shin J, Chen CH, Wang JG and Kario K. Applications of artificial intelligence for hypertension management. *J Clin Hypertens (Greenwich)*. 2021;23:568–574.

557. Narita K, Hoshide S, Tsoi K, Siddique S, Shin J, Chia YC, Tay JC, Teo BW, Turana Y, Chen CH, Cheng HM, Sogunuru GP, Wang TD, Wang JG and Kario K. Disaster hypertension and cardiovascular events in disaster and COVID-19 pandemic. *J Clin Hypertens (Greenwich)*. 2021;23:575–583.

558. Tomitani N, Hoshide S, Buranakitjaroen P, Chia YC, Park S, Chen CH, Nailes J, Shin J, Siddique S, Sison J, Soenarta AA, Sogunuru GP, Tay JC, Turana Y, Zhang Y, Wanthong S, Matsushita N, Wang JG and Kario K. Regional differences in office and self-measured home heart rates in Asian hypertensive patients: AsiaBP@Home study. *J Clin Hypertens (Greenwich)*. 2021;23:606–613.

559. Verma N, Rastogi S, Chia YC, Siddique S, Turana Y, Cheng HM, Sogunuru GP, Tay JC, Teo BW, Wang TD, Tsoi KKF and Kario K. Non-pharmacological management of hypertension. *J Clin Hypertens (Greenwich)*. 2021, 23:1275-1283.

560. Shin J, Chia YC, Heo R, Kario K, Turana Y, Chen CH, Hoshide S, Fujiwara T, Nagai M, Siddique S, Sison J, Tay JC, Wang TD, Park S, Sogunuru GP, Minh HV and Li Y. Current status of adherence interventions in hypertension management in Asian countries: a report from the HOPE Asia Network. *J Clin Hypertens (Greenwich)*. 2021;23:584–594.

561. Tomitani N, Wanthong S, Roubsanthisuk W, Buranakitjaroen P, Hoshide S and Kario K. Differences in ambulatory blood pressure profiles between Japanese and Thai patients with hypertension /suspected hypertension. *J Clin Hypertens (Greenwich)*. 2021;23: 614–620.

562. Kotruchin P, Pratoomrat W, Mitsungnern T, Khamsai S and Imoun S. Clinical treatment outcomes of hypertensive emergency patients: results from the hypertension registry program in Northeastern Thailand. *J Clin Hypertens (Greenwich)*. 2021;23:621–627.

563. Lin JY, Kuo KL, Kuo YH, Wu KP, Chu KC, Jiang YC, Chuang YF and Cheng HM. Association between real-world home blood pressure measurement patterns and blood pressure variability among older individuals with hypertension: a community-based blood pressure variability study. *J Clin Hypertens (Greenwich)*. 2021;23:628–637.

564. Chia YC, Devaraj NK, Ching SM, Ooi PB, Chew MT, Chew BN, Mohamed M, Lim HM, Beh HC, Othman AS, Husin HS, Mohamad Gani AH, Hamid D, Kang PS, Tay CL, Wong PF and Hassan H. Relationship of an adherence score with blood pressure control status among patients with hypertension and their determinants: findings from a nationwide blood pressure screening program. *J Clin Hypertens (Greenwich)*. 2021;23:638–645.

565. Shima D, Ii Y, Higa S, Kohro T, Hoshide S, Kono K, Fujimoto S, Niijima S, Tomitani N and Kario K. Validation of novel identification algorithms for major adverse cardiovascular events in a Japanese claims database. *J Clin Hypertens (Greenwich)*. 2021;23: 646–655.

566. Chuang SY, Chang HY, Tsai TY, Cheng HM, Pan WH and Chen CH. Isolated systolic hypertension and central blood pressure: implications from the national nutrition and health survey in Taiwan. *J Clin Hypertens (Greenwich)*. 2021;23:656–664.

567. Watanabe H, Kabutoya T, Hoshide S and Kario K. Atrial fibrillation is associated with cardiovascular events in obese Japanese with one or more cardiovascular risk factors: the Japan Morning Surge Home Blood Pressure (J-HOP) Study. *J Clin Hypertens (Greenwich)*. 2021;23:665–671.

568. Mitsungnern T, Srimookda N, Imoun S, Wansupong S and Kotruchin P. The effect of pursed-lip breathing combined with number counting on blood pressure and heart rate in hypertensive urgency patients: a randomized controlled trial. *J Clin Hypertens (Greenwich)*. 2021;23:672–679.

569. Kotruchin P, Imoun S, Mitsungnern T, Aountrai P, Domthaisong M and Kario K. The effects of foot reflexology on blood pressure and heart rate: a randomized clinical trial in stage-2 hypertensive patients. *J Clin Hypertens (Greenwich)*. 2021;23:680–686.

570. Fujiwara T, Hoshide S, Tomitani N, Kanegae H and Kario K. Comparative effects of valsartan plus cilnidipine or hydrochlorothiazide on nocturnal home blood pressure. *J Clin Hypertens (Greenwich)*. 2021;23:687–691.

571. Sato M, Takahashi M and Kario K. Critical angioedema induced by a renin angiotensin system blocker in the contemporary era of increasing heart failure: a case report and commentary. *J Clin Hypertens (Greenwich)*. 2021;23:692–695.

572. Kario K, Tomitani N, Buranakitjaroen P, Chen CH, Chia YC, Divinagracia R, Park S, Shin J, Siddique S, Sison J, Soenarta AA, Sogunuru GP, Tay JC, Turana Y, Wang JG, Wong L, Zhang Y, Wanthong S, Hoshide S, Kanegae H and HOPE Asia Network. Rationale and design for the Asia BP@Home study on home blood pressure control status in 12 Asian countries and regions. *J Clin Hypertens (Greenwich)*. 2018;20:33–38.

573. Kario K, Tomitani N, Buranakitjaroen P, Chia YC, Park S, Chen CH, Divinagracia R, Shin J, Siddique S, Sison J, Ann Soenarta A, Sogunuru GP, Tay JC, Turana Y, Zhang Y, Nailes J, Wanthong S, Hoshide S, Matsushita N, Kanegae H, Wang JG and HOPE Asia Network. Home blood pressure control status in 2017–2018 for hypertension specialist centers in Asia: results of the Asia BP@Home study. *J Clin Hypertens (Greenwich)*. 2018;20:1686–1695.

574. Ueshima H, Sekikawa A, Miura K, Turin TC, Takashima N, Kita Y, Watanabe M, Kadota A, Okuda N, Kadowaki T, Nakamura Y and Okamura T. Cardiovascular disease and risk factors in Asia: a selected review. *Circulation*. 2008;118:2702–2709. https://www.ahajournals.org/journal/circ.

575. Perkovic V, Huxley R, Wu Y, Prabhakaran D and MacMahon S. The burden of blood pressure-related disease: a neglected priority for global health. *Hypertension*. 2007;50:991–997.

576. Lawes CM, Rodgers A, Bennett DA, Parag V, Suh I, Ueshima H, MacMahon S and Asia Pacific Cohort Studies Collaboration. Blood pressure and cardiovascular disease in the Asia Pacific region. *J Hypertens*. 2003;21:707–716. https://journals.lww.com/jhypertension/pages/default.aspx.

577. Ishikawa Y, Ishikawa J, Ishikawa S, Kayaba K, Nakamura Y, Shimada K, Kajii E, Pickering TG, Kario K and Jichi Medical School Cohort Investigators Group. Prevalence and determinants of prehypertension in a Japanese general population: the Jichi Medical School Cohort Study. *Hypertens Res*. 2008;31:1323–1330.

578. Greenlund KJ, Croft JB and Mensah GA. Prevalence of heart disease and stroke risk factors in persons with prehypertension in the United States, 1999–2000. *Arch Intern Med*. 2004;164:2113–2118.

579. Katsuya T, Ishikawa K, Sugimoto K, Rakugi H and Ogihara T. Salt sensitivity of Japanese from the viewpoint of gene polymorphism. *Hypertens Res*. 2003;26:521–525.

580. Powles J, Fahimi S, Micha R, Khatibzadeh S, Shi P, Ezzati M, Engell RE, Lim SS, Danaei G, Mozaffarian D, Global Burden of Diseases N and Chronic Diseases Expert Group. Global, regional and national sodium intakes in 1990 and 2010: a systematic analysis of 24 h urinary sodium excretion and dietary surveys worldwide. *BMJ Open*. 2013;3:e003733.

581. Toriumi S, Kabutoya T, Hoshide S and Kario K. Different age-related impacts of lean and obesity on cardiovascular prognosis in Japanese patients with cardiovascular risks:

the J-HOP (Japan Morning Surge-Home Blood Pressure) Study. *J Clin Hypertens (Greenwich)*. 2021;23:382–388.

582. Omboni S, Aristizabal D, De la Sierra A, Dolan E, Head G, Kahan T, Kantola I, Kario K, Kawecka-Jaszcz K, Malan L, Narkiewicz K, Octavio JA, Ohkubo T, Palatini P, Siegelova J, Silva E, Stergiou G, Zhang Y, Mancia G, Parati G and ARTEMIS Investigators. Hypertension types defined by clinic and ambulatory blood pressure in 14 143 patients referred to hypertension clinics worldwide. Data from the ARTEMIS study. *J Hypertens*. 2016;34:2187–2198. https://journals.lww.com/jhypertension/pages/default.aspx.

583. Hoshide S, Kario K, de la Sierra A, Bilo G, Schillaci G, Banegas JR, Gorostidi M, Segura J, Lombardi C, Omboni S, Ruilope L, Mancia G and Parati G. Ethnic differences in the degree of morning blood pressure surge and in its determinants between Japanese and European hypertensive subjects: data from the ARTEMIS study. *Hypertension*. 2015;66:750–756. https://www.ahajournals.org/journal/hyp.

584. Kario K, Bhatt DL, Brar S and Bakris GL. Differences in dynamic diurnal blood pressure variability between Japanese and American treatment-resistant hypertensive populations. *Circ J*. 2017;81:1337–1345.

585. Li Y, Wang JG, Gao P, Guo H, Nawrot T, Wang G, Qian Y, Staessen JA and Zhu D. Are published characteristics of the ambulatory blood pressure generalizable to rural Chinese? The JingNing population study. *Blood Press Monit*. 2005;10:125–134. https://journals.lww.com/bpmonitoring/pages/default.aspx.

586. Imai Y, Ohkubo T, Sakuma M, Tsuji II, Satoh H, Nagai K, Hisamichi S and Abe K. Predictive power of screening blood pressure, ambulatory blood pressure and blood pressure measured at home for overall and cardiovascular mortality: a prospective observation in a cohort from Ohasama, northern Japan. *Blood Press Monit*. 1996;1:251–254. https://journals.lww.com/bpmonitoring/pages/default.aspx.

587. Fujiwara T, Hoshide S, Kanegae H, Nishizawa M and Kario K. Reliability of morning, before-dinner, and at-bedtime home blood pressure measurements in patients with hypertension. *J Clin Hypertens (Greenwich)*. 2018;20:315–323.

Index

Note: Page number followed by f indicates figure and t indicates table.

Essential Manual of 24-Hour Blood Pressure Management: From Morning to Nocturnal Hypertension, Second Edition. Kazuomi Kario.

© 2022 John Wiley & Sons Ltd. Published 2022 by John Wiley & Sons Ltd.